BIOLOGY LAB BOOK

Fourth Edition

Michael B. Clark

and

Michael R. Riddle

D1451162

Suspended Animations, Publisher
Jamul, CA

BIOLOGY LAB BOOK
Fourth Edition

Illustrations: Sandra Schiefer, © 1994, 1995, 1996, & 2006, *Schiefer Enterprises*

Layout Design, Editing: Sandra Schiefer

Editing, Electronic Typesetting and Layout:

> Lily Splane
> *Cyberlepsy Media*
> 2739 Wightman Street
> San Diego, CA 92104

This book is printed by:

> *Print Books*
> 43550 Dash For Cash Circle
> Temecula CA 92592

ISBN 978-1-885380-01-2

Printed in the United States of America by:

> ***Suspended Animations***
> 20275 Deerhorn Valley Road
> Jamul, CA 91935

September 2011

Foreword

Everyone likes to look through *Biology Lab Book*. And why not, it looks like fun! But it's more than student-friendly. This manual covers all of the topics expected in a traditional lab class for non-majors, and yet is clear, direct, and easy to understand. Furthermore, the labs have been classroom tested by over 50,000 students. The changes suggested by those students, their teachers, and the lab technicians have been incorporated into the third edition of *Biology Lab Book*.

Our goal is to provide basic labs that are self-contained and totally dependable. Other lab manuals usually require that the organizational work be handled by the teacher and the lab technician. They provide only a skeletal set of instructions and guiding questions, leaving most of the technical problems and student questions unaddressed. The teacher and the lab technician are in service to these books. In our opinion, that idea is exactly backwards. A good book should serve the students, the lab technician, and the teacher who adopts it. *Biology Lab Book* and its supplementary materials were created with

that in mind. Because our labs are easy to understand, students can become self-directed. The open-ended format of each lab activity allows teachers to expand a favorite topic and add their own experiments to the lab without disrupting the overall organization.

The lab technician will be pleased to discover that our labs are easy to set up and maintain during the week. All experiments are written with supply budgets and safety in mind. The labs contain reminders to the students about proper lab procedures. However, those statements are not meant to replace the thorough discussions of safe lab behavior and proper equipment handling that are a necessary part of every lab class.

Finally, *Biology Lab Book* owes its success to many people. We would like to thank the teachers and students and lab technicians at all the schools who have used our lab books. And we offer a very special thank you to those on the following campuses whose comments and suggestions have helped us to make *Biology Lab Book* better every year.

Suspended Animations, Publisher, 20275 Deerhorn Valley Road, Jamul CA 91935

Notes To The Student
Welcome to *Biology Lab Book*

This book was written for you—the non-major biology student. *Biology Lab Book* uses an approach that is easy to understand. It allows you to build your knowledge of science one step at a time, no matter what your previous background.

A lab class is quite different from a lecture class. Mostly, it is more "doing" than listening, and more "looking" than taking notes. Some students are apprehensive because of these differences, and they worry about their chances of success. The comments and suggestions below should answer most of your questions about how to succeed in your lab class.

1. We use words sparingly, constructing each sentence as a clue to something important about the topic. Read carefully, and work step-by-step through the instructions and explanations.

2. Always practice safety in the lab classroom. Make sure that you understand the instructions for properly using lab equipment, lab materials, and chemical solutions. Ask your instructor when you have a question or any confusion about safe lab procedures.

3. Be prepared. Briefly read the lab activities *before* you come to class. If you and your lab partner are prepared, you will learn more during the lab and will finish the work before the end of class.

4. Pay particular attention to the ***bold-italics*** terms and concepts. These designate the central themes and definitions of words used in the lab. They are important ideas and many will be found on your lab tests.

5. Take time to review your work. Most students leave as soon as they finish the lab. Later, they are surprised when their answers are incorrect. Take advantage of the last half-hour of each lab. It is an excellent opportunity for checking your understanding of the topic with your instructor and other students.

6. Your instructor will have more time to give study hints near the end of the lab class when the less interested students have already left. This is the perfect opportunity for you to ask what will be emphasized on the lab test.

7. Come early to the first day of lab class. Check out the other students. One (or more) of them is going to be your lab partner. Pick a good one! Some students are not interested in learning biology, and will make you do all the work. Find someone who is serious about success. Be a good partner for them. Look for several other students who are good lab partners and form a study group for tests.ivivChapter 1Measurement

Finally, have fun! Taking an active interest in the lab activities will make the time pass quickly, and will increase your chances for success in biology lab class. Good luck to you, and let us know how *Biology Lab Book* has helped you. We welcome your comments and suggestions.

Suspended Animations, Publisher

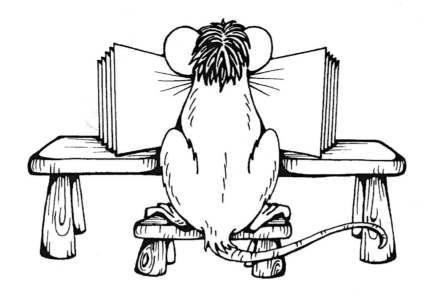

BLB Table Of Contents

MEASURE MENT

Ancient measurement of length was based on the human body. For example, the length of a foot, the length of a stride, the span of a hand, and the breadth of a thumb sufficed as general standards. There were many different measurement systems developed in ancient times, most of them used in only a small locality. One measurement that gained universality was the Egyptian *cubit* around 3000 B.C.E. The cubit was the approximate length of an arm from the elbow to the extended fingertips, or roughly 18 inches.

—HTTP://WWW-HISTORY.MCS.ST-AND.AC.UK/HISTTOPICS/MEASUREMENT.HTML

Number systems are typically based on the number 10, uncoincidentally the number of fingers humans normally possess. There are, however, many number systems in use throughout the world. Our time measurement is founded on base 10 *and* base 6. Computers employ hexadecimal (base 16; all numerals past 10 are represented by the letters A, B, C, D, E, and F) in programming, but utilize binary (base 2, representing "on" and "off" circuits) in operation.

—HTTP://WWW.HELIUM.COM/ITEMS/1255107-UNDERSTANDING-BASE-NUMBER-SYSTEMS

Zero is the universal placeholder in which "nothing" means "something." For most of human history, zero didn't exist! We can thank India for inventing the zero. Zero was discovered independently somewhere between the 4th and 9th century CE by the Mayans.

—"THE STORY OF 1," PBS HOME VIDEO, PRODUCED FOR THE BBC, 2005

What we usually refer to as the Arabic numeral system actually heralds from India around 500 BCE.

—"THE STORY OF 1," PBS HOME VIDEO, PRODUCED FOR THE BBC, 2005

MEASUREMENT

INTRODUCTION

Some people insist that measuring things is the only way to get a fair deal from another human being. But it is also said that the measuring of things is at the heart of all mistrust between people. Whatever the correct judgment may be, historians tell us that measurement systems are based on political and economic needs, and can be found wherever humans have a network of dealing with each other.

Originally, measurement systems depended on the type of material being exchanged. For example, a farmer selling apples would price them by the cart-load, not by the bucket. But when selling milk, a cart-load of liquid would have been ridiculous, and a bucket more appropriate. These kinds of systems developed and changed as they were used. To prevent squabbles among merchants and buyers, *standard* "cart-loads" and "buckets" were determined, and these became the basis for the systems of measurement we use today.

As science developed, the need for scientific measurement began to overlap the measurement systems used for trade. But there are problems with adapting trade measurement systems for use in science. In grade school children are taught the English System which uses inches, feet, yards; cups, pints, quarts, gallons; ounces, pounds, tons. However, a quart in Canada is equal to 1.136 liters. A quart in the United States is equal to 0.946 liters. And in Mexico there are no quarts, only liters. For trade purposes, these inequities can be worked out, but in science or industry where precision is important, the English System simply will not do.

Then, 100 years ago, the International Metric System was devised to standardize measurement around the world. This system provides exact precision in **powers of 10**. There is a standard reference unit used in each measurement category. On either side of the reference unit, the units increase by 10, 100, and 1000 or decrease by $\frac{1}{10}$, $\frac{1}{100}$, and $\frac{1}{1000}$.

The universal standard unit for weight is the **gram** (g). The standard for volume is the **liter** (l). The standard unit for length is the **meter** (m).

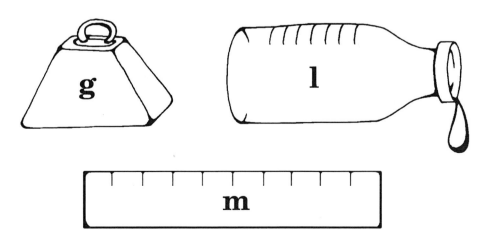

Science embraced the Metric System and so did the majority of the countries in the world. It was anticipated that the United States would be converted to the Metric System by now. It is unfortunate that so much confusion is created by converting quarts to liters, pounds to grams, and inches to meters. The solution is familiarity and practice until the United States completely adopts the Metric System.

In today's lab you will be introduced to the Metric System. You will learn to use simple measuring equipment that will help you remember the different units of the Metric System.

ACTIVITIES

ACTIVITY #1

"SOME BASICS OF THE METRIC SYSTEM"

REVIEW

FRACTIONS

Fractions represent parts of a whole, and there are two methods of expressing them:

> *First*—Simple Fractions
> Examples are $\frac{1}{4}$, $\frac{1}{2}$, $\frac{9}{25}$, etc.

> *Second*—Decimal Fractions
> Examples are 0.25, 0.50, 0.36, etc.

FRACTION CONVERSION

RULE 1 — *If you want to convert a simple fraction into a decimal fraction, then divide the top number of the simple fraction by the bottom number.* Therefore, the simple fraction $\frac{9}{25}$ is converted into decimal form by:

$$25 \overline{\smash{\big)}\ 9.00} = 0.36$$

RULE 2 — *If you must convert a decimal fraction into a simple fraction, then put the decimal fraction over 1.00 (this represents the whole), and reduce the top and bottom numbers to the simplest fraction.* Therefore, the decimal fraction 0.36 converts into:

$$\frac{0.36}{1.00} \quad \text{or} \quad \frac{36}{100} \div \frac{4}{4} \quad \text{or} \quad \frac{9}{25} \quad \text{expressed as a simple fraction.}$$

? QUESTION

Show your work in figuring out the following problems.

1. $\frac{3}{4} =$ _____ (decimal fraction)

2. $\frac{9}{20} =$ _____ (decimal fraction)

3. $0.4 =$ _____ (simple fraction)

4. $0.15 =$ _____ (simple fraction)

In the previous discussion we saw that fractions are *parts* of the number *1*. Percents (%) are *parts* of the number *100*. Therefore, in order to convert a decimal fraction into a percent, we must first *multiply* the decimal fraction by 100.

The decimal fraction 0.23 is equal to 23%. (See the factors of 10—Multiplication Rule below if you need help with this.)

? QUESTION

Convert the following decimal fractions into percents, and show your work.

1. $0.79 =$ _____ %
2. $0.07 =$ _____ %
3. $0.18 =$ _____ %
4. $0.001 =$ _____ %
5. $0.809 =$ _____ %

FACTORS OF 10

Because the Metric System is based on units that differ from each other by factors of 10, we need to review how the decimal position *moves* when converting within metric units.

MULTIPLICATION RULE

When multiplying a number by 10, 100, 1000, etc., move the decimal position *to the right* by the number of 0's (zeros) in the multiplier. For example:

$$25 \times 10 = 25.0 = 250$$

$$25 \times 100 = 25.0\,0 = 2500$$

$$25 \times 1000 = \underline{\hspace{3cm}}$$

$$2.5 \times 100 = \underline{\hspace{3cm}}$$

$$0.25 \times 1000 = \underline{\hspace{3cm}}$$

$$0.002507 \times 100,000 = \underline{\hspace{3cm}}$$

By the way, you add 0's as you move the decimal point to an empty space.

Try these for practice.

This rule allows you to convert *large* metric units like meters into *small* metric units like millimeters.

DIVISION RULE

When dividing a number by 10, 100, 1000, etc., move the decimal position **to the left** by the number of 0's (zeros) in the divisor. For example:

$$25 \div 10 = 2\,5. = 2.5$$

$$25 \div 100 = 2\,5. = 0.25$$

$$25 \div 1000 = 0\,2\,5. = 0.025$$

Again, you add 0's as you move the decimal point to an empty space.

See the Important Message below.

$$0.25 \div 10 = \underline{\hspace{2cm}}$$

$$2.5 \div 10 = \underline{\hspace{2cm}}$$

$$2.5 \div 1000 = \underline{\hspace{2cm}}$$

Try these for practice.

This rule allows you to convert **small** metric units like millimeters into **large** metric units like meters.

IMPORTANT MESSAGE

In science, the rule about decimal fractions like .025 is that you always put a "0" (zero) in front of the decimal point so that there is no confusion about the number being smaller than one. Therefore, we write the above example as 0.025.

METRIC PREFIXES

The Metric System is a standardized method for defining **length**, **volume**, and **weight**.

The standard metric units are **meter** (m), **liter** (l), and **gram** (g).

There are over a dozen prefixes used with each of these standard units that define "portions" of units and differ from each other by factors of 10. In this lab you will need to use only **three** of the metric prefixes. **Memorize them now!**

Prefix	Abbreviation	Compared to Standard	Examples
Milli	m	$\frac{1}{1000}$	mm, ml, mg
Centi	c	$\frac{1}{100}$	cm, *, *
Kilo	k	1000	km, *, kg

* cl, cg, and kl won't be used in this lab.

1. If you convert from a *centi* metric unit to a *milli* metric unit, are you going to a smaller unit or a larger unit in size?

2. How much difference is there between a *centi* unit and a *milli* unit?

3. How many decimal positions would you move for a conversion from *centi* to *milli*?

4. Converting from *centi* to *milli*, would you be moving the decimal position to the left or to the right? _____ You would be using the _____ rule.

5. Let's review your answers with an example.
   24.5 centimeters = _____ millimeters

6. Now, let's try it in reverse.
   53 millimeters = _____ centimeters

There will be more practice on these conversions as you go through the next sections on *standard* metric units.

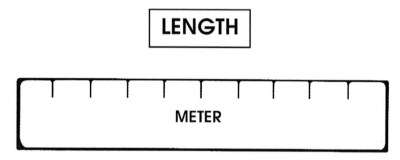

LENGTH

METER

The standard reference for *length* in the Metric System is the *meter* (abbreviated as m). You will be using three prefixes with this standard metric unit: milli ($\frac{1}{1000}$), centi ($\frac{1}{100}$), and kilo (1,000).

Remember to use the rules pertaining to the movement of the decimal point.

? QUESTION

1. The abbreviation for millimeter is **mm**. How many millimeters are in a meter? _____

2. The abbreviation for centimeter is **cm**. How many centimeters are in a meter? _____

3. The abbreviation for kilometer is **km**. How many kilometers are in a meter? _____
   (Did you get tricked by this question?)

4. How many meters are in a kilometer? _____

5. How many mm are in 1 cm? _____

6. How many cm are in a mm? _____

7. 40 cm = _____ m.

8. 40 cm is what fraction of a meter? _____

9. 40 cm is what % of a meter? _____

10. $\dfrac{32 \text{ m}}{10 \text{ mm}}$ = _____   *Hint:* You must have the same units on the top and bottom before doing the division.

11. 1.2 m x 30 = _____ m = _____ cm.

VOLUME

The standard value for *volume* in the Metric System is the *liter* (abbreviated as **l**).

The prefixes used for metric length units also apply to volume units. However, milli is the only prefix that we will use during this lab. The milliliter (**ml**) is a very common unit for the scientific measurement of small volumes of liquid.

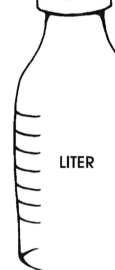

LITER

? QUESTION

1. How many milliliters are in a liter? _____

2. How many liters are in a milliliter? _____

3. 355 ml = _____ l (This is a familiar volume for a canned soda.)

4. 750 ml = _____ l (This is a familiar volume for wine bottles.)

5. 15 ml = _____ l (This volume is used in cooking—one tablespoon.)

6. What % of a liter is 15 ml? _____

7. $\frac{1}{2}$ liter = _____ ml

WEIGHT

The standard reference for **weight** in the Metric System is the *gram* (abbreviated as **g**).

The metric prefixes that we will use during this lab are *milli* and *kilo*.

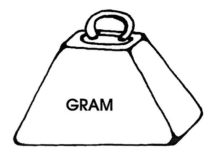

GRAM

? QUESTION

1. How many grams are in a kilogram? _____

2. How many kilograms are in a gram? _____

3. How many milligrams are in a gram? _____

4. How many milligrams are in a kilogram? _____

5. 454 g = _____ kg (This is a familiar weight for a small loaf of bread.)

6. What % of a kilogram is 454 g? _____

7. 2.265 kg is the weight for a small bag of sugar. You are baking cupcakes for a school fund drive. It takes 100 g of sugar to make one batch of cupcakes. How many batches of cupcakes can you make with one small bag of sugar? (Show your work.)

ACTIVITY #2

"CONVERSIONS: METRIC ←→ ENGLISH"

You are familiar with the English System of measurement. In this Activity we will review some conversions between the English and Metric Systems.

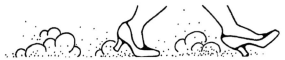

LENGTH

GO GET

A combination meterstick/yardstick.

NOW

1. Make a line on a piece of paper exactly 10 inches long.

2. Measure that same line in centimeters. 10 inches = _____ cm.

? QUESTION

1. How many centimeters are in one inch? _____ cm = 1 inch

2. How many centimeters are in one foot? _____ cm = 1 foot

3. How many centimeters are in one yard? _____ cm = 1 yard
   (Check your answer with the measuring stick.)

VOLUME

GO GET

1. A 1-liter graduated cylinder.

2. A 10-milliliter graduated cylinder.

3. A 1-quart graduated cylinder.

4. An eyedropper.

5. A teaspoon.

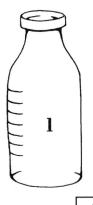

1. Fill the container marked "1 quart" with water. (There may be a painted line indicating the exact 1-quart amount.)

2. Pour the 1 quart of water into a graduated cylinder for measuring liters.

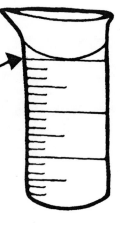

The curve of the water line is called the *meniscus*.

? QUESTION

1. How many ml are there in a quart? _____ ml = 1 quart

2. Which is the greater volume? (circle your choice)   4 Liters   or   1 Gallon

NOW

1. Count the number of drops of water it takes to fill the small graduated cylinder to the 1-milliliter mark.

    1 ml = _____ drops

2. Fill the 10-milliliter cylinder to the 5-milliliter mark. Pour that amount into the teaspoon.

    5 ml = _____ teaspoon

WEIGHT

? QUESTION

Try this weight problem. Home Depot bought sacks of cement from a company in Mexico. The sign above the cement display reads: "100 lb $4.95." The 100-lb cement sacks were also marked "45 kg."

1. How many sacks of cement can you buy for $4.95? _____

2. How many pounds are in one kilogram? _____

3. How much do you weigh in kilograms? _____

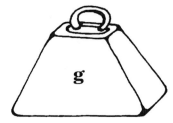

TEMPERATURE

The English measurement of temperature is in degrees Fahrenheit (°F). Using this scale, water freezes at 32°F and boils at 212°F.

There is a scientific temperature scale that is more like a metric scale. It uses Celsius (°C), and on this scale water freezes at 0°C and boils at 100°C.

This scale was copied from a dual scale thermometer. Using this illustration, answer the questions below.

? QUESTION

1. How many °F are there between the 0°C mark and the 100°C mark? _____
   Therefore, how many °F are there in one °C? _____

2. Water freezes at what temperature in °F? _____
   At what temperature in °C? _____

3. Water boils at what temperature in °F? _____
   At what temperature in °C? _____

4. What is your favorite air temperature in °F? _____
   What would that be in °C? _____

5. What is your idea of a "hot day" in °F? _____
   What temperature is that in °C? _____

6. Your normal body temperature is 98.6°F. Your child's forehead seems to be hot. You grab a Celsius thermometer by mistake and take her temperature. It reads 37°. Should you rush her to the hospital? _____ (The formula for converting °C into °F is: **°F = °C x 1.8 + 32**.) Why must the number 32 must be added?

7. Your cookbook says that roast beef is rare at 140°, medium at 160°, and well done at 170°. You like your beef cooked medium-rare and only have a meat thermometer in °C. What temperature will the thermometer have to reach for the roast to be done the way you like it?

8. The water temperature gauge on you new Volkswagen reads 85°C. Are you overheating your engine? _____ Explain.

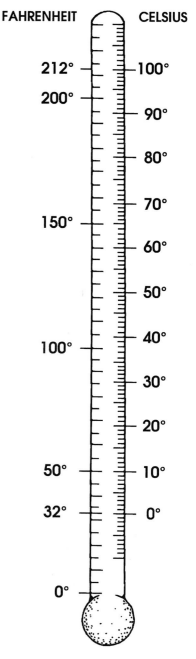

FAHRENHEIT   CELSIUS

212° — 100°
200° — 90°
— 80°
— 70°
150° — 60°
— 50°
— 40°
100° — 30°
— 20°
50° — 10°
32° — 0°

0°

ACTIVITY #3

"PERSONAL LIST OF METRIC REFERENCES"

Think of something easy to remember that you can associate with each of the metric units below.

Perhaps a centimeter might be the width of one of your fingernails.

Share your ideas among other members of your group. Be specific.

Whatever you choose as a reference, *make sure it's something you won't forget!*

MY METRIC LIST

Name: _____

Metric Unit   **My Personal Reference**

Length:

    mm _____

    cm _____

    m _____

    km _____

Volume:

    ml _____ (How many drops?) _____

    l _____

Weight:

    mg _____

    g _____

    kg _____ (How many pounds?) _____

ACTIVITY #4

"A TEST OF YOUR MEASURING SKILLS"

HOW TO WEIGH AN OBJECT

Weighing balances are used to measure the weight of an object. It is important that the object to be weighed is put inside a weighing container so that the material is not spilled on the balance pan.

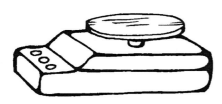 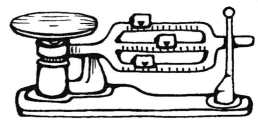

STEP 1 "Zero" the scale. (Your instructor will show you how to do this.)

STEP 2 Then, weigh the weighing container.
Why is it important to weigh the container first?

STEP 3 Put the substance or object into the weighing container, and weigh them together.

STEP 4 Determine the difference between the weights for Step 1 and Step 2.

GO GET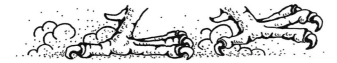

Some table salt.

NOW

Your instructor will give you specific directions for using each type of weighing scale. Make sure that you "zero" the scales before weighing.

1. Weigh 2.7 g of table salt, and put that amount onto a piece of paper. This is the recommended daily intake of salt in your diet.

2. Weigh 11.6 g of table salt, and put that amount next to the other pile. This is the typical daily salt intake by people in our society.

ACTIVITY #5

"A SIMPLE SCIENTIFIC EXPERIMENT"

The scientific method begins with observation. There is something in the world we want to understand, and this is followed by a possible explanation based on our observations. That explanation is called the hypothesis. Although the hypothesis is actually a question, it is written as a declarative statement related to an experiment designed to test whether the hypothesis is true or not. For example, the question, "Are pennies before 1982 the same weight as pennies after 1982?" can be changed into an experimental hypothesis: "Pennies before and after 1982 are the same weight."

NOW

1. There are 20 pennies in each date category on the lab table.

2. Weigh a group of 10 coins from each date category to get a better estimate of the weight of a single coin (divide the group weight by 10).

3. Record the results.   Before 1982 pennies: _____ g   After 1982 pennies: _____ g

So, did the experiment tell us the hypothesis is true or false?

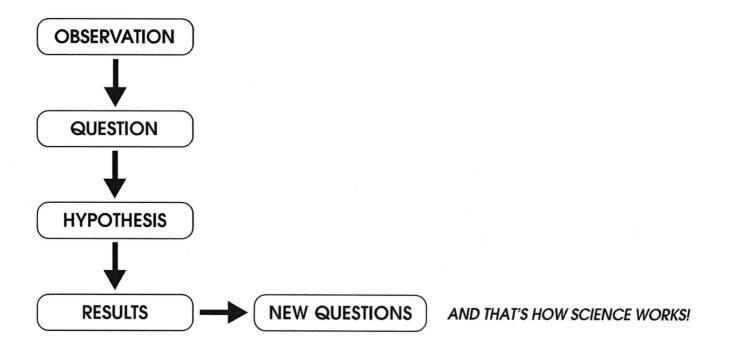

This leads to another question. You have observed that older pennies (before 1982) seem to be a different weight from more recent pennies (after 1982). You wonder why. Is the difference in weight of the pennies because they are not the same size, or because they are not made of the same metals? Now, it's your job to test the next hypothesis.

THEN

1. Determine how you would estimate the size of the coins by measuring the volume of water displaced by the coins.

2. Use the graduated cylinder on the lab table and 10 coins together to get a better estimate of water displacement and the individual coin size. Do this for both pre- and post-1982 pennies.

3. A simple answer to the question of differences in metal is revealed when pennies are cut in half. Ask your instructor to show you those pennies.

4. Complete the lab report for this activity below.

LAB REPORT

Question:

Hypothesis:

Experimental Design:

Results:

Conclusions:

MICROSCOPE

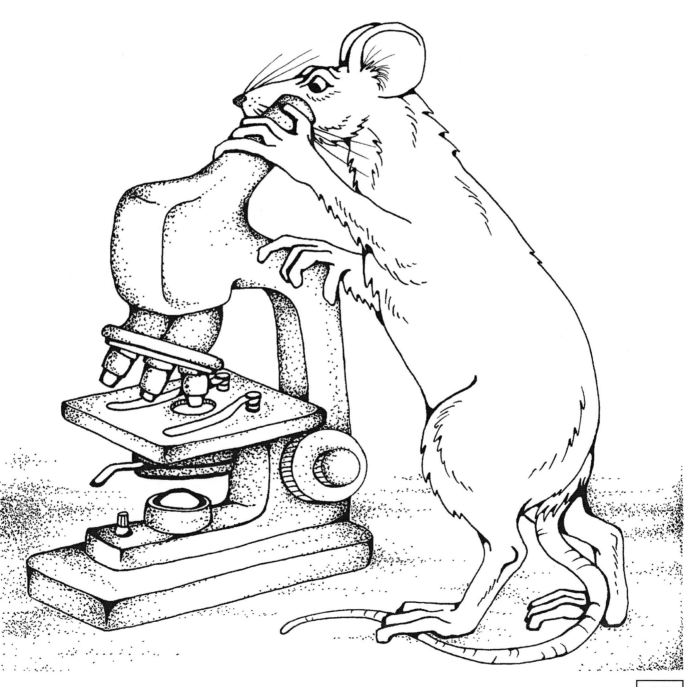

The microscope was invented in the Netherlands by Anton Van Leouwenhoek in 1608.

—HTTP://WIKI.ANSWERS.COM/Q/WHAT_R_THE_TEN_MOST_INTERESTING_FACTS_ABOUT_MICROSCOPES#IXZZ1RYOQXGSZ

The maximum useful magnification of a standard microscope is 1200x with an oil-immersion lens (without oil immersion, it is about 800x). The scanning electron microscope has a magnification range from 15x to 200,000x (achieved in 25 steps) and a resolution of 5 nanometers.

—HTTP://EN.WIKIPEDIA.ORG/WIKI/MAGNIFICATION

—HTTP://WIKI.ANSWERS.COM/Q/
WHAT_IS_THE_MAXIMUM_MAGNIFICATION_OF_THE_SCANNING_ELECTRON_MICROSCOPE#IXZZ1RYTQDPJ6

The Canadian Center for Electron Microscopy has developed the world's most powerful electron microscope to date—the Titan 80-300 Cubed. The power of this microscope can be thought as equivalent to "taking the Hubble Telescope and aiming it at the atomic level." This microscope is so powerful that it can easily probe the electrons that bind atoms together. The Titan stands about 5½ feet tall (plus several desktops of auxiliary equipment) and costs $15 million to build.

—HTTP://WWW.TECHNOSPIKES.COM/2010/07/MOST-ADVANCED-MICROSCOPE-OF-WORLD.HTML

The world's smallest scanning electron microscope is the Phenom, about the size and shape of a desktop computer, It can magnify up to 20,000x, while costing a mere $72,000.

—HTTP://WWW.POPULARMECHANICS.COM/TECHNOLOGY/GADGETS/4218957

For home microscopy enthusiasts, an LED-illuminated pocket microscope that can provide 45x magnification and measures less than 7½ inches long by 1½ inches wide, sells for $4.57 on Amazon.com.

—HTTP://WWW.AMAZON.COM/SE-MINI-45X-MICROSCOPE-ILLUMINATOR/DP/B002E0MU70/
REF=WL_IT_DP_O?IE=UTF8&COLIID=I97GYKY6YGRXQ&COLID=6T58DINJ57UQ

A new X-ray microscope can image details as small as a billionth of a meter—without using a lens. The new microscope uses a powerful computer program to unscramble and convert patterns from X-rays bouncing off materials into images of objects as small as one nanometer across—on the scale of a few atoms.

—HTTP://WWW.LIVESCIENCE.COM/15661-SUPERMAN-RAY-MICROSCOPE-ENABLES-NANOVISION.HTML

THE MICROSCOPE

INTRODUCTION

Physical reality is easiest to comprehend when we can see it. But, humans can't see very small or very far away things. We had to discover and explore the smaller world of atoms and the larger world of the universe by using indirect observations and our imaginations.

It wasn't until the inventions of the microscope and the telescope in the 1600's that humans were able to directly observe the worlds of the very small and the very large. Because of those inventions, biology and astronomy became major arenas of scientific exploration.

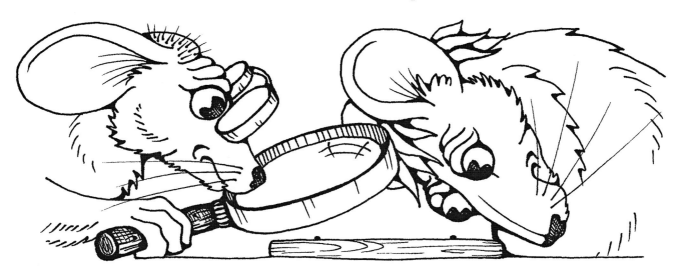

Your naked eye cannot see an object that is less than $\frac{1}{10}$ of a millimeter in length. But with a compound or dissecting microscope, small objects seem huge. The microscope is an extension of your visual sense. And this week, you will learn to use this tool and study the structure of organisms that ordinarily you cannot see.

ACTIVITIES

ACTIVITY #1

"FILM ON THE MICROSCOPE"

You will hear a short lecture or watch a film on the microscope before answering the questions below.

| GO GET | 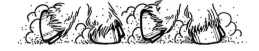 |

A compound microscope. Unless you are extremely rich, *be sure to carry it with both hands!*

| NOW |

Work in groups of 3 or 4 to answer the questions below. Refer to Figures 1 through 6 on the following pages to help you in your discussions.

| ? QUESTION |

1. What happens to a beam of light when it passes through a lens? _____

2. If the light rays from an object enter the eye at a small angle, then the object will cover a _____ (smaller or larger) portion of the back of the eye.

3. The closer you move an object to your eye, the _____ (smaller or larger) the angle of light from that object entering your eye. Therefore, the object appears to be _____ (smaller or larger).

4. The magnifying lens _____ (increases or decreases) the angle of light coming from the object viewed. This results in _____ (increased or decreased) spread of the image at the back of the eye.

5. What is resolution?

6. Is resolution the same as magnification? _____

7. What is the total magnification if the objective lens is 4x and the ocular lens is 10x? _____

8. What is the field of view? Be specific.

9. What happens to the size of the field of view as you change magnification? _____

10. Which objective lens gives the greatest magnification? _____

11. Which objective lens gives the greatest field of view? _____

12. When you search for a specimen, which lens should be used first? _____

13. What is the depth of focus? Be specific.

14. How does depth of focus change with magnification? Be specific.

FIGURE 1

CLOSE vs. FAR IMAGES

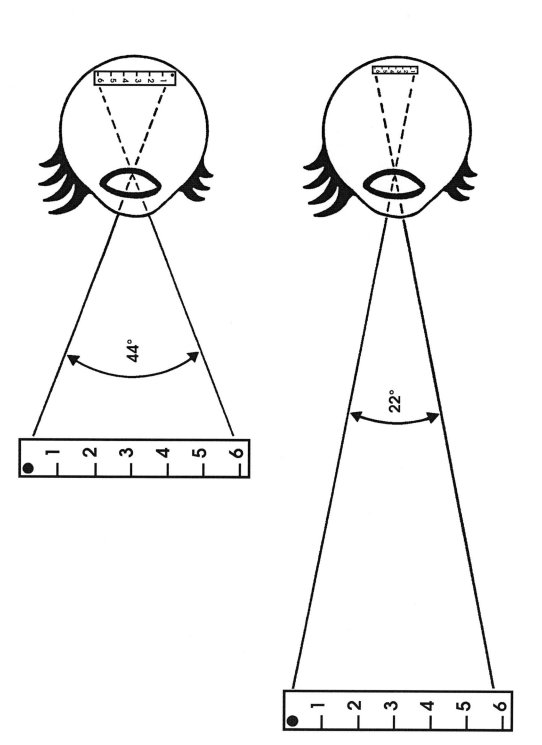

The light rays from a big object take up more of the surface at the back of the eye than the light rays from a small object. This is one way that our brains distinguish between small and large objects. Likewise, the light rays from a near object take up more of the surface at the back of the eye than the light rays from a distant object. This is why distant objects appear small compared to close objects.

It is the *angle* of light entering the eye that determines the amount of light spreading on the back of the eye. Big objects have a greater angle of spread than small objects. And near objects have a greater angle of spread than far objects.

FIGURE 2

CLOSE VS. MAGNIFIED IMAGE

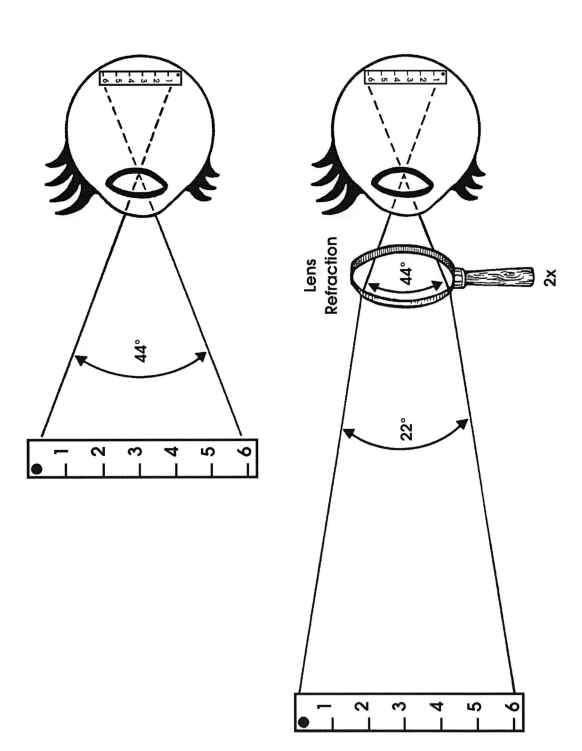

A magnifying lens bends the light rays traveling through it and *increases the angle* of light entering the eye, resulting in a bigger spread of the image at the back of the eye. Therefore, the object seems twice as close.

Because the image is spread over the entire back surface of the eye, more nerve cells are activated and much more *clarity of image* is sent to the brain. We see the object as bigger and we have excellent resolution at the same time.

FIGURE 3

RESOLUTION: SEEING IN FINE DETAIL

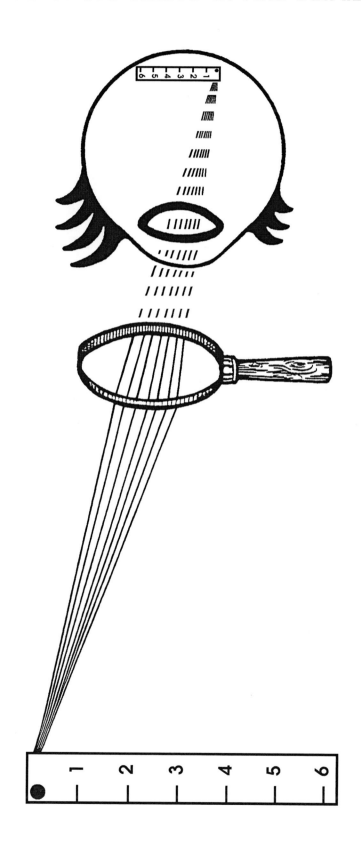

Resolution is the clarity of image produced by the microscope lenses. It is influenced by several factors. Shorter wavelengths of energy passing through the object result in better resolution. Electrons have a much shorter wavelength than visible light, which is why electron microscopes produce the best resolution. Also, a thin layer of oil between the object and the lens produces less random scattering (blurring) of light rays. Finally, excellent quality lenses refocus "stray" light rays from each point of the viewed object, which greatly improves resolution.

FIGURE 4

COMPOUNDED IMAGE

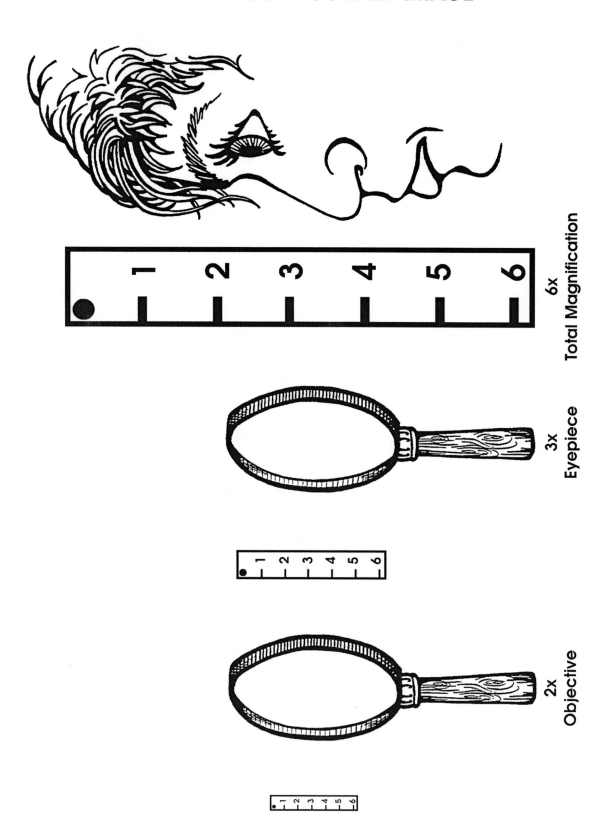

6x
Total Magnification

3x
Eyepiece

2x
Objective

When there are *two* lenses in a sequence, the image of the object is magnified *twice* before entering the eye. In this example, the first lens magnifies the object 2x, and the second lens magnifies that 2x image by 3x more. This results in a *compounded* magnification of 6x the original size.

FIGURE 5

MAGNIFICATION VS. FIELD OF VIEW

(Inverse Proportionality)

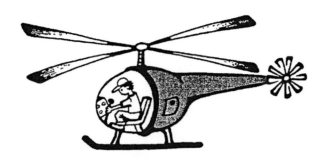

Less Magnification

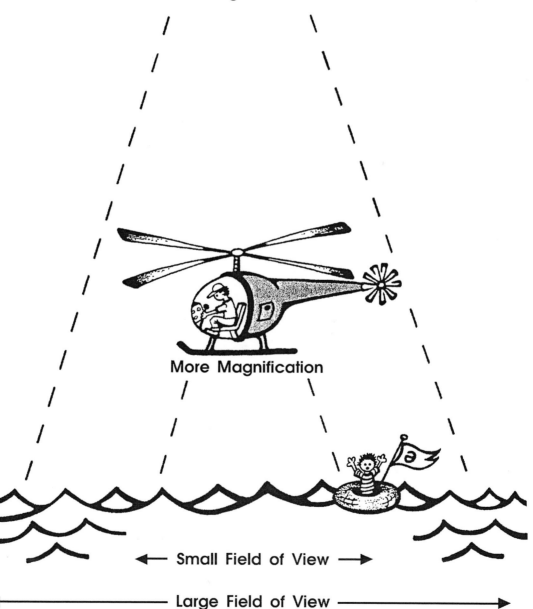

More Magnification

← Small Field of View →

← Large Field of View →

FIGURE 6

MAGNIFICATION vs. DEPTH OF FOCUS

(Inverse Proportionality)

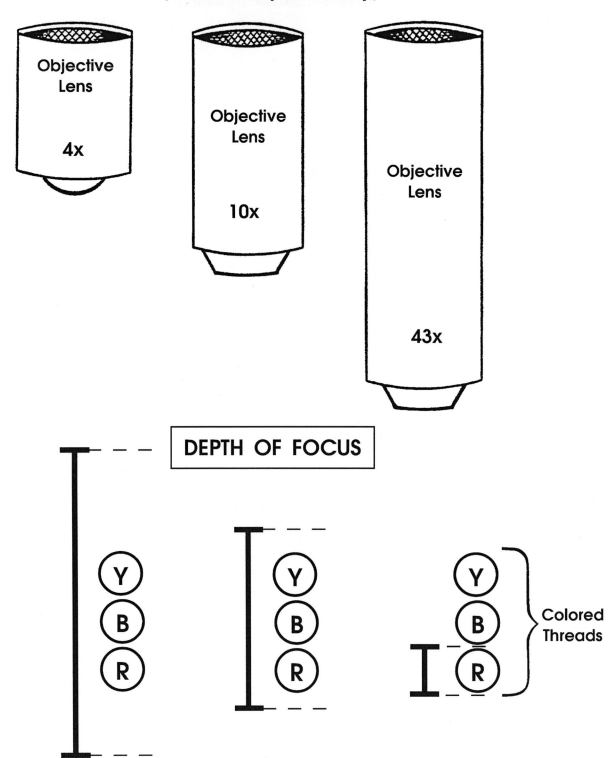

The *more* the magnification the *less* the depth of focus.

Get familiar with the parts of a microscope by referring to the picture below and looking at your microscope. (Be able to name the parts and their functions on a Lab Test.)

Parts	Function
1. **Nosepiece**	A circular plate with 3 or 4 objective lenses that can be rotated into viewing position for different magnifications.
2. **Objective Lens**	This is the first lens that magnifies the image, and it is positioned just above the object being viewed.
3. **Ocular Lens**	This is the second lens that magnifies the image, and it is the one closest to your eye when you are looking through the microscope tube.
4. **Coarse Focus Knob**	Turning this knob decreases the distance between the objective lens and the stage, and allows you to focus the image entering your eye.
5. **Fine Focus Knob**	Use this knob to fine-focus the image and when viewing through the higher magnifications.
6. **Iris Diaphragm**	This lever (or rotating disk) adjusts the amount of light shining through the object. Use just enough light to illuminate the object and give good contrast.
7. **Condenser**	Some microscopes have a light condenser with an iris diaphragm lever. The condenser focuses light on the microscope slide. It should be positioned the same distance below the slide as the objective lens is above the slide. To achieve the clearest image, adjust the condenser each time you change the objective lens.
8. **Stage**	This is the platform designed to hold the microscope slide.

ACTIVITY #2

"A PINHOLE MICROSCOPE"

The pinhole microscope will demonstrate how the control of light rays determines your ability to see very small and close-up objects.

GO GET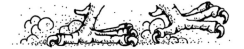

1. An 8" x 8" piece of black paper with a pinhole in the center.
2. A piece of paper with typed words on it.
3. A metric ruler.

NOW

In the first trial, don't use the pinhole paper. Hold the typewritten page in your left hand and slowly move it towards your eye. At some point the words on the page will become blurry. Have your lab partner measure the distance from the typed page to your eye. _____ cm.

? QUESTION

1. As you moved the printed page closer to your eye, did the *size* of the letters appear to change?

2. The words became blurry at some point close to your eye. What *quality* of your vision is being lost up close? _____ (We used this term to describe the clarity of the image.)

THEN

Repeat the experiment using the pinhole paper. Hold the pinhole paper with your right hand, and position the hole as close to your eye as possible. Move the typed page closer to your eye, and notice that the words which were blurry at _____ cm in the first trial are now readable at _____ cm this time.

? QUESTION

1. What *quality* of your vision has been improved by the pinhole paper?

2. Can you figure out how the pinhole microscope works? (Refer back to Figure 3 to help you with your answer.)

ACTIVITY #3

"FINDING AND FOCUSING"

 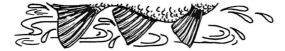

GO GET

1. A compound microscope, one microscope slide, and one coverslip.

2. A cutout of the letter "**e**" from a piece of newspaper.

NOW

1. Turn on the microscope light.

2. Use the coarse focus knob to move the nosepiece all the way "up," and "click" the 4x objective lens into position. (Some microscopes raise the nosepiece, and others lower the stage. Check to see which microscope type you have.)

3. Get a prepared slide of the letter "e" or make a slide with the letter "e". Cut out a magazine letter "e" and place the letter on the glass slide. Slowly lower a coverslip over the letter to hold it in place. *Use no water.*

4. Place the slide on the stage, position the letter "**e**" over the stage hole, and secure the slide.

5. Look through the ocular lens and slowly turn the coarse focusing knob so that the distance between the lens and the slide decreases. The letter "**e**" will come into view.

6. Center the letter "**e**" in your field of view, and use the fine focus.

7. Adjust the iris diaphragm until you have the proper amount of light with good contrast. It is very important that you reduce the light so that the details of the object can be seen. *Using too much light is the most common mistake that students make when working with the microscope.*

? QUESTION

1. Draw the letter "**e**" as it is positioned on the stage. Then draw the orientation of the letter "**e**" as it appears when viewed through the microscope.

2. What has happened to the orientation of the image as it passes through the lenses of the microscope?

3. When you move the slide forward on the stage, in what direction does the "**e**" appear to move when viewed through the microscope?

4. When you move the slide to the right, in what direction does the "**e**" appear to move?

5. What are your conclusions about the appearance and movement of an object when viewed through a microscope?

Normal View

Microscope View

ACTIVITY #4

"DEPTH OF FOCUS: CROSSED THREADS"

Think back to the photographs that you have taken and looked at. There always seems to be a zone of sharp focus in the picture, with objects out of focus in front of and behind the sharp focus zone.

The sharp focus zone is called the *depth of focus*. This can become a serious problem when using a microscope as you increase the magnification. In fact, when looking through a microscope, the zone of sharp focus can be a major limitation in viewing the whole object. But, you can make use of that restriction as a tool to inspect *different layers* of the object being viewed.

Depth of focus is inversely proportional to magnification. In other words, as the magnification of the object increases, the depth of focus decreases. (Don't confuse this with *resolution,* which is a function of lens quality.)

GO GET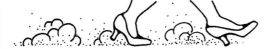

A prepared microscope slide of three crossed and colored threads.

NOW 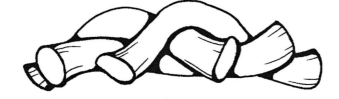 Crossed Threads

1. Review the directions in Activity #3 for finding and focusing with the 4x objective lens.

2. Once you have the crossed threads in focus—with proper contrast—be sure the point where the threads cross is *centered* in your field of view.

3. Turn the nosepiece until the 10x objective lens "clicks" into place. If you did a good job of centering the cross of the threads at low power, then the cross should be in your field of view at higher power. If not, go back to step #1 and try again.

4. Focus using the fine focusing knob, and adjust the contrast if necessary. Again, center the crossing threads in the field of view.

5. Turn the nosepiece until the high power (40x or 43x, depending on microscope brand) objective lens "clicks" into place, and focus using the fine focusing knob. Adjust the contrast if necessary. Properly position the condenser if your microscope has one.

IMPORTANT MESSAGE

Do not make the mistake of raising the nosepiece before switching to the 43x objective lens!

If your threads were in focus at 10x, then the high power lens will *not* hit the slide.

6. Now, use the fine focusing knob to move the zone of sharp focus below the threads so that all the threads are blurred and slightly out of focus.

7. Then, reverse the direction you were turning the fine focusing knob. Watch the crossed threads until the *first* thread comes into focus. That will be the *bottom* thread.

   Hint: If you start out of focus *above* the threads, and move the lens closer to the slide, then the first thread to come into focus will be the top thread. However, if you start out of focus *below* the threads, and move the lens away from the slide, then the first thread to come into focus will be the bottom thread. Focus back and forth until you can determine the arrangement of the crossed threads.

Normally, focusing the highest power objective lens should be started slightly below the object (out of focus) and moved away from the stage so that you don't accidentally crunch the lens into the glass slide, cracking it and scratching the lens. After you become very practiced with a microscope, you won't make this mistake, but for now *please be very careful*.

? QUESTION

1. What color is the thread that is on the bottom, the middle, and the top?

   _____ top

   _____ middle

   _____ bottom

2. What microscope part is used to change the light intensity? (Answer may differ depending on your microscope model)

3. What happens to the light intensity as you increase or decrease magnification of the objective lens?

4. When you switch to higher magnification, what should you do to the light intensity?

5. Describe the proper focusing technique in terms of moving the lens (especially the high-power lens) up and down when you first look at an object.

6. Why is this focusing technique so important?

ACTIVITY #5

"ESTIMATING THE SIZE OF AN OBJECT"

In order to estimate the size of an object, it is absolutely necessary to have an idea of the size of your field of view.

This applies to estimating the size of *any* object. For instance, if a person was standing next to a tree and you knew the size of the tree, then you would have a standard against which you could estimate the size of the person.

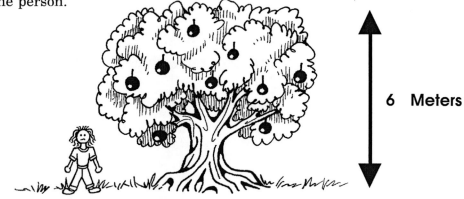

6 Meters

The person is about _____ (what fraction) the size of the tree. Therefore, the person is about _____ meters tall.

The standard we use to estimate the size of an object when viewed under the microscope is the *diameter* of the *field of view*.

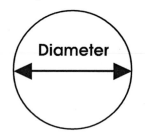

Diameter

The field of view looks like this.

And the *diameter* of the field of view is the length of a straight line through the center of the circle.

GO GET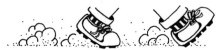

A transparent 15-centimeter ruler.

NOW

1 mm

1. Each dash on the metric side of this ruler is a millimeter unit. Under the microscope these dashes appear wide. To properly measure the diameter of the field of view under a microscope, you must measure a millimeter as the distance from one side of a mark to the same side of the next mark.

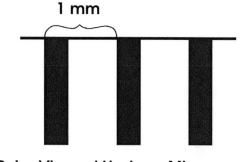

Ruler Viewed Under a Microscope

2. Using the ruler, measure the diameter of the field of view with the 4x objective lens in position. Estimate this diameter to the nearest $\frac{1}{10}$ of a millimeter.

Diameter of 4x field of view = _____ mm.

3. Since the diameter of the field of view is *inversely proportional* to the magnification, we can use this knowledge to estimate the diameter for the other two higher power lenses.

Remember: As magnification *increases*, the field of view *decreases*.

? QUESTION

1. If the diameter of the field of view through the 4x lens is 4mm, then under 10x it will be

Larger than 4mm   or   Smaller than 4mm

2. What is the diameter of the field of view you measured through the 4x lens?

_____ mm

3. Instead of physically measuring the diameter of the 10x view, you can use a calculation to give you the answer. Because the 10x objective lens provides $2\frac{1}{2}$ times *more* magnification than the 4x objective lens, its field of view is $2\frac{1}{2}$ times *smaller* ($10 \div 4 = 2\frac{1}{2}$).

So, use the above calculation to figure out how big the diameter of the field of view would be through the 10x lens. *Remember:* The field will be $2\frac{1}{2}$ times smaller than at 4x.

_____ mm

4. The calculation method used for the 10x lens in the previous question above also applies to the 43x objective lens. 43x is _____ times more magnification than the 4x objective. So, the diameter of the field of view using the 43x objective lens will be _____ times smaller than at 4x.

Note: If your microscope has a 40x objective or some other number, substitute the magnification of the lens that you do have for all of the calculations above where the number "43x" occurs.

5. What is the diameter of the field of view for your microscope through the 43x lens?

_____ mm

GO GET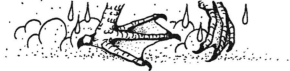

1. A glass slide and a coverslip.

2. The small letter "**i**" cut from a newspaper. Be sure to include the dot.

1. After making a slide of the "i" like you did in Activity #3, look at it under low power and center the dot in your field of view. Switch to the 10x objective lens, center the dot, then go to the 43x lens. Estimate how much of the field of view is occupied by the dot through the 43x lens.

_____ %

2. If the dot is about _____ % of the 43x diameter of view, then the diameter of the dot is approximately _____ mm.

ACTIVITY #6

"SEARCHING THE FLY WING"

This Activity will test your ability to look for something specific under the microscope.

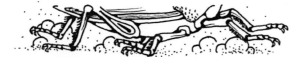

GO GET

A prepared microscope slide of a fly wing.

NOW

1. Look at the picture of the fly wing at the front of the lab. Study it carefully. A particular vein intersection will be marked on the picture.

2. If it helps you to remember, draw a simple sketch from the picture.

   Be sure to indicate the field of view as it appears in the picture.

3. Find the *exact* vein intersection in your microscope slide *under the same magnification* as you see in the picture.

4. Be able to do this exercise on a Lab Test.

Fly Wing Veins

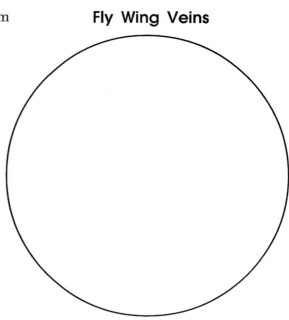

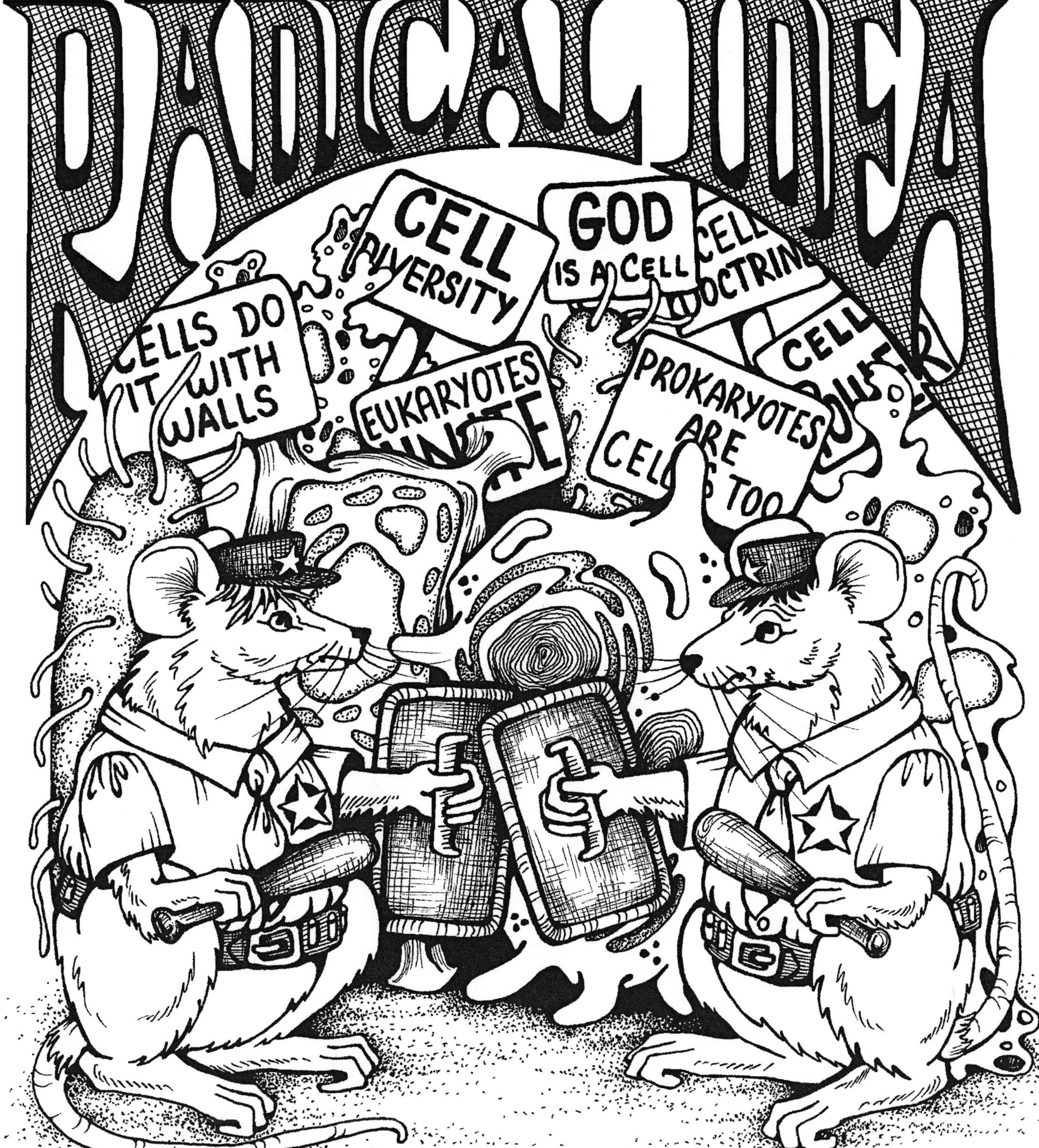

DYNAMIC DEVELOPMENTS
AND
FASCINATING FACTS
IN BIOLOGY

Cells may have first evolved from simple chemical structures known as *liposomes* or *micelles*. Micelles are formed when fatty substances such as phospholipids are added to water, allowing a fatty soap bubble to form a thin membrane that has the ability to envelope and accommodate chemical compounds such as DNA. These "proto-cells" can replicate and begin other chemical processes that help them maintain their fragile membranes.

—MODEL OF SELF-REPLICATING CELL CAPABLE OF SELF-MAINTENANCE, BY NAOAKI ONO AND TAKASHI IKEGAMI,
—HTTP://ARXIV.ORG/PS_CACHE/ADAP-ORG/PDF/9905/9905002V2.PDF

When a cell becomes damaged or undergoes some type of infection, it will self destruct —commit suicide—by a process called *apoptosis*. Apoptosis (also called programmed cell death, or PCD) works to ensure proper development and to keep the body's natural process of mitosis in check. It is such a precise process that it is as intrinsic as is mitosis. A cell's inability to undergo apoptosis can result in the development of cancer.

—HTTP://USERS.RCN.COM/JKIMBALL.MA.ULTRANET/BIOLOGYPAGES/A/APOPTOSIS.HTML

Researchers at the Craig Venter Institute, have synthesized the first self-replicating artificial cell. The cell was not made "from scratch," but was derived from the genome of a simple bacterium, *Mycoplasma mycoides*. Nucleotides were added until an entire copy of the genome could produce daughter cells that self-replicated.

—HTTP://WWW.POPULARMECHANICS.COM/SCIENCE/HEALTH/BREAKTHROUGHS/SYNTHETIC-CELL-BREAKTHROUGH#IXZZ1JI43SE24

A cell has been genetically engineered to emit laser light. Expressing green fluorescent protein (GFP), the cell can amplify photons into pulses of laser light. A living laser is especially unusual, because typical bioluminescence employs a diffuse light mixture of many frequencies, while laser light is "coherent" light of a single frequency (also known as "monochromatic"). The spherical shape of the cell itself acts as a lens, refocusing the light and inducing emission of laser light.

—HTTP://WWW.NATURE.COM/NPHOTON/INDEX.HTML

Cells have been revealed to communicate through the exchange of photons. Living cells in culture synchronize their internal chemical processes, even though they are mechanically, chemically, and electrically isolated from one another. Biologists have long known that photons play a central role in the biochemistry of many plant and bacterial cells. This is the basic theory behind photosynthesis, but photon exchange and stimulation is now understood to occur in animal cells as well. Optical or UV photons enter a cell and stimulate the creation of *excitons* (a species of electron) on certain long-chain molecules. The exciton travels along the molecule, influencing the way it reacts with molecules in other cells. This discovery generates more questions than answers. For example, how do cells discriminate between biophotons and background light? And what to make of other evidence that the photons can sometimes be coherent, as in a laser beam?

—HTTP://WWW.PHOTOBIOLOGY.COM/PHOTOBIOLOGY99/CONTRIB/APPLEGATE/INDEX.HTM

CELLS: A RADICAL IDEA

INTRODUCTION

Educated people of the early 1800's had the belief that some invisible force was responsible for life in all its growing and changing forms. In 1839, Schleiden and Schwann presented the idea that *cells* were the creative force responsible for living organisms. Even though it was a radical change from the beliefs of the time, their ideas were accepted almost without question. The logic and proofs presented made perfect sense. Many puzzling questions were now answered.

The *Cell Law* states:

1. all of life consists of cells,
2. all cells come from previous cells, and
3. all life processes derive from cellular activities.

The implications of this principle are profound. It means that:

1. all life forms are related to each other at the cellular level,
2. all functions of organisms (including humans) are based on individual cell activities, and
3. all cellular activities are based on chemical processes.

Yet, in spite of what it implied, scientists and laymen were in agreement about cells. How different was the reception of Schlieden and Schwann when compared to other pioneers in biology, like Gregor Mendel in genetics research, and Charles Darwin in concepts of evolution.

This week you will look at cells and discover some of their general features.

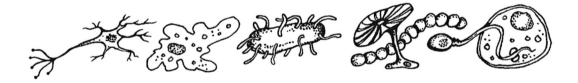

ACTIVITIES

ACTIVITY #1

"HOW TO MAKE A WET MOUNT SLIDE"

In order to observe cells, you will have to become good at the technique of making a slide. This requires patience and careful handling of equipment. Take your time.

IMPORTANT MESSAGE

Whenever you make a slide of something during this semester, you should use the wet mount method. It is the very best way to get a clear view of the object, and it prevents the specimen from drying out.

| STEP 1 | You will need a microscope slide and a coverslip. |

| STEP 2 | Put a *drop* of water on the slide. |

| STEP 3 | Put the object into the drop of water. The object must be *very* thin. You will see the importance of this when you make a wet mount of onion cells. |

| STEP 4 | Place the coverslip over the object by first placing one edge down, and then slowly lowering the other side so that you don't trap air bubbles. Air bubbles will look like discarded tires, and are actually quite interesting in appearance, but they will interfere with your view of the object you really want to see. |

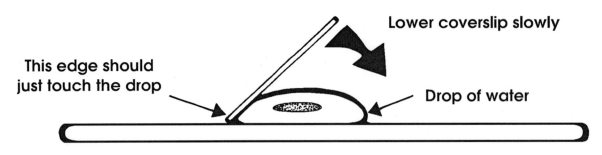

Lower coverslip slowly

This edge should just touch the drop

Drop of water

SIDE VIEW OF SLIDE

ACTIVITY #2

"HUMAN CHEEK CELLS"

There are two types of cells: *prokaryotic* and *eukaryotic*. All of the cells you look at in the lab today are of the type called **eukaryotic** (true nucleus). The eukaryotic type of cell is the basic component of all multi-celled life forms. Some eukaryotic cells, such as the *Paramecium*, are single-celled organisms.

However, the largest number of single-celled organisms are the bacteria and their relatives, and they are of another cell type called **prokaryotic** (before nucleus). You will have the opportunity to investigate them later in the semester.

Now you will begin your journey into the world of cells by looking at *human cheek cells*.

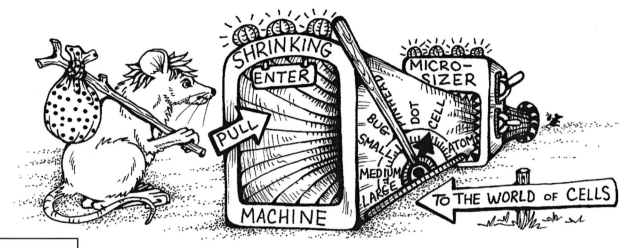

GO GET

1. A compound microscope.
2. A microscope slide and coverslip.
3. A toothpick.
4. Methylene Blue stain

NOW

1. Put a small drop of water on the microscope slide.

2. *Gently* scrape the inside of your cheek with the blunt end of the toothpick. You will have collected hundreds of eukaryotic cells on the toothpick.

3. Pay attention to exactly where you put the cells on the slide. They are hard to find. *Throw away the toothpick into the special waste container or disinfectant solution.*

4. Cover the drop with a coverslip.

5. Look at the cells under high power with your compound microscope. ***Remember:*** They will be very hard to see.

6. Now, put a drop of *methylene blue* stain at the edge of the coverslip. Use a small piece of tissue paper at the other edge of the coverslip to absorb the excess fluid and pull the stain across the slide. This method allows you to apply a stain without removing the coverslip.

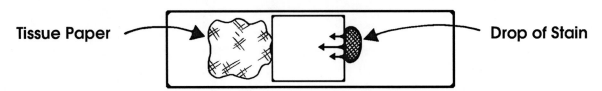

Tissue Paper →   ← **Drop of Stain**

Applying stain to the object will darken some cell structures, allowing you to see them better. Experiment with the iris diaphragm, light intensity, and condenser (if your microscope has one) to get more contrast and clarity.

7. Look at the cells again under high power. You should be able to see the **nucleus** and the **cell membrane**. The nucleus controls the cell functions, and the cell membrane controls what molecules go into and out of the cell.

Human Cheek Cells

8. The advantage of stains is that we can see structures better. The disadvantage is that stains kill the cells. *Never use a stain if you want to see living cells!*

9. Draw a simple sketch of your cheek cells. Label the cell membrane and the nucleus.

? QUESTION

1. How do you know that your cheek cells are *eukaryotic* cells?

2. You may be asked on a Lab Test to make a wet mount of cheek cells, and find them under the microscope. Can you do it?

3. Point out the cell membrane and cell nucleus to your lab partner. Be able to do the same for your instructor on a test.

FINALLY

Use alcohol or disinfectant solution to clean your slide before reuse in the next Activity. Follow the directions from your instructor.

ACTIVITY #3

"ONION CELLS"

In this Activity, you will be examining a plant cell. As you work through the steps, notice a difference between plant and animal cells (human cheek cells).

GO GET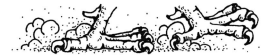

1. Cutting board and knife.

2. Cut an onion into "onion rings."

NOW

1. The cut onion will come apart into $\frac{1}{8}$"-thick rings. Make your peel from the inside (not the outside) of one of the onion rings. You should be able to peel off a one-cell-thick layer of tissue. It will look like a piece of plastic wrap. You can use a razor blade or forceps to start the peel. But don't slice off a piece; that will be many cell layers thick. You need a one-cell layer.

2. Place the onion peel into a drop of water on the slide, trying not to fold it over on itself.

3. Finish the wet mount, and look at the cells under the compound microscope (low power first, then high power).

4. Now, put a drop of *iodine* stain at the edge of the coverslip. Use the tissue paper to draw the stain across.

5. Look at the cells again. You should be able to see the ***nucleus*** and the ***cell wall***. The nucleus controls cell functions, and the cell wall is a little box made of cellulose (wood) produced by the cell for support. *Draw a simple sketch of the onion cells at high power. Label the cell wall and the nucleus.*

Onion Cells

? QUESTION

What differences and similarities did you observe between the onion (plant) cells and the cheek (animal) cells?

FINALLY

Wash off the slide and coverslip so that you can use them for the next Activity. Don't throw them away. They can be used over and over again.

ACTIVITY #4

"PARAMECIUM"

A *Paramecium* is a one-celled organism. Because it must do everything in its life as only one cell, it is far more complex than any single human cell.

 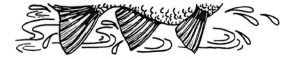

A drop of water from the bottom of the *Paramecium* culture (these organisms usually settle near the bottom), and put the drop on your slide.

NOW

1. Make a wet mount, and find the *Paramecium* under the 10x objective lens (that will be 100x magnification).

2. Your job is to train your hands to be able to follow this organism under the microscope. *Hint:* Don't think! Let your hands work by themselves.

3. Practice your quick-vision skills by making a simple sketch of the *Paramecium*. Label the nucleus and the cell membrane.

Paramecium

4. *Optional:* We have a product called Protoslo® that can be added to the water drop sample. It will dramatically slow the movements of the *Paramecium* because it thickens the water. However, Protoslo® will also push the one-celled organisms to the outside perimeter of the water drop. You have to first mix the Protoslo® with the drop of sample.

? QUESTION

1. What obvious differences did you observe in the one-celled organism as compared to one cell of a multi-celled organism (cheek or onion cells)?

2. If you were asked on a test to find a *Paramecium* in "pond water," could you do it? *Remember:* Pond water will contain many different organisms.

3. How do you think a *Paramecium* eats? (Refer to your textbook for the answer.)

FINALLY

Wash off the slide and coverslip in preparation for the next Activity.

ACTIVITY #5

"*ELODEA* LEAF"

Elodea is found in freshwater ponds, and is commercially grown and sold as an aquarium plant. Pay attention to the differences between the *Elodea* cells and the onion cells that you observed in Activity #3.

 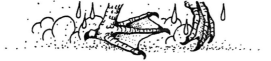

An *Elodea* leaf from near the tip of a healthy plant. Use forceps to pluck the leaf. Keep track of which side is the *upper* side of the leaf.

NOW

1. Make a wet mount with the upper side of the leaf facing up, and find the *Elodea* cells under the 10x objective. Look near the tip of the leaf. These are often very active cells. Then switch to high power magnification.

2. You will know that the cells are alive and active if you can see **chloroplasts** moving around the cell. It may take a few minutes of warming under the microscope light before the chloroplasts begin to move. Chloroplasts are the cell structures (organelles) that do *photosynthesis* (food production) in plants.

3. There is a large sac of fluid inside the *Elodea* cell called the **central vacuole**. Imagine a swimming pool that has a huge clear sac of water floating in it. You can't actually see the sac of water, but the movements of everyone in the pool will be influenced as they bump into that large clear sac.

   Now watch the movement of chloroplasts. See if you can observe the indirect evidence that the central vacuole is in the cell and is influencing the movement of those chloroplasts.

   Draw a sketch of the *Elodea* leaf cell and label the central vacuole and the chloroplasts.

Elodea Cells

4. During the Microscope Lab you used the fine focus at high power to determine which color of thread was on top of the others.

   An *Elodea* leaf is two cells thick. You should be able to decide whether the top layer is made of bigger or smaller size cells than the bottom layer. Do this now.

1. What color are the chloroplasts?

2. When you see the color of plants, what *structures* are you actually seeing?

3. What does the *movement* of the chloroplasts tell you about the cell?

4. If you can't actually see the central vacuole inside the *Elodea* cell, then how do you know that it is there?

5. *Elodea* leaves are two cells thick. One of the layers has thick cell walls. Those cells are in the . . . (circle your choice)

         Top layer   or   Bottom layer

6. What is the most obvious difference you observed between the *Elodea* cell and the onion cell?

    What does that observation tell you about the activity of food production in the onion cell?

    Where is food produced in the onion plant?

FINALLY

*Save this **Elodea** slide for the next Activity. You will look at the cells one more time.*

ACTIVITY #6

"COMPARISON OF COLOR IN FLOWER PETAL, RED-ONION SKIN, AND *ELODEA* LEAF"

The color of plant parts is determined by various *pigments* inside the cells. In some cells the color is inside organelles called **plastids**. Chloroplasts are one kind of plastid. There are other plastids that contain different colored pigments.

In other cells the pigment is distributed throughout the *water* of the central vacuole. Your task in this Activity, is to determine and compare where the color is located in an *Elodea* leaf, red-onion skin, and yellow flower petal.

In order to determine whether a pigment is in the central vacuole or inside the plastids, you must look at one cell layer, and note the distribution of the color within the individual cells.

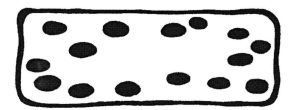

A color distribution like this indicates that the pigment is inside the plastids.

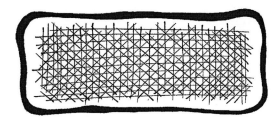

A color distribution like this indicates that the pigment is in the water of the central vacuole.

GO GET

1. A small piece of red onion.

2. A yellow flower petal. (Your lab may substitute red bell pepper.)

3. Your *Elodea* leaf slide from Activity #5.

4. Two more slides and coverslips.

NOW

1. Make a wet mount of a one-cell-thick layer of the red-onion skin. Peel a layer from the inside red part of the onion (not from the dry outside skin).

2. Determine whether the red color is inside the plastids or distributed throughout the water of the central vacuole.

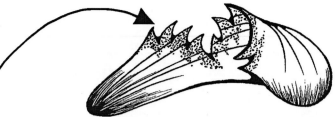

THEN

1. Make a tearing peel of the yellow flower petal.

   The ragged edge will be one cell thick.

2. Make a wet mount of the yellow flower petal, and look at the *one-cell-thick* area on the ragged edge of the tearing peel.

3. Determine whether the yellow color is inside of the plastids, or distributed throughout the water of the central vacuole.

   Note: If your lab is using red bell pepper, then cut a very small piece (without the skin) and crush it on your slide with a razor blade. Apply a drop of water and coverslip.

? QUESTION

1. Look again at your slide of the *Elodea* leaf. Where is the green color in *Elodea* cells?

2. Where is the red color in the red-onion skin cells?

3. Where is the yellow color in the yellow flower petal cells (or red bell pepper cells)?

4. If you were asked on a Lab Test to determine where the color is in red rose petal cells, or orange flower petals, could you do it and show your evidence (including your skill at making a *one-cell-thick* wet mount)?

FINALLY

Wash off your slides and coverslips. Save one for the next Activity.

ACTIVITY #7

"*ZEBRINA* LEAF EPIDERMIS WITH STOMATA"

Most animals have some method of breathing. Do plants have any such equivalent process?

Scattered throughout the *underside* skin of the *Zebrina* leaf are small openings called **stomata**. Stoma is the Greek word for "mouth." These openings look like green lips.

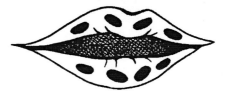

The stomata regulate the flow of air into and out of the leaf. Your job is to find these stomata.

GO GET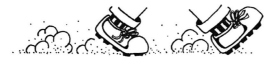

A *Zebrina* leaf.

NOW

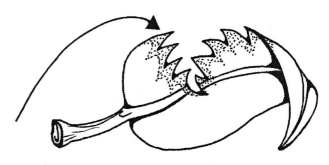

1. Make a leaf peel with the leaf upside down so that you can get a one-cell-thick peel of the **underside** of the *Zebrina* leaf. (The top side of the leaf does not have stomata.) A thin layer will peel off the bottom of the leaf as you tear if you are doing the procedure correctly. Cut off the thin layer piece with a razor blade. Don't try to make a thin slice with your razor blade. You won't get a single-layer slide. Always use the tear/peel technique.

2. Make a wet mount and look for the stomata.

3. Look closely at the structure of the stomata. Notice whether you can identify the organelles inside of the two cells that make up the stomata. These two stomata cells are called *guard cells* because they "guard" the opening. (Your textbook discusses the details of the chemical processes by which the stomata are opened and closed.)

4. Look at the skin cells around the stomata. Notice what cell organelles they *don't* have.

5. Draw a simple sketch of the *Zebrina* leaf stomata and the surrounding cells.

Stomata

1. *Zebrina* leaf stomata perform a specific function. What is it?

2. What organelles do the guard cells contain that are absent in the skin cells of the leaf?

3. Why would the guard cells have chloroplasts when the other skin cells of the leaf don't have chloroplasts?

4. If you were asked on a Lab Test to make a *one-cell-thick* wet mount of leaf stomata, could you do it?

FINALLY

Wash off your slide and coverslip, and return them to the supply table. Return your compound microscope to the cabinet.

CHEMISTRY CONCEPTS

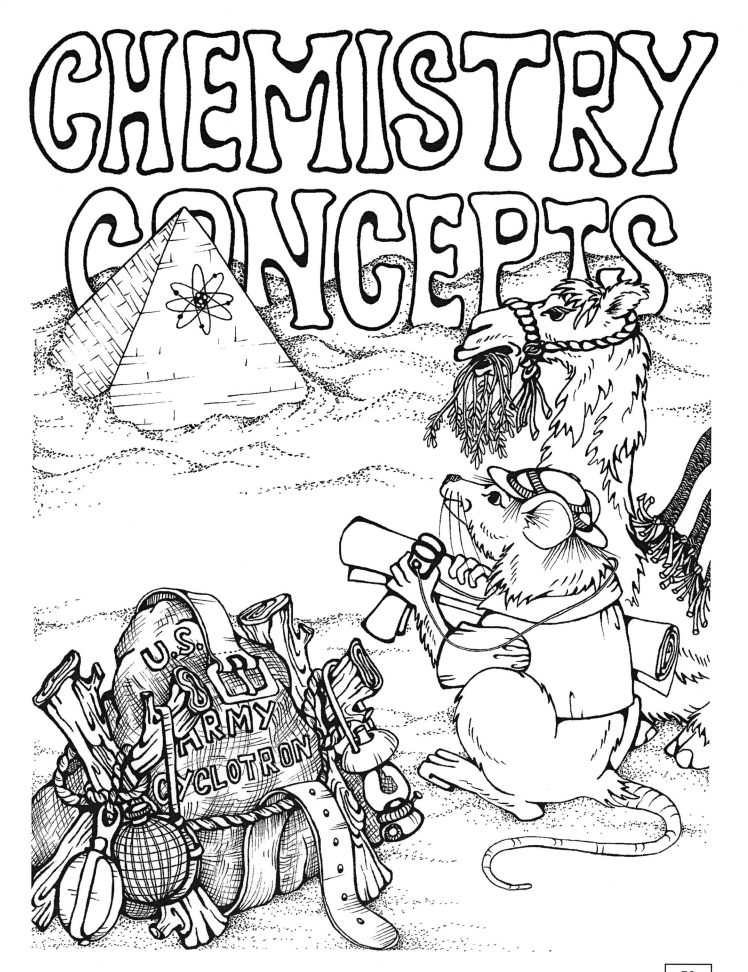

DYNAMIC DEVELOPMENTS AND FASCINATING FACTS IN BIOLOGY

The only letter not appearing on the Periodic Table is the letter J.

On average, the Universe contains one atom for every 88 gallons of space.

—HTTP://WWW.SKYGAZE.COM/CONTENT/FACTS/UNIVERSE.SHTML

Hydrogen is the most abundant element in the Universe (75%).

Oxygen is the most abundant element in the earth's crust, waters, and atmosphere (about 49.5%).

Graphite (as found in a pencil lead) can be transformed into diamond by applying a temperature of 3000 °C and pressure of 100,000 atmospheres. Get to work....

Twenty percent (20%) of Earth's oxygen is produced by the Amazon rain forest.

Aluminum is the most common metal in the Earth's crust—8% by weight.

The element Californium-252 is the most expensive substance in the world: as much as $68 million for one gram.

Francium is the rarest element on Earth. Approximately 30g (about one ounce) exist on Earth at any one time (in uranium deposits), as it decays in 20 minutes.

—HTTP://WWW.APS.ORG/PUBLICATIONS/APSNEWS/199607/FRANCIUM.CFM

A plastic container can resist decomposition for as long as 50,000 years.

Tungsten has the highest melting point at 3410 °C (6170 °F).

—HTTP://WWW.SCIENSATIONAL.COM/CHEMISTRY.HTML

CHEMISTRY CONCEPTS

INTRODUCTION

The first principles of the universe are atoms and empty space;
everything else is merely thought to exist.

—Democritus (~ 400 B.C.)

Chemistry is the science that deals with the nature of and the changes in the composition of matter. The relationship of particles within the atom, and the interactions between the atoms account for everything that we call "matter" in our world. At first it seems impossible to believe that air, liquid, and solid could be made of the same basic particles. But when we watch a cube of ice melt in a pool of water, then drip onto a hot plate and become vapor, we are forced to conclude that there is something going on that we can't explain in any other way.

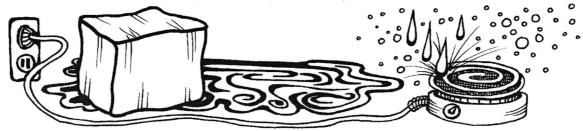

Our eyes can't see the particles but we know they must be there—in another world—in a world of atoms.

This lab is meant to be an aid to your understanding of some of the chemical processes and interactions that will be discussed throughout your study of biology. Here we will start the discussion. And we hope this lab will encourage you to continue your exploration into the science of chemistry.

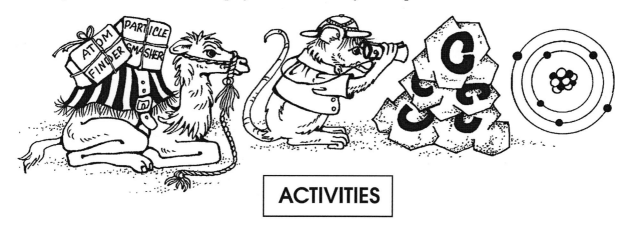

ACTIVITIES

ACTIVITY #1

"THE PERIODIC TABLE OF ELEMENTS"

The word *element* originally came from a Latin word meaning "first principle." In Roman times, people thought that the universe was made up of four basic elements: earth, air, fire, and water.

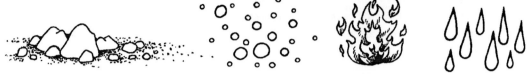

Today, the modern chemist defines an *element* as the most basic kind of substance which cannot be broken into simpler substances by ordinary chemical processes. Over the years, more than 100 elements have been discovered and described.

Water is the most abundant material on the surface of the earth. However, using our definition, we don't call water an element because it can be broken down into two simpler substances: *hydrogen* and *oxygen*. Hydrogen and oxygen cannot be broken down into simpler substances, so we conclude that they are elements.

OBSERVE

Study the "Abbreviated" Periodic Table of Elements on the next page for a few minutes. Notice how the different elements are listed, grouped, and numbered.

All living things are chemical combinations based on the lighter elements. These are shown in this "Abbreviated" Periodic Table. (A complete Table of Elements can be found in your textbook or the lab room.)

During the formation of the earth, heavy elements sank into the inner molten core and were not available for use in chemical processes taking place on the surface of the planet. Look again at the Table of Elements. These are the common elements that were available in the "Soup of Life" from which you came.

? QUESTION

1. Do you know what the numbers on the periodic chart mean?

2. Do you know why the elements are listed in certain groups?

3. Do you recognize the names of any elements on the chart by their alphabetical symbols?

4. Use your textbook or a lab chart to access a complete periodic table. Notice that the element symbol is not always an abbreviation of the name of that element. What are the common names for the element symbols Na and K?

"ABBREVIATED" PERIODIC TABLE OF ELEMENTS

Group I	Group II	Group III	Group IV	Group V	Group VI	Group VII	Inert Gases
1 **H** 1							2 **He** 4
3 **Li** 7	4 **Be** 9	5 **B** 11	6 **C** 12	7 **N** 14	8 **O** 16	9 **F** 19	10 **Ne** 20
11 **Na** 23	12 **Mg** 24	13 **Al** 27	14 **Si** 28	15 **P** 31	16 **S** 32	17 **Cl** 35	18 **Ar** 40
19 **K** 39	20 **Ca** 40						

ACTIVITY #2

"ATOMS AND ISOTOPES"

ATOMIC STRUCTURE

One of the most important questions in chemistry is: What makes one element different from another element?

The smallest particle of an element that can exist and still retain the chemical properties of that element is called an *atom*. Today we know that there are particles even smaller than atoms called *protons*, *neutrons*, and *electrons*. It is the various combinations of these subatomic particles that control the chemical properties of the different elements.

All atoms consist of an inner core that contains most of the mass of the atom, and an outer zone in which there are very light particles, called electrons, that are either like energy waves or like particles, depending on how they are studied. If you monitor electrons with a machine that looks for particles, they will appear to be particles. And if you try to find them as energy waves, that machine will record them as energy waves. Their nature is both particle and wave.

The inner core is called a *nucleus*, and it is made up of two kinds of particles: *protons* and *neutrons*. The outer zone of the atom is filled with those tricky, high energy particles called *electrons*.

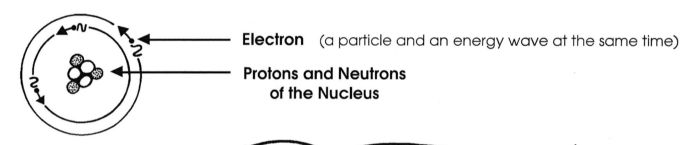

Electron (a particle and an energy wave at the same time)

Protons and Neutrons of the Nucleus

Atom Facts

1. A proton has a mass of 1 atomic mass unit.
2. A neutron has a mass of 1.
3. An electron has a mass of almost 0 (zero).

4. A proton has an electrical charge of +1.
5. A neutron has an electrical charge of 0 (neutral).
6. An electron has an electrical charge of –1.

In this lab we must simplify definitions and explanations. A chemistry class would look at the concepts of weight and mass with important differences. Here, we consider them as equals. (This is, in fact, not true.)

ATOMIC NUMBER AND ATOMIC MASS

The Periodic Table of Elements contains the atomic mass and atomic number of each element. These numbers indicate the number of protons, neutrons, and electrons in each element's basic structure.

OBSERVE

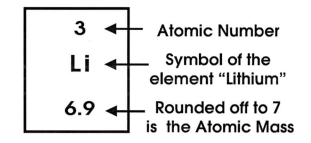

1. Each square in the Periodic Table represents an *element*.

2. There are two numbers in each square.

   a. The smaller number at the top of the box is the ***atomic number***.

   b. The number at the bottom of the box is the average of all isotopes of the element. If you "round off" this value to the nearest whole number, then that number is the ***atomic mass***. On your "Abbreviated" Periodic Table we have provided the rounded off atomic masses.

INFORMATION

Atomic Number = # of Protons

Atomic Mass = # of Protons + # of Neutrons

A single atom has an overall neutral charge because the number of + charges (protons) is equal to the number of − charges (electrons) in the atom.

Hint: If you know the atomic number, then you automatically know how many protons or electrons are in that atom. This is because the number of protons is equal to the number of electrons.

? QUESTION

1. Using the "Abbreviated" Periodic Table of Elements, put the appropriate symbol by the element's name, and determine the number of protons, electrons, and neutrons.

Element	Symbol	# of Protons	# of Electrons	# of Neutrons
Lithium				
Beryllium				
Boron				
Carbon				
Nitrogen				
Oxygen				
Fluorine				

2. Use the chart you just completed to answer the following questions.

    a. What is the atomic number for carbon? _____

    b. What is the atomic mass for lithium? _____

    c. What is the atomic number for nitrogen? _____

    d. What is the atomic mass for oxygen? _____

    e. Fe is the symbol for the element ferrous, commonly known as iron. Knowing that information, what is the name for the chemical structure pictured here?

                       Answer: a ferrous wheel.

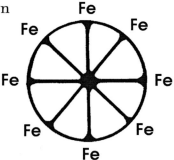

ISOTOPES

The Periodic Table of Elements lists each element with its number of protons (which is also the same as the number of electrons) and its atomic weight. In an accurate Periodic Table, those atomic weights are not whole numbers. This is because each element has several different forms called isotopes. Isotopes have the same number of protons (and electrons), but have different numbers of neutrons. That means they will have slightly different atomic weights. Isotopes usually have identical chemical properties because those properties are dependent on the number of electrons, which remains the same number in the isotopes of any particular element. You may have heard of radioactive iodine which is used in medicine, heavy water which is used in nuclear reactors, or carbon 14 which is used in paleontology to date fossils. All of these are isotopes of the elements iodine, hydrogen, and carbon, respectively.You may have heard of radioactive iodine which is used in medicine, heavy water which is used in nuclear reactors, or carbon 14 which is used in paleontology to date fossils. All of these are isotopes of the elements iodine, hydrogen, and carbon, respectively.

The mass (protons + neutrons) of individual isotopes is not included in the Periodic Table, but instead is indicated by putting a number to the upper left of the element's symbol. For example, ^{12}C is an isotope of carbon and is called carbon twelve because its atomic mass is twelve. ^{14}C has an atomic mass of 14; it is called carbon fourteen. Because of its radioactive properties, ^{14}C can be put into a sugar molecule, and that molecule can be "followed" through your metabolism to determine how you process your food Calories.

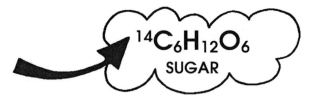

$$^{14}C_6H_{12}O_6$$
SUGAR

Isotopes are often used as a chemical "tag" to follow the molecules of a particular substance through a biochemical process. For example, in medicine, radioactive iodine is injected into the the bloodstream and the isotope is tracked with special machines as it filters into the patient's kidney and urine. It is used to discover kidney disease or kidney malfunction.

1. How many neutrons are in ^{14}C ? _____ Its atomic mass is _____.

2. How many neutrons are in ^{12}C ? _____ Its atomic mass is _____.

3. ^2H is called deuterium. It is the isotope of hydrogen that is used to make heavy water for nuclear power plants.

   How many neutrons are in ^2H ? _____

   Its atomic mass is _____.

4. Why do the isotopes of an element have the same basic chemical properties?

5. What is the primary use of isotopes in medicine and biological research?

ACTIVITY #3

"MOLECULAR FORMATION"

THE EIGHT GROUPS OF ELEMENTS

Look at your "Abbreviated" Periodic Table of Elements. About 150 years ago, chemists discovered that all of the known elements could be arranged from low atomic weight to high atomic weight. And, when they were put in this order, it was noticed that there were repeating physical and chemical properties. It was amazing! There is a recognizable pattern in the structure of all matter.

The design of the Periodic Table of Elements is based on those repeating patterns. The elements in Groups I, II, and III are all *metals* (except for hydrogen, which chemically reacts like a metal but is a gas). The other groups are called the *non-metals*.

Metals easily *release* electrons to other groups. The *group number* of the metals indicates *how many electrons* can be released: 1, 2, or 3.

The non-metal elements in Groups IV through VII *attract* or *share* electrons from other elements. Now, if you take the group # of a non-metal element and subtract it from the number *eight*, then you will know the *number of electrons* that this element will attract or share.

For example, the element oxygen will attract two electrons when it combines with other elements to form molecules.

$$(8 - \text{Group VI} = 2)$$

To complete our discussion of the groups in the Table, the *inert gases*—the final group—get their name because they *do not* react with any other element.

The key to understanding *chemical bonding* comes from understanding the interactions between the electrons of different elements when they bump into each other. Do they create a chemical reaction, or is there no chemical reaction? The number "8" turns out to be a very important clue in predicting molecular formations in chemistry.

NOW

Keeping in mind what you have just learned about the Periodic Table of Elements, answer the following questions.

? QUESTION

1. Does sodium (Na) attract or release electrons? _____

    How many electrons are involved in the transfer? _____

2. Does chlorine (Cl) attract or release electrons? _____

How many electrons are involved in the transfer? _____

3. What do you think would happen if a sodium atom and a chlorine atom bumped into each other?

4. Welders use helium (He) and argon (Ar) gases to blow over the metal during the welding process. Why would they want to use these gases?

5. If 10 magnesium (Mg) atoms and 10 chlorine (Cl) atoms were allowed to bump into each other, could they combine to form a substance? _____

How many molecules would be made? _____

Would there be any atoms left over? _____

Which ones? _____ How many? _____

6. My friend, the inventor, says that she has just made a translucent, light-weight metal by combining aluminum with helium and silicon. She wants me to invest $10,000 in the process, and promises that we will be millionaires in only six months. What do you think I should do? Why?

IONS

An atom has the same number of positive charges (protons) as negative charges (electrons). Some atoms can lose electrons (Groups I, II, and III), and other atoms can gain electrons (Group VII). An ion is an atom that has lost or gained electrons, and thereby becomes charged (either + or −) An ion that has gained an electron will acquire an excess negative electric charge, and the ion formed by losing an electron will have a positive charge. These ions are very important in our life processes, and we would all die without them. (More about that later.)

Ions act differently from uncharged atoms. Think of them as being like magnets + and −, and other atoms as being like non-magnets.

The "Abbreviated" Periodic Table of Elements provides some information about the formation of ions. As we discussed before, Group I elements can lose one electron, and Group II elements can lose two electrons. Guess what Group III elements can lose? Three electrons!

So, when atoms in Groups I, II, and III become ions, they will have a _____ charge.

Groups IV, V, and VI elements usually *share* electrons with other elements, and don't form ions. These elements will have a neutral charge.

Group VII elements attract and *gain one* electron. They can form ions, and they will have a _____ charge.

1. What is the electrical charge of an electron? _____

2. Fluorine is in Group VII. What would be the electrical charge of a fluorine (F) atom that gained an electron? _____

3. What would be the electrical charge of a sodium (Na) atom that lost an electron? _____

4. Refer to your "Abbreviated" Table of Elements, and determine whether the following atoms would form ions by losing or gaining electrons.

	Lose Electrons	Gain Electrons	Ion Electrical Charge
Cl			
Be			
Al			
Mg			
H			

CHEMICAL BONDS

Chemical bonds hold molecules together in living organisms. Furthermore, energy for the biological processes in living things is provided by the breaking and forming of chemical bonds in the molecules that drive our metabolism.

Two important types of chemical bonds are produced by the interactions between the electrons of different atoms: ionic bonds and covalent bonds.

IONIC BONDS

What do you think would happen if a + ion of lithium got very close to a − ion of fluorine? (Remember to think about ions as behaving like the + and − ends of magnets.)

The atoms of some molecules are held together by the attraction between oppositely charged ions. That force of attraction is called an *ionic bond*.

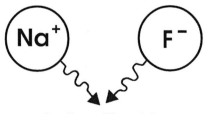

Sodium Fluoride
to prevent tooth decay

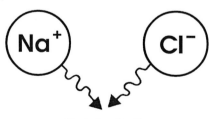

Table Salt

Ions are essential in many of the physiological processes of organisms such as nerve conduction and muscle contraction. Because ionic bonds are easily broken by water, the ions can be dissolved and moved throughout the fluids of an organism and delivered to every part of the body.

COVALENT BONDS

Elements in Groups IV, V, and VI *share* electrons with other atoms when bonding. The atoms of some molecules are held together by this mutual sharing of electrons. This cohesive force is called a *covalent bond*.

Covalent bonds are important to living organisms because they are strong enough to hold together the molecular structure of the organism. However, these bonds aren't so strong that they can't be broken and "remodeled" into other molecules that the organism needs.

The covalent bonds in glucose are strong enough to make wood (cellulose).

The covalent bonds in glucose have enough energy to "drive" our metabolic processes (cell respiration).

The covalent bonds in glucose can be "remodeled" into other organic molecules that the organism needs.

Glucose Molecule

? QUESTION

Based on what you know about elements in the Periodic Table, determine whether the following elements would interact to form ionic or covalent bonds.

Elements Reacting	Type of Bond
Na and Cl	
H and O	
H and Cl	
C and H	

ACTIVITY #4

"THE RULE OF EIGHT IN MOLECULAR FORMATION"

Remember: The elements in the Periodic Table of Elements are listed in vertical *groups* that have Roman numbers I through VII plus a group called the "inert gases." We have been discussing each group # with a special description of the behavior of electrons in the atoms of that group.

NOW

Whenever chemists observed atoms reacting with each other, they noticed that the *sum of their group numbers* usually equalled eight, or multiples of 8 (16, 24, 32, 40, etc.). This is called **"The Rule of Eight."** Let's see how this "Rule of Eight" works in understanding *chemical formulas.*

Chemical formulas are written to show how many atoms of each element are bonded together to make a molecule of a substance. For example $C_6H_{12}O_6$ is the chemical formula for one molecule of sugar.

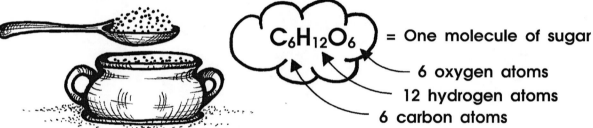

$C_6H_{12}O_6$ = One molecule of sugar

— 6 oxygen atoms
— 12 hydrogen atoms
— 6 carbon atoms

Let's look at water: H_2O. By looking at this formula, you know that it takes _____ hydrogen atom(s) to bond with _____ oxygen atom(s).

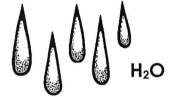

H_2O

Now, add the group numbers. Hydrogen has a group # of I (1). Oxygen has a group number of VI (6). Two hydrogens (1 + 1) and one oxygen (6) equals a total of 8. *"The Rule of Eight!"*

Try another simple one—table salt (sodium chloride): NaCl. The formula tells you that it takes _____ sodium atom(s) to bond with _____ chlorine atom(s). Add the group numbers: The group # of sodium is I (1) and the group # of chlorine is VII (7).

$$1 + 7 = 8.$$ There's that *"Rule of Eight"* again!

Try this one on your own. Go back to the sugar molecule: $C_6H_{12}O_6$.

6 atoms of carbon (group # _____) 6 x _____ = _____

12 atoms of hydrogen (group # _____) 12 x _____ = _____

6 atoms of oxygen (group # _____) 6 x _____ = _____   (Sum of all group

Total = _____   numbers)

Is the total of _____ a multiple of 8?_____ *"The Rule of Eight"* again!

1. Determine the sum of the group numbers for the atoms in each of the molecules below, and see if your answer still agrees with the "Rule of Eight."

	Sum of Group #'s	Rule of 8?
NH_3 (ammonia)		
$CaCl_2$ (calcium chloride)		
Al_2O_3 (aluminum oxide)		

2. Let's see if you can use this "Rule of Eight" to write a chemical formula by determining how many *atoms* of one element would be necessary to combine with how many *atoms* of another element to form a particular molecule.

$1\ Mg +$ _____ $Cl \longrightarrow MgCl$ _____ (magnesium chloride)

$2\ H + 1\ S +$ _____ $O \longrightarrow H_2SO$ _____ (sulfuric acid)

$1\ C +$ _____ $H \longrightarrow CH$ _____ (methane)

$2\ H +$ _____ $O + 1\ C \longrightarrow H_2CO$ _____ (carbonic acid)

FINALLY

Chemists explain this "Rule of Eight" phenomenon by saying that all atoms (except for the inert gases) have *incomplete* outer electron shells. When atoms react with each other, each atom ends up with a compete outer shell of 8 electrons. This principle they call "The Rule of Eight" or "The Octet Rule."

There is much more to this idea, but we'll have to leave that to your further explorations into chemistry. For instance, if you consider the different molecules of gas in the air you breathe: H_2, O_2, or N_2, do their sum of group numbers equal 8? What's going on? Why?

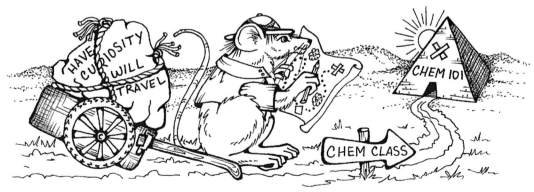

For now, you will just have to be content with scratching the surface of chemistry. Understanding atoms, molecules, and the bonding of elements that make up all of the different substances that you are and you see on this planet will require a class in chemistry.

Chapter 4

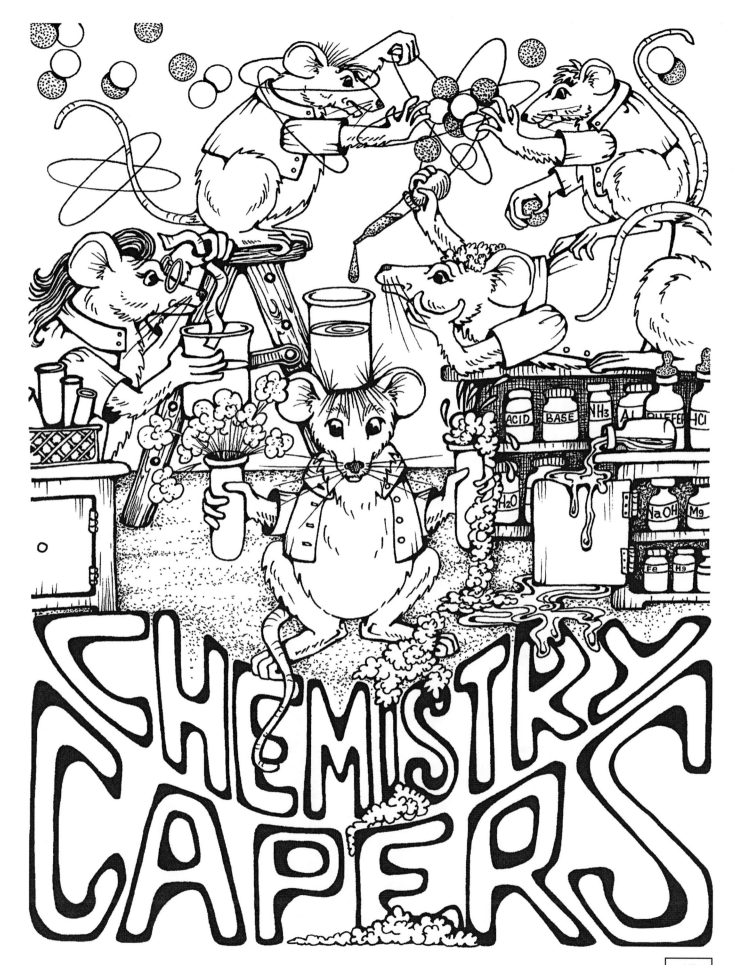

Much more fresh water is stored underground in aquifers than on the earth's surface. Because of the hydrologic cycle, the same water that existed on the earth millions of years ago is still present today—and in your body!

—HTTP://WWW.ALLABOUTWATER.ORG/WATER-FACTS.HTML

Water is *incompressible,* meaning that it can't be squeezed to fit into a smaller volume. Change the *phase state* of water to ice or gas, and the rule no longer applies!

—HTTP://SCIENCEDEMONSTRATIONS.FAS.HARVARD.EDU/ICB/ICB.DO

One inch (2.5 cm) of rain is equal to 10 inches (25 cm) of snow.

—HTTP://WWW.SCIENSATIONAL.COM/CHEMISTRY.HTML

Hot water freezes faster than cold water! Water's strange behavior was dubbed the *Mpemba Effect,* after a Tanzanian cooking class student who brought it to the world's attention in 1969. It is even possible to make snow by tossing a bucket of hot water into subzero temperature air. The factors leading to the anomaly are many, including speed of evaporation, supercooling effects , convection, conduction, dissolved gases, ordered clustering, surface tension, and a myriad of other influences.

—HTTP://SASUKE.ECON.HC.KEIO.AC.JP/~KEN/PHYSICS-FAQ/HOT_WATER.HTML

How many phases of water are there? If you answer three—liquid, gas, and solid—you'd be wrong. There are at least five different phases of water and fourteen different phases (that scientists have discovered so far) of ice.

—HTTP://WWW.NEATORAMA.COM/2008/08/22/5-REALLY-WEIRD-THINGS-ABOUT-WATER/

Freezing very pure water past its freezing point at standard pressure, it is possible to *supercool* water so that it never forms ice crystals to become solid. Ice crystals need *nucleation points*—gas bubbles, impurities, or the rough surface of the container—to start forming. Without these conditions, water can exist as a supercooled liquid well below its freezing point.

—HTTP://WWW.NEATORAMA.COM/2008/08/22/5-REALLY-WEIRD-THINGS-ABOUT-WATER/

Even weirder water antics: At -38 °C even the purest supercooled water spontaneously turns into ice (with a little audible "bang," no less). But, what happens if you continue to lower the temperature? At -120 °C something strange starts to happen: The water becomes *ultraviscous,* or thick like molasses. Below -135 °C, it becomes "glassy water," a solid with no crystal structure.

—HTTP://WWW.NEATORAMA.COM/2008/08/22/5-REALLY-WEIRD-THINGS-ABOUT-WATER/

At the molecular level, water is stranger still. In 1995, physicists found that when neutrons were aimed at water molecules, they observed 25% fewer hydrogen protons than expected. At the attosecond (10–18 second) level, weird quantum effects dominate and the chemical formula for water isn't H_2O. It's actually $H_{1.5}O$!

—HTTP://WWW.AIP.ORG/ENEWS/PHYSNEWS/2003/SPLIT/648-1.HTML

CHEMISTRY CAPERS

Life first evolved in water, and most life on this planet lives in water. Furthermore, plant and animal forms are 70% to 90% water. These facts clearly establish the importance of this substance to all living beings. Water is rare in the universe, and because of this, life is also rare.

In this lab we will investigate some of the unique chemical properties of water: the most essential substance for living organisms.

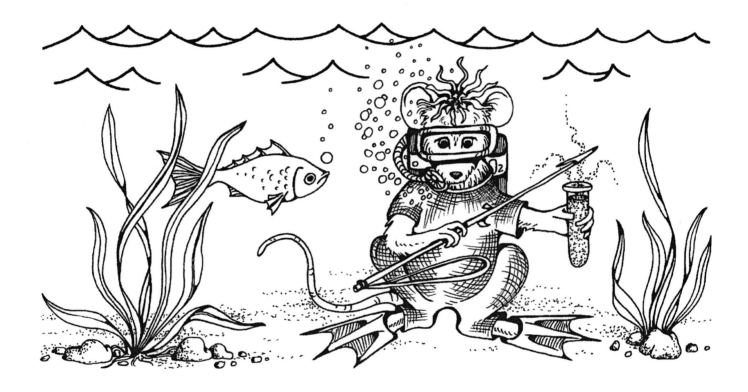

ACTIVITIES

ACTIVITY #1

"PROPERTIES OF WATER"

In this Activity you will investigate some of the physical properties of water. A more thorough discussion of water's characteristics can be found in your textbook.

HYDROGEN BONDS

When two hydrogen atoms react with an oxygen atom to form water, there is an *unequal sharing* of electrons among the atoms. This creates a slightly negative charge on the side of the water molecule that has more of the "electron cloud."

Water molecules act like a bunch of magnets holding on to each other by the attractions between the + and − ends.

The force created by those attractions is called a **hydrogen bond**, and it is the secret to all of water's special properties.

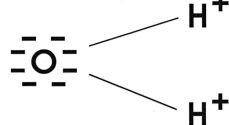

? QUESTION

1. As water falls from the clouds, what force keeps the water in drops?

2. In order for the liquid water to evaporate and become steam, heat must be added. In a pan of boiling water, what bond is being broken by the heat of the stove?

3. So, if heat is required to evaporate water, then what is released when water condenses?

4. On a calm, but rainy day, the temperature rises slightly when it starts to rain. Explain.

WATER ADHESION

Adhesion occurs when two or more different substances are stuck together as if by glue. Water has some interesting adhesion properties.

GO GET

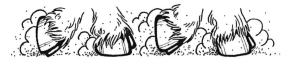

1. A small container of water.

2. An eyedropper.

3. Four microscope slides.

1. Put several drops of water on one slide, then place the other slide directly on top of the wet slide.

2. Try to pull apart the glass slides *without* sliding them past each other.

3. Repeat this experiment with the two dry slides.

? QUESTION

1. How strong is the force of attraction between the two dry slides?

2. How strong is the force of attraction between the two wet slides?

3. What is the name of the force that holds the two slides together?

4. A freeze-dried anchovy is fairly easy to break between your fingers. Yet, when the fish is allowed to sit in water for a while, it only bends with the same effort. Explain.

5. Based on your answer to #4, what is one important role of water in living organisms?

CAPILLARITY

GO GET
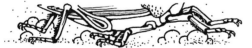

1. A glass capillary tube.

2. A small container of water.

NOW

Hold the capillary tube vertically between your fingers, and put the bottom end just below the surface of the water. Water holds onto itself (cohesion) and holds onto the glass (adhesion).

The process you have just observed is called *capillarity*.

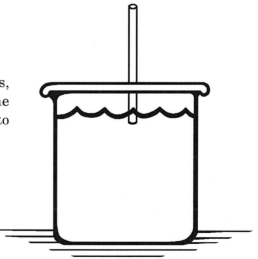

1. What happened when you did this experiment?

2. Draw a simple sketch of the results.

3. Explain your results. What is it about water that makes it do this? (Be specific about the forces of attraction.)

4. How is this property of water important to plants?

HEATING PROPERTIES OF WATER

The difficulty of heating water reveals the strength of the hydrogen bonds and the *temperature stabilizing role* of water within living organisms.

When a substance (like water) is heated, the rate of temperature increase depends on how easy it is for heat energy to increase the speed of molecular motion in that substance. If it doesn't require much heat to increase the motion, then we say that the substance is "easy to heat up."

You can apply this idea to the heating of water, and answer the question: ***"Are the hydrogen bonds between water molecules strong enough to make water a substance that is hard to heat up?"***

GO GET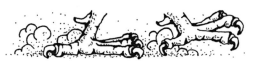

1. A hot plate.

2. A chunk of metal.

3. A beaker (the 100-ml size is best).

4. A container of water.

5. Tongs to remove weight.

The cooling rate of an object is directly related to the amount of heat energy absorbed by that object. If an object cools quickly, then it didn't absorb much heat energy to start with. If water is slow to cool, then it absorbed a lot of energy to heat it up.

1. Weigh the piece of metal.

2. Put an amount of water equal to the weight of the metal object into the beaker.

3. Put the piece of metal into the water, and heat the container until it just begins to steam.

4. Immediately remove the piece of metal from the beaker, and put both the beaker of water and the piece of metal onto the table. (Your results are more accurate if you pour the hot water into a room temperature beaker at the same time you put the metal on the table.)

5. Repeatedly touch both the water and the piece of metal until both are approximately the same temperature. Keep track of how long it takes for each to cool.

> Time for the water to cool = _____
>
> Time for the metal to cool = _____

? QUESTION

1. Which substance cooled the slowest? (circle your choice)

   Metal   or   Water

2. Which substance would require more heat energy to heat it up? Remember that the amount of heat given off by a substance equals the amount of heat absorbed by that substance when it was heated. (circle your choice)

   Metal   or   Water

3. We experience sitting in 70°F water as much more chilling to the body than sitting in room air at 70°F. Explain why.

   It is estimated that you lose heat to cold water four times faster than to cold air. Your body is mostly water. What if your body had much less water in it, and the rest of it consisted of substances that heated and cooled as easily as metal. Would a cold environment be more chilling or not? Explain.

4. What bond gives water its unique property of being slow to heat up and slow to cool down?

5. Is water a temperature-stabilizing substance for living organisms?

EVAPORATION OF WATER

Heating water from 0° to 100°C just "shakes" the molecules. As you continue to heat water at 100°C, hydrogen bonds begin to break. The heat of vaporization is the amount of energy needed to break hydrogen bonds. It can be measured if you know how much heat is used to boil away 10 ml of water already at 100°C.

GO GET

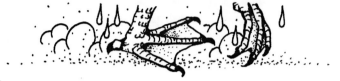

1. A hot plate.

2. Three equal-size beakers (the 250-ml size is best).

3. A thermometer. *Be careful, please!* This equipment is fragile.

NOW

1. Fill Beakers Ⓐ and Ⓑ with the proper amounts of water, and put them in the freezer or into special "ice tubs" for Beakers Ⓐ and Ⓑ to stay cold.

   Beaker Ⓐ is the heat meter. It will be heating during the experiment. Each 1°C increase in Beaker Ⓐ means that 100 calories of energy has left the hot plate and entered each of the three beakers.

   Beaker Ⓑ is a comparison to see which takes more energy—heating water or boiling water. **Note:** Heating water increases the movement of water molecules. This is difficult because the hydrogen bond is so strong. Boiling liquid water into steam requires breaking hydrogen bonds.

   Beaker Ⓑ is the experiment. How much energy is required to break (boil away) all of the hydrogen bonds in 10 ml of water?

2. Prepare a large container of boiling water. *Use the special measuring pipettes for safely removing 10 ml of boiling water.* You must prepare Beaker Ⓒ at the last minute just before you start the experiment. Read on.

3. Preheat your hot plate at a setting that you know will boil water moderately. (*Not the highest setting!*)

4. It is important that you start all three beakers at *exactly the same time*, without time for the beakers to change temperature before heating on the hot plate. Record the starting time as soon as all beakers are on the hot plate.

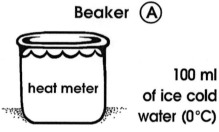

Beaker Ⓐ
heat meter
100 ml of ice cold water (0°C)

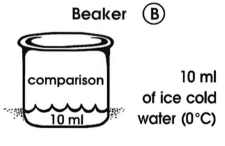

Beaker Ⓑ
comparison
10 ml
10 ml of ice cold water (0°C)

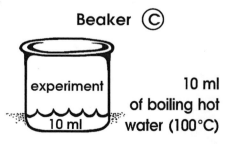

Beaker Ⓒ
experiment
10 ml
10 ml of boiling hot water (100°C)

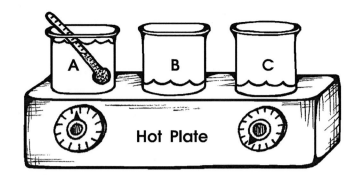

Hot Plate

5. *There are three events that you must record during this experiment.*

    a. How many minutes does it take for Beaker Ⓑ to go from 0°C to 100°C (little bubbles form at the bottom)?

          _____

    b. How many minutes does it take for all of the water in Beaker Ⓒ to boil away?

          _____

    c. You must watch very carefully to determine the exact temperature of the water in Beaker Ⓐ at the exact time when all of the water finally boiled out of Beaker Ⓒ.

          _____ °C in Beaker Ⓐ

? QUESTION

1. What takes more energy? (circle your choice)

    To heat 10 ml of water   or   To boil away (*evaporate*) 10 ml of water that
      from 0°C to 100°C.   is already at boiling temperature (100°C).

2. When water evaporates (boils away), explain what happens to the hydrogen bonds between molecules.

3. Beaker Ⓐ (Heat Meter) tells us how much heat energy left the hot plate and entered the Experiment Beaker Ⓒ. One calorie of energy is the amount of heat required to increase the temperature of 1 ml of water 1°C. How much did the temperature change in Beaker Ⓐ? _____°C. (Subtract the starting temperature if it was above 0°C.)

4. Now, calculate the total calories of heat recorded by the Heat Meter (Beaker Ⓐ) considering both the amount of water in it and the temperature change of the water.

          _____ calories

5. The answer to question #4 is the amount of energy to vaporize 10 ml of water in Beaker Ⓒ. How many calories would be required to evaporate only 1 ml of water?

          _____ calories

6. When water evaporates (boils away), explain what happens to the hydrogen bonds between molecules.

ACTIVITY #2

"WHAT THE HECK IS pH?"

HYDROGEN IONS

An ion is an atom that has lost or gained electrons, and thereby has become electrically charged (either + or −). Ions act differently from uncharged atoms. (It's like comparing magnets with non-magnets.)

These ions are very important in our life processes, and we would die without them. Table salt is an example of two essential ions—sodium and chloride.

Of all the ions in your body, none is more important than the **hydrogen ion, H+**. The term *"pH"* refers to the concentration of H+ ions in water. Biologists are interested in H+ concentration because it affects chemical reactions so greatly.

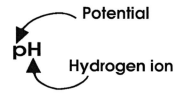

A small change in this ion can dramatically affect life. Acid rain and acid stomach are two expressions of the concentration of H+ ions. Also, the blood of a human is so sensitive to H+ concentration that a small pH change from your normal of **7.4** can result in your death.

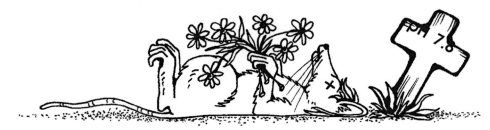

We monitor the pH of our fish aquariums and our swimming pools in order to avoid potential problems. In the case of the aquarium, we are trying to maintain a good environment for micro-organisms, whereas, in the swimming pool, we are trying to prevent micro-organisms from growing.

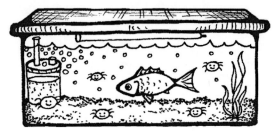 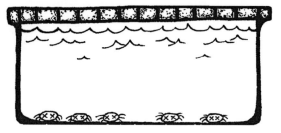

? QUESTION

1. Knowing how important pH can be to living organisms, what effect does acid rain have on forests?

2. What does the "p" stand for in the term pH?

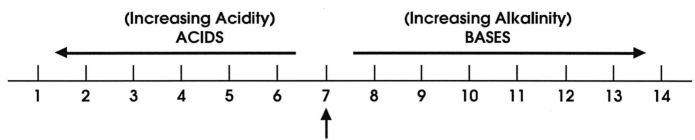

pH SCALE

(Increasing Acidity)
ACIDS

(Increasing Alkalinity)
BASES

1 2 3 4 5 6 7 8 9 10 11 12 13 14

Neutral pH

▶ The pH scale ranges from 1 to 14.

▶ Each H_2O molecule can form two opposite ions: H^+ and OH^-.

▶ Different substances (acids and bases) when added to water will change the balance of H^+ and OH^-.

pH = 7

The concentration of H^+ is equal to the concentration of OH^- at pH = 7

▶ Each step *up* the pH scale means that there is 10 times more OH^- (base) and 10 times less H^+ (acid) than the step below.

▶ Each step *down* the pH scale means that there is 10 times more H^+ (acid) and 10 times less OH^- (base) than the step above.

▶ A water solution with a pH of 7 is ***neutral*** because the concentration of the H^+ ions (acid) is equal to the concentration of the OH^- ions (base).

▶ If the pH is less than 7, then there are more H^+ (acid) ions than OH^- (base) ions, and the solution is called an ***acid***.

▶ If the pH is more than 7, then there are more OH^- (base) ions than H^+ (acid) ions, and the solution is called a ***base***.

? QUESTION

1. pH is a measure of _____ ion concentration.

2. A pH of 3 would be . . . (circle your choice)

        Acid   or   Base

3. A pH of 11 would be . . . (circle your choice)

        Acid   or   Base

4. What is the relationship between H^+ and OH^- at a pH of 7?

5. How much more H^+ is in water at a pH of 3 when compared to a pH of 6?

6. How much more OH^- is in water at a pH of 11 when compared to a pH of 7?

HOW TO MEASURE pH

The pH can be measured with a machine or with special color indicators. A pH machine directly reads the H^+ concentration and displays the pH on a screen. A color indicator is a special molecule that changes color at a particular pH level.

Follow the directions given by your instructor if you are using a pH machine. Otherwise, follow these instructions.

GO GET

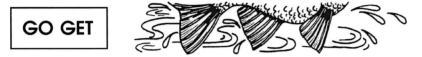

A pH paper test kit.

NOW

1. Use the pH paper test kit to determine the pH of the *three unknown solutions* on the demonstration table.

2. Tear off a 1" strip of pH test paper, and squirt a drop on it from the test solution. Compare the color of the pH test paper to the pH color chart. That's the pH!

The Unknown Solutions

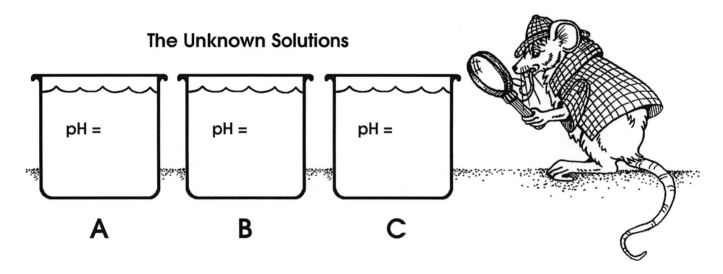

? QUESTION

1. Is solution A acid or base or neutral? _____

2. Is solution B acid or base or neutral? _____

3. Is solution C acid or base or neutral? _____

BUFFERS

A *buffer* is a chemical substance that can be added to water, and will make that solution *resist* a pH change.

 GO GET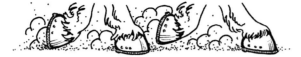

1. 25 ml of *Sample X* in a small beaker.
2. 25 ml of *Sample Y* in a small beaker.

} *Mark both of the beakers!*

3. A dropper-bottle of phenol red.

4. A dropper-bottle of acid.

NOW

1. Set up two beakers: one with 25 ml of Sample X and one with 25 ml of Sample Y. Label each.

2. Put 5 drops of *phenol red* into each beaker.

   Phenol red is a pH color indicator. It turns *yellow* in *acid*, and it turns *red* in *base*.

3. Counting the drops, add acid one drop at a time until each beaker turns yellow. *Gently shake* the beakers after each drop in order to mix the acid into the test solution. (If either solution hasn't changed to yellow after 25 drops of acid have been added, then stop adding acid and assume that it will take many more drops to change the pH.)

? QUESTION

1. Which solution contains a buffer? (circle your choice)

   Sample X   or   Sample Y

2. How many *more* drops of acid did it take to change the buffered solution compared to the nonbuffered solution?

   _____ more drops.

3. Why do you think that one of the brands of aspirin is called "Bufferin"?

ACTIVITY #3

"MOLECULAR MOTION"

All atoms and all molecules move! They are bouncing off of each other at an incredible speed. (It's a good thing that O_2 and N_2 molecules are so small, because they would "sandblast" your skin if they were bigger.)

Chemists discovered that the speed of molecular motion is influenced by several factors, and we will investigate two of them. Also, we will look at a couple of special effects created by molecular motion.

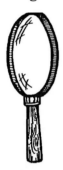

CAN YOU SEE MOLECULAR MOTION?

Actually, molecules are too small to see. But a clever physicist calculated the energy in moving water molecules, and has determined that those molecules have enough energy to bump into and move some very small particles, like carmine dye. When viewed under a microscope, this movement can be seen.

GO GET

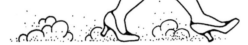

1. A slide and coverslip.
2. A compound microscope.
3. A drop of *carmine dye* particles.

NOW

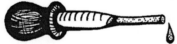

1. Make a wet mount of the carmine particles.

2. Look at the *very very* smallest particles that you can see. Show your instructor.

3. The vibrating motion of these particles suspended in water is called **Brownian Motion**. (Named after guess who?) The tiny particles move whenever a water molecule (which you can't see) bumps into the carmine particle. Observe.

? QUESTION

1. When you watch *Brownian Motion* are you actually seeing *molecules* move? Explain.

2. What do you think would happen if you held a flame under the slide? Explain.

3. What would happen if you held an ice cube under the slide? Explain.

LIGHT MOLECULES VS. HEAVY MOLECULES

The weight (from the Periodic Table) of all the atoms in one molecule of a substance is called the molecular weight. Methylene Blue dye has a molecular weight of 374. The purple dye Potassium Permanganate has a molecular weight of 158. If molecular weight makes any difference in the speed of motion, then we should be able to measure that difference.

You will need to work as a class for this experiment. Assign one member of your group to work with members from other groups.

 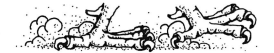

1. Two agar plates.

2. Put *one* crystal of *Methylene Blue* in the middle of the agar plate. (Your instructor may have you put a drop of Methylene Blue solution into one of the small depressions in the agar.)

3. Put *one* crystal of the *Potassium Permanganate* in the middle of the other agar plate. (If you are using solutions, put a drop of Potassium Permanganate into the other agar depression.)

NOW

1. Record the starting time for this experiment.

2. At 30 minutes and one hour, come back to the agar plates and measure the *diameter* of the spreading colors. Record your measurements in the chart below.

RATE of SPREAD (Diameter of Color)

Test Molecule	In 30 Minutes	In One Hour
Potassium Permanganate (molecular weight 158)		
Methylene Blue (molecular weight 374)		

3. Share the results with the other members of your lab group.

? QUESTION

1. Which molecules move faster? (circle your choice)

   Potassium Permanganate   or   Methylene Blue

2. What does this experiment tell you about the speed of movement of different-sized molecules?

ACTIVITY #4

"DIFFUSION OF WATER INTO AND OUT OF CELLS"

The movement of molecules from where they are in high concentration to an area where they are in low concentration is called *diffusion*. Because *all* molecules move, they also *diffuse!*

When a cube of sugar is put into a cup of coffee we know that the sugar will diffuse from where it is in high concentration (the cube) to where it is in low concentration (the hot coffee).

However, we don't normally think about what the water molecules are doing in that same cup of coffee.

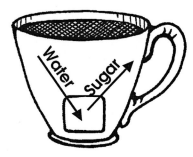

The rules of diffusion apply to water concentration just like they do to the sugar. Water will diffuse from where it is in high concentration (the hot coffee) to where it is in low concentration (the sugar cube).

We can observe the effects of water diffusion in living cells. The diffusion of water through a cell membrane is called *osmosis*. This is a very important process involving the movement of water throughout the cells of all living organisms.

GO GET	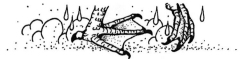

1. A slide and coverslip.
2. A leaf from the *Elodea* plant.
3. An eyedropper of salt water.

NOW

1. Make a wet mount of the *Elodea* leaf and look at the leaf cells under high power. Draw a picture of the distribution of chloroplasts within a typical cell.

2. Work with another lab group. One group is to leave their normal *Elodea* slide under the microscope. The other group is to add salt water to their *Elodea* slide.

3. Put one drop of salt water at the edge of the coverslip. Use a piece of tissue paper on the opposite side of the coverslip to absorb and pull the salt water across the slide. The salt water will soon surround all the leaf cells.

4. Wait 10 minutes. Look back and forth between the two microscopes. Draw a picture of the distribution of chloroplasts in the normal Elodea cell. Then, draw the distribution of chloroplasts in the salt water cell. *Be sure to clean the microscope stage if you got any salt water on it.*

Elodea Cell

Salt Water Added

Let this picture represent one *Elodea* cell surrounded by salt water. The small circles are the water molecules and the larger circles are the salt molecules.

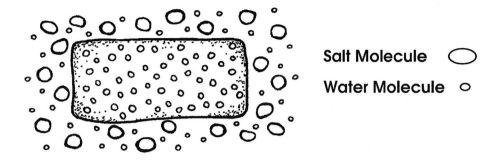

Salt Molecule

Water Molecule

1. Where is the *water* in high concentration? (circle your choice)

   Inside of the cell   or   Outside of the cell

2. Where is the *water* in low concentration? (circle you choice)

   Inside of the cell   or   Outside of the cell

3. In what direction will *osmosis* (water diffusion) occur? (circle your choice)

   Into the cell   or   Out of the cell

4. Explain what you saw in your second picture of the *Elodea* leaf cells. (What is the membrane surrounding the grouped chloroplasts? What happened to the central vacuole?)

5. When you eat a lot of highly salted food (a bag of potato chips, for example), what happens?

   Why?

6. People with high blood pressure or heart problems are told to be careful about their intake of salt. Why?

FINALLY

Under normal conditions root hair cells are relatively low in water molecules and high in other kinds of molecules (cell salts and nutrients). *Draw arrows* to show water movement between the soil water, the root hair cell, and the water transporting tube.

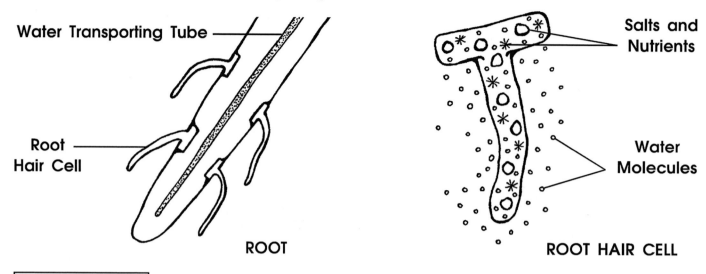

Water Transporting Tube

Root Hair Cell

ROOT

Salts and Nutrients

Water Molecules

ROOT HAIR CELL

? QUESTION

1. What would happen to the water movement if you put salt or a lot of fertilizer in the soil?

2. Explain how the properties of water investigated in Activity #1 and Activity #4 assist a plant in the movement of water from the soil, into the root hair, and throughout the structure of the plant.

OPTIONAL

Water is a most unusual substance. It changes volume at different temperatures. Try this surprising experiment.

1. Very accurately mark the water level in a beaker of cool water.

2. Heat the beaker of water to just before steaming (when bubbles start to appear) and record the water level.

3. Refill the beaker with ice cubes and enough water to match your first water level mark. (Push all the ice below the water surface.)

4. Allow the ice to melt, and record the water level.

5. Compare your results. Surprised?

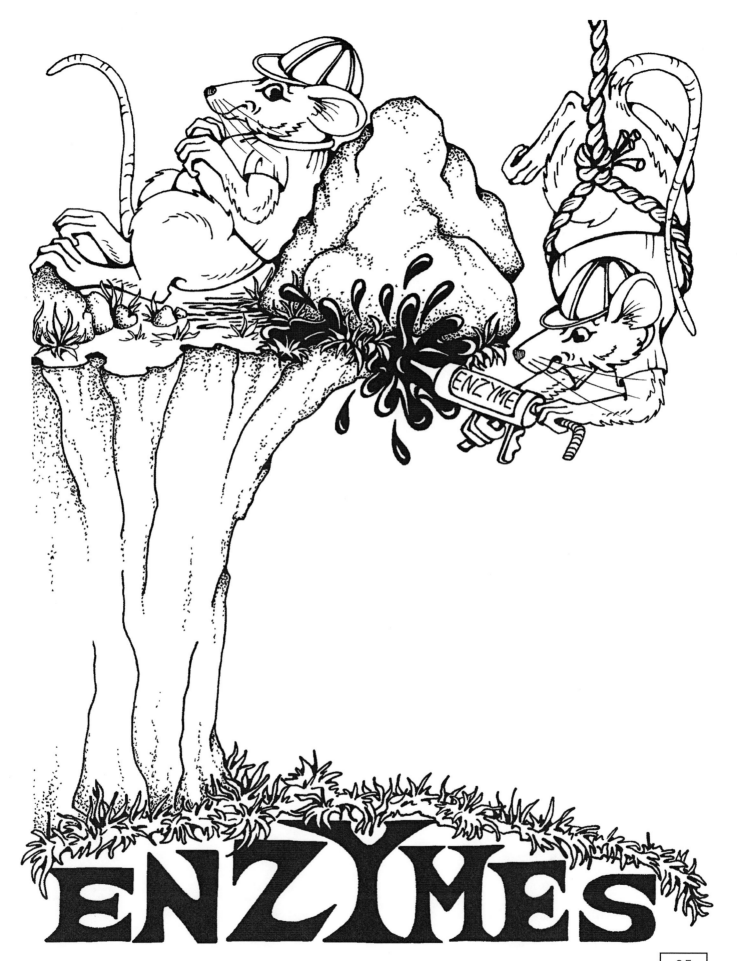

ENZYMES

Not only proteins, but vitamins and minerals comprise enzymes. Vitamins are considered enzyme precursors (or *coenzymes*), and are essential to enzyme systems in the chemistry of life. Familiar examples of coenzymes from the Citric Acid cycle include NAD—nicotinamide adenine dinucleotide integrating niacin (vitamin B3), and pantothenate (B5) in α-ketoglutarate and pyruvate dehydrogenases.

—"Vitamin & Mineral Fact Sheets," *Nutritional Self-Defense: Better Health in a Polluted, Over-Processed, and Stressful World*, Lily Splane, M.N., Anaphase II Publishing, 2003, p. 267

The human body contains more than 50,000 enzymes in three classes: metabolic, digestive, and food. Food enzymes are derived from fresh, raw produce and are required to replenish and augment the enzymes we manufacture in our bodies.

—http://www.enzymedica.com/what_are_enzymes.php

Genetic disorders are caused by mutations resulting in deficiencies of important enzymes. Humans suffer from many genetic enzyme disorders, some of which are fatal. G6PD (glucose-6-phosphate dehydrogenase) deficiency is in fact the most common genetic enzyme deficiency, triggered by ingestion of drugs, food and other substances and causing hemolytic anemia. G6PD enzyme deficiency affects an estimated 600 million (about 10% of the population) people worldwide. Tay-Sachs disease, an affliction of Ashkenazi Jews, results in mutations in the HEXA gene on chromosome 15, which disrupts the activity of the enzyme beta-hexosaminidase A, preventing the breakdown of the fatty substances that accumulate and damage the brain and nervous system. Phenylketonuria (PKU) is an inherited deficiency of phenylalanine hydroxylase, the enzyme that breaks down the amino acid phenylalanine; the disease is treatable with a low-phenylalanine diet. Trimethlyaminuria (TMAU), or "fish odor syndrome," is a rare genetic enzyme disorder in which the body is not able to break down trimethylamine. Without this oxidation process, food and other organic compounds essentially decompose in the body, leading to a fishy-smelling body odor and breath.

—http://g6pddeficiency.org/index.php

—http://nervous-system.emedtv.com/tay-sachs-disease/treatment-for-tay-sachs.html

—http://www.ncbi.nlm.nih.gov/pubmedhealth/PMH0002150/

—http://www.bizarremedical.com/

ENZYMES

INTRODUCTION

Living cells need to build molecules and break molecules. *Enzymes* are special proteins made by the cell, and they greatly speed up the chemical processes of molecular making and breaking.

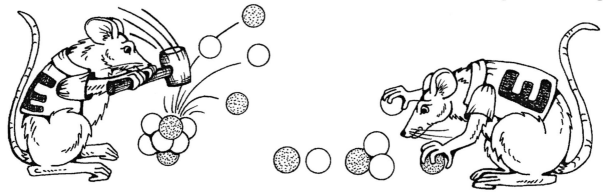

If cells did not have enzymes, then high amounts of heat energy would be required to perform the necessary chemical reactions. That quantity of heat would destroy most structures in the cell, and therefore would be detrimental to the life processes of the whole organism.

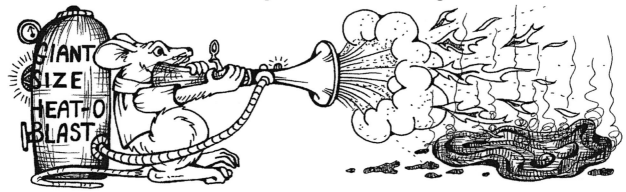

Because enzymes are so important to life, our genetic systems have evolved special genes to control their production. Biochemists tell us that the differences between one species and another species are the kinds of enzymes produced and the genetic sequence of that production.

This lab is designed to help you develop a general understanding of how enzymes operate, and appreciate some of the environmental factors that influence their operation.

ACTIVITIES

ACTIVITY #1

"ENZYME ACTION"

THE ROLE OF HEAT IN CHEMICAL REACTIONS

Heat energy can be used to break the chemical bonds holding big molecules together, producing smaller molecules. Heat also speeds up molecular motion, thereby increasing the frequency of molecular collisions. Collisions of small molecules can result in the spontaneous formation of larger molecules.

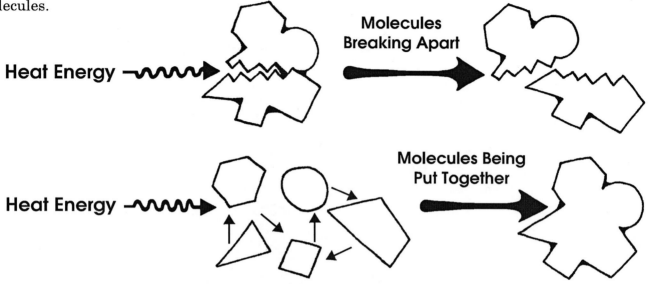

Because of these two properties of heat, molecules can be created and restructured into new substances. However, a problem arises when you need to do both jobs at the same time. In a big chemical factory, reactions can be separated so that the heat needed to drive one process won't interfere with the other processes. Because of its structure and size, a cell isn't able to do this. Therefore, a cell needs another solution for the control of biochemical events—*enzymes*.

? QUESTION

1. When you add *heat* energy to a chemical system, what happens to the speed of molecular reactions?

2. But, if too much *heat* energy is added to a system, what happens?

ENZYME SHAPE

Enzymes have unique **shapes** and **reactive sites** that allow them to break apart molecules or put together molecules without using very much heat energy. The special shape of a particular enzyme will attract and hold two molecules close to each other until they chemically bond. Or, a slightly *different* enzyme will break a large molecule into smaller molecules.

$$A + B \longrightarrow AB$$

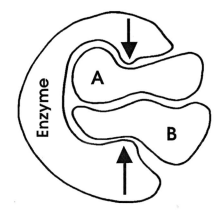

OR

$$AB \longrightarrow A + B$$

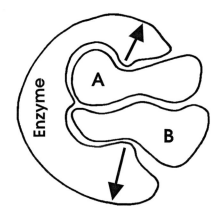

? QUESTION

1. What do you think creates the unique shape of an enzyme?

2. What would happen to a normal chemical process in your cells if the shape of the enzyme controlling that process was changed by an environmental toxin?

ENZYMES AND ENERGY OF ACTIVATION

All reactions need a "push" to get started. This push is called the *energy of activation*. Sometime the "push" involves quite a lot of energy. If the cell was dependent only on heat to supply the energy of activation, then the cell would soon *overheat*, and molecules would be *destroyed* by that heat energy. Enzymes radically decrease the "push" required to start a reaction.

Another way of thinking about enzyme function is to imagine that they are like the grease in the picture. And, like grease, enzymes can be used over and over, because they aren't actually changed by the chemical reaction.

Any substance that speeds reactions and is not used up during the process is called a *catalyst*. Enzymes are catalysts.

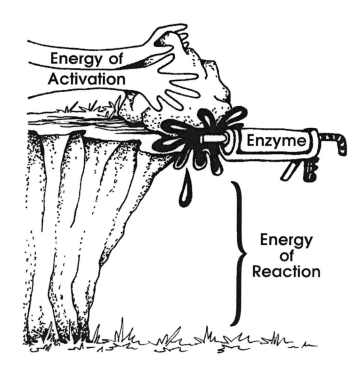

1. What do enzymes change about the *amount* of energy required to make chemical reactions occur?

2. Are enzymes destroyed or used up during the chemical reaction?

3. What is another term for a substance that speeds a reaction but is not part of the end product?

GENES AND ENZYMES

There are many thousands of different chemical reactions that occur during the life of an organism. Each of these reactions is controlled by its own enzyme.

Obviously, every organism must possess the ability to manufacture these enzymes. Each enzyme is created under the direction of a cluster of *genes*, and you have many, many genes (50,000 or so in a human). You need lots of genes because many different enzymes are necessary to perform all of the biochemical processes that make up your life as a complex organism.

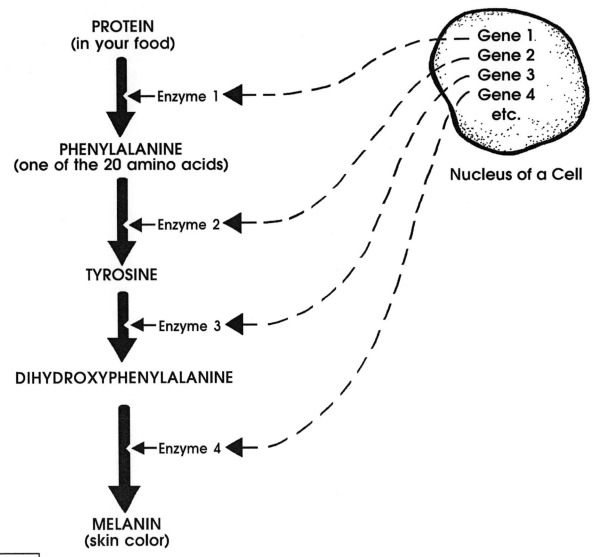

1. Why does your body need so many different enzymes?

2. What component in the nucleus is responsible for synthesizing a particular enzyme?

3. What kind of molecule is an enzyme?

4. If a gene were changed by "mutation," then what do you think would happen to the shape of the enzyme built by that gene?

5. Based on your answer to question #4, what would be the consequence to the organism affected by those "mutations"?

6. 98.3% of all human genes also occur in the chimpanzee. What does this suggest about the similarity of chemistry in these two species?

7. There is only a 0.4% genetic difference among all humans. What does this suggest about the similarity of chemistry among humans as compared to that between humans and chimpanzees?

ACTIVITY #2

"EXPERIMENTAL DESIGN"

In science, we try to make sure that the work done during the day gets us a little closer to understanding what is really going on in the world. *Experimental Design* is the planning of an experiment so that we get a *yes* or a *no* answer to a question we are asking.

THE EXPERIMENTAL CONTROL

The scientific method begins with a possible explanation of something we are observing. That explanation is a called the *hypothesis*. It generates the questions we are trying to answer in an experiment.

For example, we may think that adding more water to a lawn will make it grow faster, and we could design an experiment to test that hypothesis. In the "experimental design" we might decide to water the lawn twice as much as normal rainfall.

Let's suppose that we do this experiment for a month, and we observe that the lawn actually does grow quite a bit faster. Can we safely conclude that we have tested the hypothesis?

What if someone were to point out that the weather was warmer than normal during our experiment and that is why our *"experimental"* lawn grew faster than normal?

Or suppose that someone else said that our lawn really didn't grow any more than her lawn which was watered only by rainfall during the same month?

Because we can't answer these questions, our "experimental design" has failed. Why?

We did not control our experiment! An experimental *control* is a duplicate procedure that is set up exactly like the experiment *except* that the *factor being tested* (more water) *is left out*. So, in our experiment, we should have monitored a nearby lawn that received only normal rainfall during the same warm month. Then we could compare the growth rate of that "control" lawn to our "experimental" lawn which was receiving extra watering. The results from observing our control lawn would have answered both questions about our experiment's design.

All experiments need a control!

A SIMPLE ENZYME REACTION THAT WE WILL ALL DO TOGETHER

Work in groups of 3 or 4 people.

In simple words, an enzyme speeds up the conversion of a substance—called a *substrate*—into a *product*.

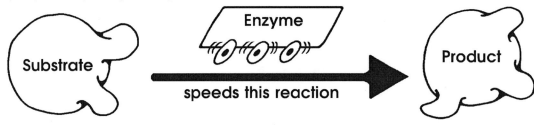

Potato juice has an enzyme that will change a colorless substrate (called catechol) into a yellow-brown product (called quinone). Forget the fancy names; we will call them substrate (colorless) and product (yellow-brown).

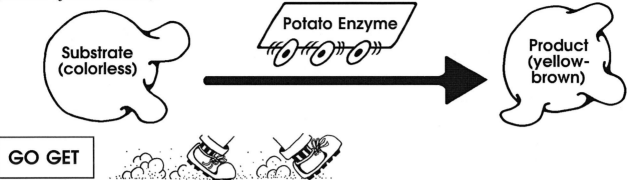

GO GET

1. Two test tubes. *Rinse them out* with tap water. They may be contaminated from the last class.

2. Colorless substrate.

3. Potato extract enzyme.

NOW

1. Work in roups of 3 or 4 people

2. Fill each tube half-full with distilled water.

3. Add 10 drops of the colorless *substrate* to one of the test tubes and shake the tube. This is the "control" for the experiment. It does not have the enzyme.

4. Add 10 drops of the colorless *substrate* plus 10 drops of the potato extract *enzyme* to the other test tube and shake the tube. This is the "experimental" tube. It has the enzyme.

5. Record how long it took (in seconds) for experimental tube turn yellow-brown.

? QUESTION

1. Why are we adding the enzyme to the second test tube?

2. Did you observe any *product* forming? (***Remember:*** A yellow-brown color means that the product has been made.)

   If so, how long did it take to form the product?

3. What observations can you make about the first test tube?

4. Why is the first test tube necessary for the validity of your experiment?

5. What are your conclusions?

ACTIVITY #3

"FACTORS AFFECTING ENZYME ACTION"

This part of the lab will help you learn how to design experiments and to observe some of the environmental factors that can affect enzyme action.

NOW IT'S YOUR TURN

1. Divide into groups of 3 or 4 people. Your instructor will assign two of the six questions to your group and to another group in the class. Each question will be tested by two lab groups in order to validate the experimental results.

2. Your group is to design an experiment with a control to answer *two* of the six questions below.

   (Your instructor may require that you test more than two of the questions. Be prepared to do so.)

3. Once your group has worked out an experimental design for the two questions, check with your lab instructor for possible suggestions. (For example, if you didn't time the reaction in Activity #2, you must do it in these experiments.)

4. Your group is to perform the experiments you design.

5. *Your group will report its results and conclusion to the rest of the class later in the lab period.* Fill out your lab report. Be sure your lab report is complete.

THE SIX ENZYME QUESTIONS

#1 *Is the speed of the reaction changed by the variation in temperature of normal environments (freezing to 120°F)?*

#2 *Is the speed of the reaction influenced by the amount of enzyme in the environment?*

> **Note:** Use the normal concentration of the enzyme, and compare that with $\frac{1}{2}$ and $\frac{1}{10}$ concentrations (10 drops, 5 drops, and 1 drop).

#3 *Is the speed of the reaction influenced by the amount of substrate in the environment?*

> **Note:** Use the normal concentration of substrate and compare it to $\frac{1}{2}$ and $\frac{1}{10}$ concentrations (10 drops, 5 drops, and 1 drop). However, less substrate means that the color change will be lighter because there is less substrate to turn color. How will you handle that problem?

#4 *Is the speed of the reaction influenced by the pH of the environment?*

> In Activity #2, you ran the experiment at pH = 7. Use the prepared acid and base solutions instead of water to test the effect of pH on the enzyme. In either case, leave the enzyme for at least 10 minutes in the test pH solution. This will allow enough time for the pH of

the environment to act on the enzymes, if it does. Then add the substrate to see if the enzyme is still active.

Be very careful when handling acids or bases. Wash your hands or eyes immediately if any solution touches them.

#5 *Are there natural substances, such as phenylthiourea, that can inhibit enzyme action?*

Note: Use the same approach as in #4 leaving the enzyme in the tube of phenylthiourea for 10 minutes before adding the substrate. *Be careful.* Phenylthiourea is a poison.

#6 *Are enzymes destroyed by high heat?*

Note: Heat the enzyme to steaming (not boiling) for 10 minutes. Let it cool to room temperature. Then do your testing.

? QUESTION

1. Sometimes raw vegetables and fruits are put into the refrigerator to slow the "browning" effect. How can you explain this based on results of experiments during this lab?

2. Sometimes lemon juice is put on raw vegetables or fruits to slow the "browning" effect. How can you explain this based on results of experiments during this lab?

3. When fruits or vegetables are left exposed to the air after they have been boiled, they don't turn brown. How can you explain this based on results of experiments during this lab?

LAB REPORT

Question # _____

Hypothesis:

Experimental Design:

Results:

Conclusions:

Question # _____

Hypothesis:

Experimental Design:

Results:

Conclusions:

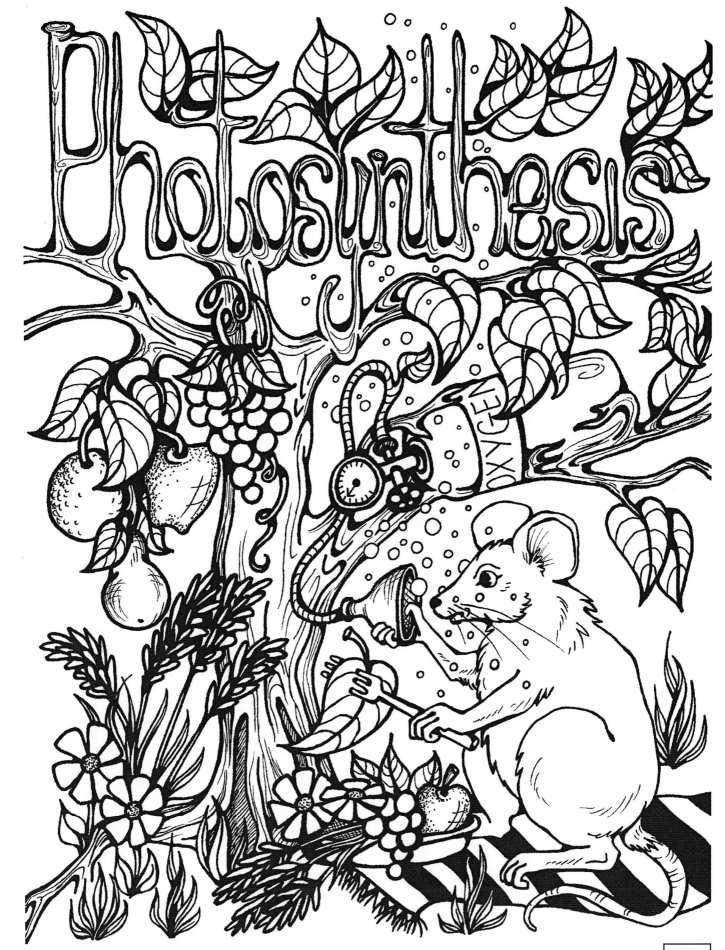

DYNAMIC DEVELOPMENTS
AND
FASCINATING FACTS
IN BIOLOGY

What turns leaves red, yellow, and purple in the autumn? When the days become shorter, photosynthesis slows, eventually stopping. Glucose is trapped in the leaves after photosynthesis stops. Waning sunlight and the cool nights of autumn cause the glucose to turn red. The brown color of trees like oaks is caused by metabolic wastes left in the leaves.

—HTTP://WWW.SCIENCEMADESIMPLE.COM/LEAVES.HTML

Elysia chlorotica, a green sea slug, is the first known animal to make proteins essential for photosynthesis, integrating genes from the algae it eats. It appears green because of co-opted chlorophyll, which makes plants green. This allows the slug to derive energy from sunlight, just like the alga does.

—HTTP://WWW.INDEPENDENT.COM/NEWS/2010/JAN/30/FIRST-KNOWN-PHOTOSYNTHETIC-ANIMAL/
—HTTP://WWW.MSNBC.MSN.COM/ID/34824610/NS/TECHNOLOGY_AND_SCIENCE-SCIENCE/T/SEA-SLUG-SURPRISE-ITS-HALFPLANT-HALF-ANIMAL

PHOTOSYNTHESIS

INTRODUCTION

Photosynthesis is the process by which plants use sunlight energy to make new plant tissue, and in doing so, they create the by-product oxygen, which is needed by animals. Sunlight activates electrons in *chlorophyll* molecules, and these "activated" electrons are used to make simple sugars. The sugars are then modified into all of the other organic molecules needed by a plant.

This week's lab on photosynthesis focuses on specific parts of the process and on the association between animals and plants. This relationship is so important, that without it, all animals (including humans) would quickly die.

 Plants change the energy of light into food energy.

 Plants also provide us with our oxygen. In the early history of our planet, 4 to 5 billion years ago, there was no oxygen in the atmosphere. Oxygen was released into the air only *after* photosynthesis evolved.

$$H_2O \quad + \quad CO_2 \xrightarrow[\text{(Chlorophyll)}]{\text{(Light Energy)}} C_6H_{12}O_6 \quad + \quad O_2$$

Water + Carbon Dioxide Gas $\longrightarrow$ Organic Molecules + Oxygen Gas

ACTIVITIES

Special Note: Activities #3 and #4 will require about an hour of your time. You should set up these two experiments *early* in the lab so that you won't run out of lab time to finish all of the Activities.

ACTIVITY #1

"LIGHT ACTIVATION OF CHLOROPHYLL"

Botanists tell us that the electrons of the chlorophyll molecule are "charged up" by light energy, and those electrons release that energy immediately to make organic molecules (food) during photosynthesis.

In this Activity, you will see for yourself whether chlorophyll can be "charged up" by light.

OBSERVE

1. Your instructor will take you into a dark room and shine a blue light on a pure chlorophyll solution. Blue light contains no other light colors in it. (Or, your instructor may use a long-wave UV light that also produces a lot of blue light.)

2. Your group is to observe. Then, go out of the room and discuss what you saw. (Your instructor may shine the blue light on green food coloring as a control experiment.)

    Hint: Pure chlorophyll cannot pass any energy onto the rest of the photosynthesis process (to make food) unless the chlorophyll is contained in the chloroplast. That does not mean that the chlorophyll can't react. It only means that it can't make food.

? QUESTION

1. When light activates the electrons of chlorophyll, then those electrons have . . . (circle your choice)

    Less energy   or   More energy

2. Physics tells us that if a substance absorbs energy, then eventually it will lose that energy in one form or another. What did you observe about the chlorophyll solution when the light was shined on it?

3. Based on the results of this experiment, fill in the empty box.

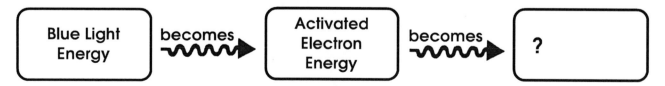

4. Plant cells, *under normal conditions*, convert activated electron energy into what?

ACTIVITY #2

"LEAF PIGMENTS"

There are many thousands of different kinds of organic molecules and sometimes they can be all mixed together in something that we want to analyze. A sample may appear to be *one* substance, but it often is a mixture of *many* different substances.

Chromatography is a very basic chemical process used to separate organic molecules from each other. During this process a solvent passes through a sample that has been impregnated on a piece of paper.

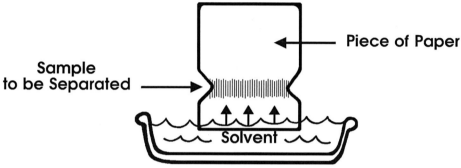

As the solvent travels up the paper, *heavier* or more chemically charged molecules will be left near the *bottom*. The other molecules (lighter or less chemically charged) will be carried *up* the paper.

The secret to understanding the results that you see here is that each *different kind* of organic molecule in the sample will be picked up by the solvent at different rates. (This depends on the individual characteristics of each substance.) Therefore, the organic molecules will be spread out along the paper according to their individual qualities.

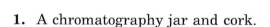

GO GET

1. A chromatography jar and cork.

2. A chromatography paper and scissors.

3. A spinach leaf and a penny.

NOW

1. Wash your hands with soap so that the substances normally on your hands (French fry grease and hamburger relish) don't become part of the chromatography separation.

2. Cut a point on the end of the chromatography paper. Cut two small notches in the sides about 1.5 cm up from the point. These notches force the solvent to go through the spinach juice.

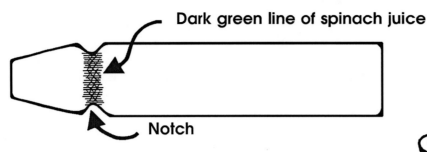

Dark green line of spinach juice

Notch

3. Roll a penny across a spinach leaf to squash a line of juice between the two notches. Make sure this line is dark green. Go over it several times. (The ridges of a quarter will work even better than a penny.)

4. Set up the chromatography jar. Place the notched paper so that when it hangs, the point *just touches* the bottom of the jar.

5. You must do the rest of the experiment *under a fume hood* or outside in the open air. ***Be careful! The solvent you are using is highly flammable!***

6. Pour the solvent into the chromatography jar to a depth of about 0.5 cm. Plug the cork with the hanging paper attached firmly into the jar. Leave the jar under the fume hood and *don't move it.*

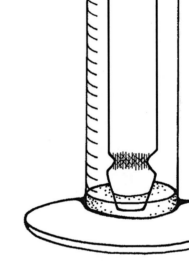

OBSERVE

During the next 10–30 minutes, the spinach juice will be separated into its individual pigments. Determine how many pigments are present. Each may be a slightly different shade, or might be the same color, but at a different location on the chromatography paper.

Present your answer, and show the evidence to your instructor.

FINALLY

When you have finished the chromatography separation, pour the solvent into the waste jar in the fume chamber, and return the chromatography setup to the lab classroom. ***Do not wash out the setup!*** Solvents collect in the air spaces of city drain systems, and can be deadly to sewer workers.

ACTIVITY #3

"CO₂ UPTAKE BY PLANTS"

The photosynthesis equation: $H_2O + CO_2 \xrightarrow[\text{(Chlorophyll)}]{\text{(Light Energy)}} C_6H_{12}O_6 + O_2$ says that carbon dioxide is used to make part of the organic molecule product (food) during the process of the reaction.

If this is true, then we should be able to observe that happening.

PHENOL RED TEST FOR CO₂

There is a very simple way to show changes in CO_2 level. Phenol red is a substance that turns yellow when CO_2 is added, and then it turns back to red when CO_2 is removed.

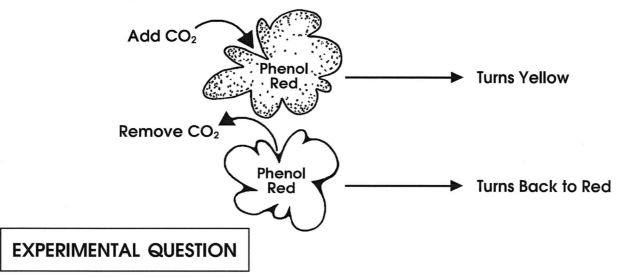

EXPERIMENTAL QUESTION

We can use phenol red as an experimental tool to answer the question: *"Do plants use CO₂ during photosynthesis?"*

EXPERIMENTAL SETUP

Don't blow through the glass tube cork.

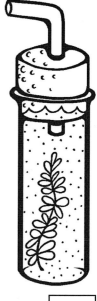

1. First, "charge up" the phenol red with CO_2 using your own breath. The easiest way is to pour one test tube full of phenol red solution into a small beaker. Blow very carefully through a straw into the solution until it turns yellow. (Don't blow so forcefully that you make a mess.)

2. Pour the yellow solution back into your test tube. Add a small piece of *Elodea* plant (about 10 cm).

3. *Carefully* put the bent glass tube cork into the test tube, leaving no *air bubbles*.

4. Put the experimental setup in front of a light source for 30 minutes. What happens?

NOW

1. Your group is to design a simple experiment that will test whether light is required by the plant during photosynthesis. Be sure to include a control.

2. Check with your instructor when you think you have a good design for the experiment.

3. Now, do it!

4. *Please put the used Elodea plants into the special container!* They have some phenol red on them that will contaminate the rest of the *Elodea* and kill it.

? QUESTION

1. If CO_2 is removed from the phenol red solution, then what process is going on in the *Elodea*?

2. Is light required by the plant during photosynthesis?

3. Describe your controls. (There are two.)

4. What is the purpose of having a control?

ACTIVITY #4

"O₂ PRODUCTION BY PLANTS"

The photosynthesis equation $H_2O + CO_2 \xrightarrow[\text{(Chlorophyll)}]{\text{(Light Energy)}} C_6H_{12}O_6 + O_2$ says that oxygen is produced.

If this is true, then we should be able to observe it.

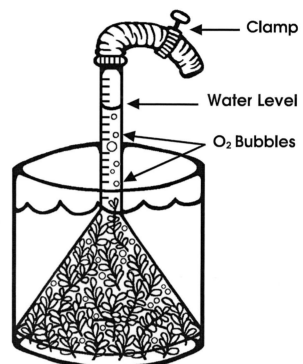

Clamp

Water Level

O₂ Bubbles

EXPERIMENTAL SETUP

Hint: There are a few tricks to this setup.

1. You need ten 2" pieces of healthy *Elodea* plants. Trim $\frac{1}{8}$" off each stem. A fresh cut will allow oxygen to bubble out of the plant.

2. You have to suck water up the funnel and up the tube, and then *clamp* the hose at the top to keep the water level from falling.

3. If the experiment is working, the oxygen bubbles will collect at the top of the tube and push the water level down. This drop in water level is what you are to measure during the experiment.

4. Set up a light source shining from the side, but make sure to put a beaker of clear water between the light and the Elodea container. (The beaker prevents the Elodea from overheating. The clear water container will absorb the heat from the light bulb, yet still allows light to pass through to the Elodea.)
   Note: If you can take the apparatus outside into the sunlight, your plants will photosynthesize much faster.

EXPERIMENTAL QUESTION

How much oxygen is produced by the Elodea plants in one hour?

NOW

1. We will do only one of these experimental setups for the whole class to observe. Select one person in your group to work with the instructor to set up the apparatus.

2. Have your group's representative record the O₂ production every 15 minutes for one hour.

3. Record the total milliliters (ml) of oxygen produced during one hour. You will use this production value during Activity #6.

   ml of O₂ produced by the plant in one hour = _____

ACTIVITY #5

"OXYGEN DEMAND FOR HUMANS"

| PROBLEM | *How much oxygen does a human need to survive one hour of biology lab class?* |

Next week we will actually measure the O_2 consumption of a mouse under different temperature conditions and compare different animals and plants.

However, this week we can borrow an estimate of human oxygen demand from experimental research.

> The O_2 used by a human in one hour can range from ¼ of a liter of O_2 per kg of body weight to as high as 8 liters. (Although that high rate of metabolism could be maintained for only about 2 minutes without total exhaustion.)

> A person in biology lab class uses about 0.4 liters of O_2 per kg of body weight in one hour as long as they aren't walking around all the time.

NOW

1. Assume that the O_2 used by a person during one hour of biology lab is about 0.4 liters (400 ml) per kg of body weight.

2. Assume that the average human weighs 60 kg.

? QUESTION

What is the oxygen demand for an average person during one hour of biology lab?

_____ = ml of O_2 used by a human in one hour

You will use this calculation again in Activity #6.

ACTIVITY #6

"HOW BIG OF A PLANT DOES IT TAKE TO KEEP YOU ALIVE?"

PREVIOUS INFO

You have an estimate of the amount of O_2 (in ml) produced during one hour by the *Elodea* Plant (see Activity #4), and you have an estimate of the amount of O_2 used by a human in one hour (see Activity #5).

NOW

1. Record the amount of oxygen that the *Elodea* plant produced in *one* hour.

   _____ ml of O_2 per hour

2. Measure the cross-sectional area of the *Elodea* plant container. If light is shining from the side, then the cross-sectional area of light on the plants is a triangle shape. (The funnel looks like a triangle when viewed from the side.)

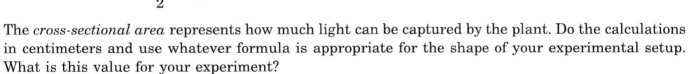

$$\text{Area} = \frac{1}{2} \text{ Height x Width}$$

The *cross-sectional area* represents how much light can be captured by the plant. Do the calculations in centimeters and use whatever formula is appropriate for the shape of your experimental setup. What is this value for your experiment?

   _____ cm² of light-catching surface

? QUESTION

How much oxygen (in ml) is produced by 1 cm² of the plant cross-sectional area?

   _____ ml of O_2 is produced per cm² of plant in one hour

Hint: You would get the correct answer by dividing your answer from question #1 above by the answer for question #2.

1. What was your calculation of the oxygen demand for a human being during one hour of lab class? (Refer to Activity #5.)

_____ ml of O_2 per hour

2. Use this formula to answer the *? QUESTION* below.

$$\text{Size of Plant Needed to Keep You Alive (in cm}^2) = \frac{\text{Human Oxygen Demand (in ml)}}{\text{Plant } O_2 \text{ Production (in ml) per cm}^2 \text{ of Plant}}$$

? QUESTION

1. What size of plant is required to keep you alive?

_____ cm^2

2. Change this plant size to m^2 by dividing your answer above by 10,000 (there are 10,000 cm^2 in one m^2). What is your answer in m^2?

Size of plant required = _____ m^2

3. If you determine the square root of the plant area above, then you will have calculated the *side measurement of a square shape* representing the plant area. Side = _____ m.

4. In the above calculations, you have determined how big a plant is required to keep you alive during daylight hours, but what will keep you alive at night? *Remember:* Plants don't photosynthesize at night.

5. Does this change your estimate of how big a plant it takes to keep you alive both day and night?

By how much?

FINALLY

Go outside and mark off on the ground how big of a plant is required to keep you alive every twelve hours.

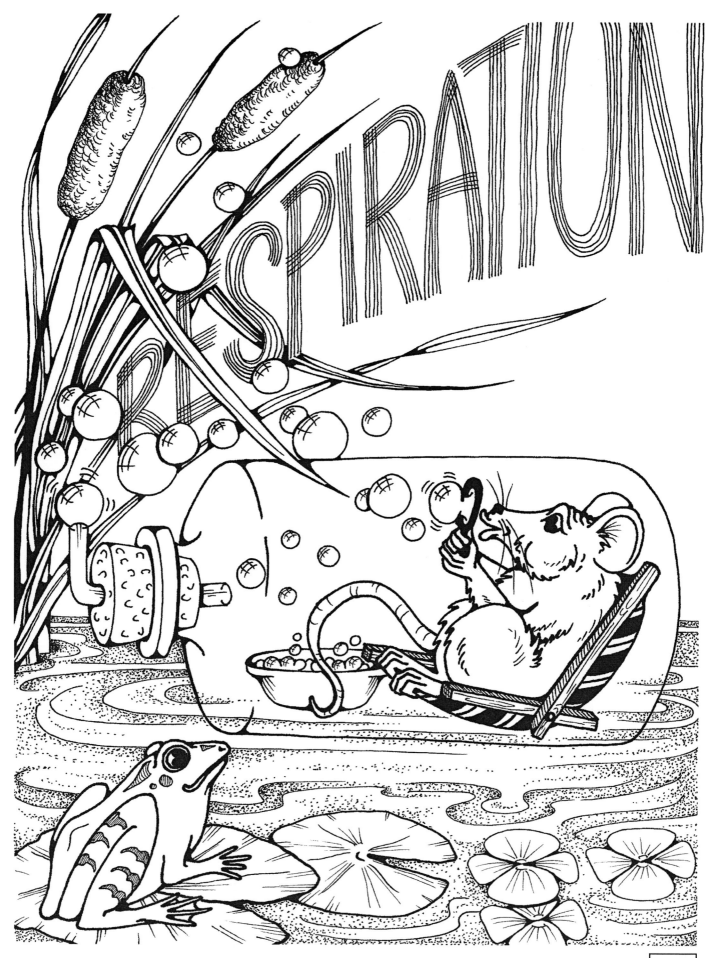

109

DYNAMIC DEVELOPMENTS
AND
FASCINATING FACTS
IN BIOLOGY

We require about the same number of calories as other primates of similar weight, but our brains require a greater percentage of those calories than brains of other species. Human brains use 25% of daily caloric intake; this percentage leaps to 87% in a newborn infant's brain. A three-pound human brain consumes up to 20 times as many calories as three pounds of muscle. Evolution advanced our brains by increasing the number of genes that code for glucose transporting proteins in the brain, but decreasing glucose transporting proteins for our muscles.

—"THE BRAIN" BY CARL ZIMMER, *DISCOVER MAGAZINE,* JULY/AUGUST 2011, P. 18–19

RESPIRATION

INTRODUCTION

Respiration is the cellular process in living organisms that extracts electron energy from the chemical bonds in *food* (organic molecules), and converts that energy into a more useful form of energy (called **ATP**) to run cell activities. This cell process uses oxygen and produces carbon dioxide. The complete equation is:

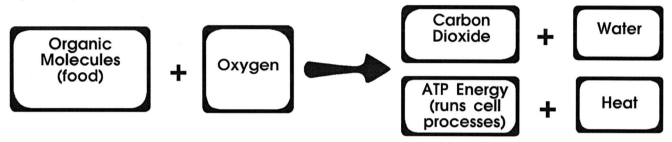

Respiration occurs inside the *mitochondria*, which are cellular organelles in both plant and animal cells. Refer to your textbook for the structural and functional description of this organelle.

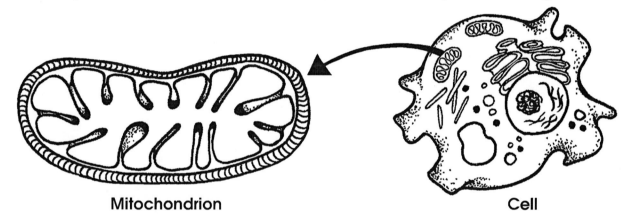

Mitochondrion   Cell

During this lab we will investigate some aspects of cellular respiration including the effects of environmental temperature on the rate of respiration in *endotherms* (internally heated animals) and *ectotherms* (externally heated animals).

ACTIVITIES

ACTIVITY #1

"HEAT PRODUCTION DURING RESPIRATION"

The Second Law of Thermodynamics states that heat is released whenever any form of energy is transformed into another form.

Since respiration is described as the conversion of food energy into usable energy for the cell, we should be able to observe heat being given off during the process.

OBSERVE

Two experimental containers were set up yesterday. One of the containers was filled with *dead seeds* killed by boiling, and the other container was filled with *live seeds*. Record the temperature of each container.

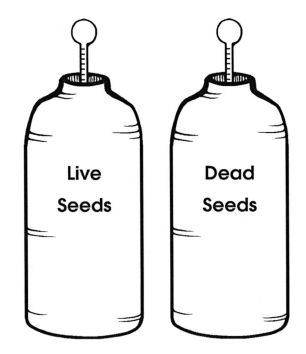

Temperature of live seeds = _____

Temperature of dead seeds = _____

These seeds demonstrate the basic respiration process that is going on in all living organisms.

? QUESTION

1. What does the equation for respiration say about *heat*?

2. What does this experiment suggest is occurring in live seeds and not in dead seeds?

3. What would happen to the respiration process in the container of live seeds if we pumped the oxygen out?

   What would happen to the temperature in that container?

ACTIVITY #2

"RESPIRATION IN AN ENDOTHERM"

Mice are **endotherms**. That is, they get most of their heat from *inside* their own body (*endo* means inside). Cellular respiration generates the heat that keeps these animals warm. (Refer to the Equation for Respiration on the first page.)

During this Activity you will monitor the **rate of respiration** (also called **metabolic rate**) in a mouse. In addition, you will investigate the *influence of environmental temperature* on the mouse's rate of respiration by comparing a mouse in a *cold environment* with a mouse in a *warm environment*.

Later, in Activity #3, you will compare the differences between an endotherm (mouse) and an ectotherm (frog).

HOW TO HANDLE MICE

Mice should be *picked up by their tail* and immediately *rested on your hand,* and then marched into the Metabolic Cage.

Do not grab them.

Grabbing scares the hell out of them, and they may bite you or pee on you because of that fear.

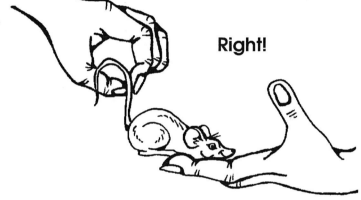

Right!

Also, *don't play with the mice* (on table tops, etc.) because there is a possibility of them getting loose on the floor.

These are professional mice. They work several years for us, and we treat them very well. So, please be careful.

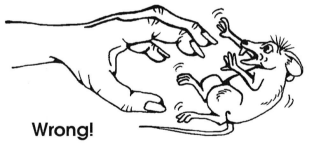

Wrong!

EXPERIMENTAL APPARATUS

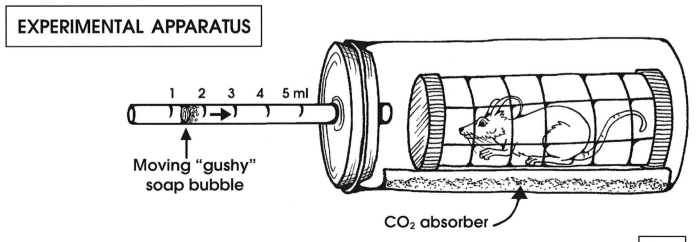

1 2 3 4 5 ml

Moving "gushy" soap bubble

CO_2 absorber

EXPERIMENTAL DESIGN

The basic question is: *What effect does environmental temperature have on the metabolic rate of an endotherm (mouse)?*

Do this experiment at two temperatures: Room Temperature and Packed in Ice.

ROOM TEMPERATURE

STEP 1

Weigh the wire cage part of the chamber: _____ grams.

STEP 2

Go get your mouse, and put it into the wire cage. Then weigh the cage with the mouse in it.

Cage + Mouse		**Cage**		**Weight of Mouse**
_____ g	−	_____ g	=	_____ g

STEP 3

Put one tablespoon of CO_2 absorber (soda lime) into the trough at the bottom of the Metabolic Rate Chamber. If your class is using small bags of CO_2 absorber instead of loose material, then place one bag on top of the mouse cage so the mouse can't pee on it.

STEP 4

Wet the inside of the glass tube with soapy water. This will help prevent the "gushy" bubble from "popping" during the experiment.

STEP 5

Put the caged mouse into the chamber and seal the cork tightly. *Don't worry! The mouse won't suffocate.* Leave the chamber alone for 10 minutes *(sealed up—cork on—no soap bubble)* to equalize the temperatures inside and outside of the chamber.

STEP 6

Use your finger to make a "gushy" soap bubble on the open end of the glass tube. Then, measure the time it takes (in seconds) for the bubble to move between the marks on the tube until 5 ml of O_2 have been consumed by the mouse. Perform three trials.

_____ seconds	_____ seconds	_____ seconds
Trial 1	**Trial 2**	**Trial 3**

1. Food + O_2 $\longrightarrow$ CO_2 + H_2O. During respiration a mouse will consume O_2, and CO_2 will be produced in its place. If no CO_2 absorber had been used in your experiment, would you have seen a change in air *volume*?

2. If you use a CO_2 absorbing substance in the Metabolic Rate Chamber, then what happens to the CO_2 that is produced during respiration?

3. Now, with the absorbing substance in the chamber, what happens to the *air volume* during your experiment as the O_2 is consumed during respiration?

PACKED IN ICE

If ice is packed around a Metabolic Rate Chamber like the type we are using, the temperature inside will stabilize at 5°C.

This cold air temperature *will not harm* the mouse as long as the mouse is removed before 45 minutes. Our experiment will take less than 20 minutes.

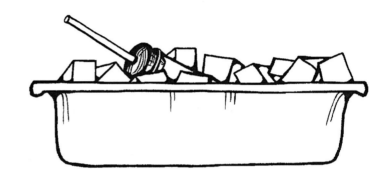

STEP 1 Now perform the "Packed in Ice" experiment. Let the chamber equalize the temperatures inside and out for 10 minutes before applying the "gushy" soap bubble.

STEP 2 After 10 minutes, apply a "gushy" soap bubble and perform the three separate measurements of the rate of respiration.

_____ seconds _____ seconds _____ seconds
      Trial 1   **Trial 2**   **Trial 3**

FINALLY

Disassemble the chamber, carefully returning your mouse to its home, and dump all CO_2 absorber and feces into the special waste jar. Don't wash the apparatus unless you are told to do so. The chamber must be dry for the next lab class.

Wash your hands!

RESPIRATION CALCULATIONS

You must convert the mouse's O_2 consumption to an hourly metabolic rate. Calculations 1 and 2 will make that conversion. This is accomplished by dividing the bubble time (in seconds) into 3,600 (the number of seconds in one hour). The resulting number is to be multiplied by 5 (5 ml of O_2 used in each trial).

CALCULATION 1

Calculate the *average* time of the three trials at room temperature.

5 ml O_2 consumed in _____ seconds (average time)

CALCULATION 2

Based on Calculation 1, how much O_2 would your mouse consume in one hour? (There are 3600 seconds in one hour.)

$$\frac{3,600}{\text{Calculation 1}} \quad \text{x} \quad 5 \quad = \quad \text{_____ ml } O_2 \text{ consumed in one hour}$$

CALCULATION 3

In order to have a metabolic rate that can be compared with an animal of different weight, we must correct the calculations considering the mouse's weight.

$$\frac{\text{Calculation 2}}{\text{Weight of Mouse}} \quad = \quad \text{_____ ml } O_2 \text{ per hour per gram of weight}$$

NOW

You have finished the calculations for room temperature. Record your answer below. Repeat the same calculations for "Packed in Ice," and record your answer below.

Metabolic rate of your mouse   =   _____   ml O_2 per hour
at room temperature (20°C)   per gram of weight

Metabolic rate of your mouse   =   _____   ml O_2 per hour
packed in ice (5°C)   per gram of weight

1. Put a dot on the graph for each of the metabolic rate values in your experiment.

2. Draw a line between those two dots, and write the word *endotherm* on the line.

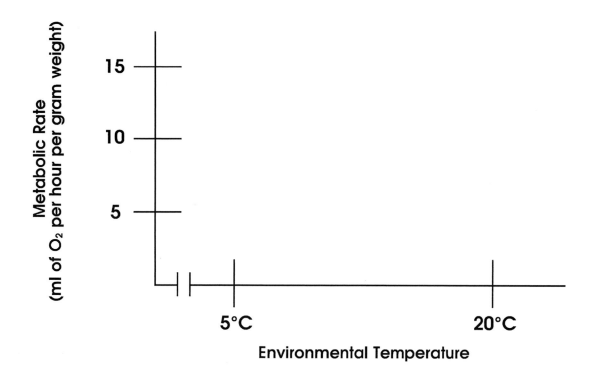

3. Check with other lab groups to see how your calculations compare with theirs.

ACTIVITY #3

"COMPARISON OF ENDOTHERM AND ECTOTHERM"

An *ectotherm* gets its heat from the environment (*ecto* means outside). The body temperature of an ectotherm is warm when the environment is warm, and the body is cooler when the environment is cold.

INFORMATION

The following results are taken from some experiments that measured the metabolic rate in a frog (*ectotherm*) of about the same size as your mouse.

	Metabolic Rate Packed in Ice (5° C)	Metabolic Rate at Room Temperature (20° C)	
Frog #1	0.05	0.30	ml O_2 per hour per gram of weight
Frog #2	0.03	0.28	
Frog #3	0.04	0.25	

NOW

1. Calculate the *average* metabolic rate for the three frogs at each of the two temperatures.

2. Put a dot on the graph for each of the average values.

3. Draw a line between those two dots, and write the word *ectotherm* on the line.

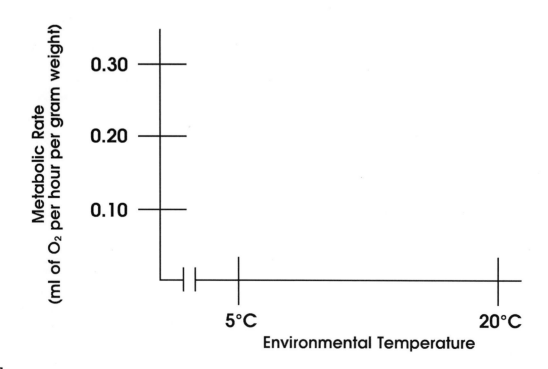

1. Which organism has the slowest rate of respiration? (circle your choice)

   Endotherm   or   Ectotherm

2. Which organism needs less food to survive? (circle your choice)

   Endotherm   or   Ectotherm

Explain why.

3. How much food does the *ectotherm* need compared to the *endotherm*? _____ %

4. Which organism would do better if the amount of food is very limited, but the environment is fairly warm? (circle your choice)

   Endotherm   or   Ectotherm

5. In what areas of the world would you expect to find ectotherms?

6. Which organism would do better in cooler environments where the food is plentiful? (circle your choice)

   Endotherm   or   Ectotherm

7. Will the organism in question #6 do fine in warmer environments if the food is plentiful?

Why or why not?

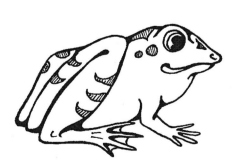
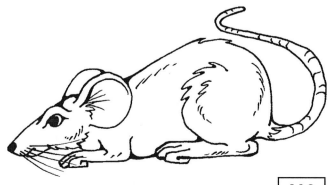

ACTIVITY #4

"FOOD DEMAND FOR HUMANS"

How much food does a human need to survive one hour of biology lab class?

We can borrow data from experimental research to help us estimate the amount of food that is required to support a human. Our calculations will be based on grams of sugar as the nutrient. Also, notice that the word *Calorie* is capitalized. When capitalized, this term represents 1000 times the value of a single calorie.

The Caloric demand for food varies greatly for a human depending on activity and environmental conditions. The energy demand might be as slow as 50 Cal per hour during sleep to as fast as 2,000 Cal per hour during extreme exercise. (Although that high rate of metabolism could be maintained for only about 2 minutes without total exhaustion.)

An average student in biology lab class uses about 100 Calories per hour as long as they aren't walking around all of the time.

INFORMATION

1. Assume a food demand of 100 Cal/hour for students.

2. A human gets about 3.85 Cal of energy from 1 gram of sugar.

? QUESTION

How many grams of sugar are required to "fuel" an average student during one hour of biology lab class?

_____ grams of sugar used in one hour

NOW

Weigh out that much sugar and show it to your lab instructor.

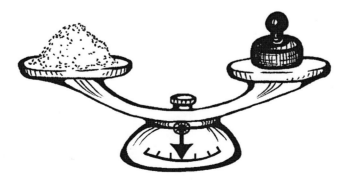

ACTIVITY #5

"RESPIRATION IN PLANTS"

The Respiration Equation states that CO_2 is produced as O_2 is used. If that is true, then we should be able to use CO_2 production as an indicator that respiration is occurring.

PHENOL RED TEST FOR CO_2

There is a very simple way to show changes in CO_2 level. Phenol red is a substance that turns yellow when CO_2 is added, and then turns back to red when CO_2 is removed.

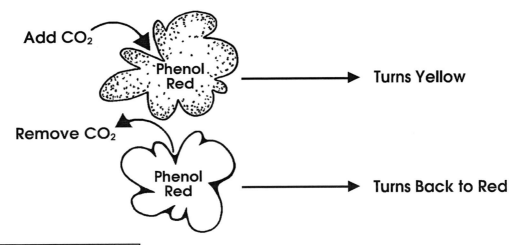

Add CO_2 → Phenol Red → Turns Yellow

Remove CO_2 → Phenol Red → Turns Back to Red

EXPERIMENTAL SETUP

Yesterday we put a small piece of *Elodea* plant into a test tube filled with dilute phenol red solution. The tube was red because the water had very little CO_2 in it.

We put this experimental setup into a closed cabinet until today.

Ask your instructor where the plant is, and make your observations.

? QUESTION

What do you conclude about plants in the dark?

SAMENESS &

VARiETY

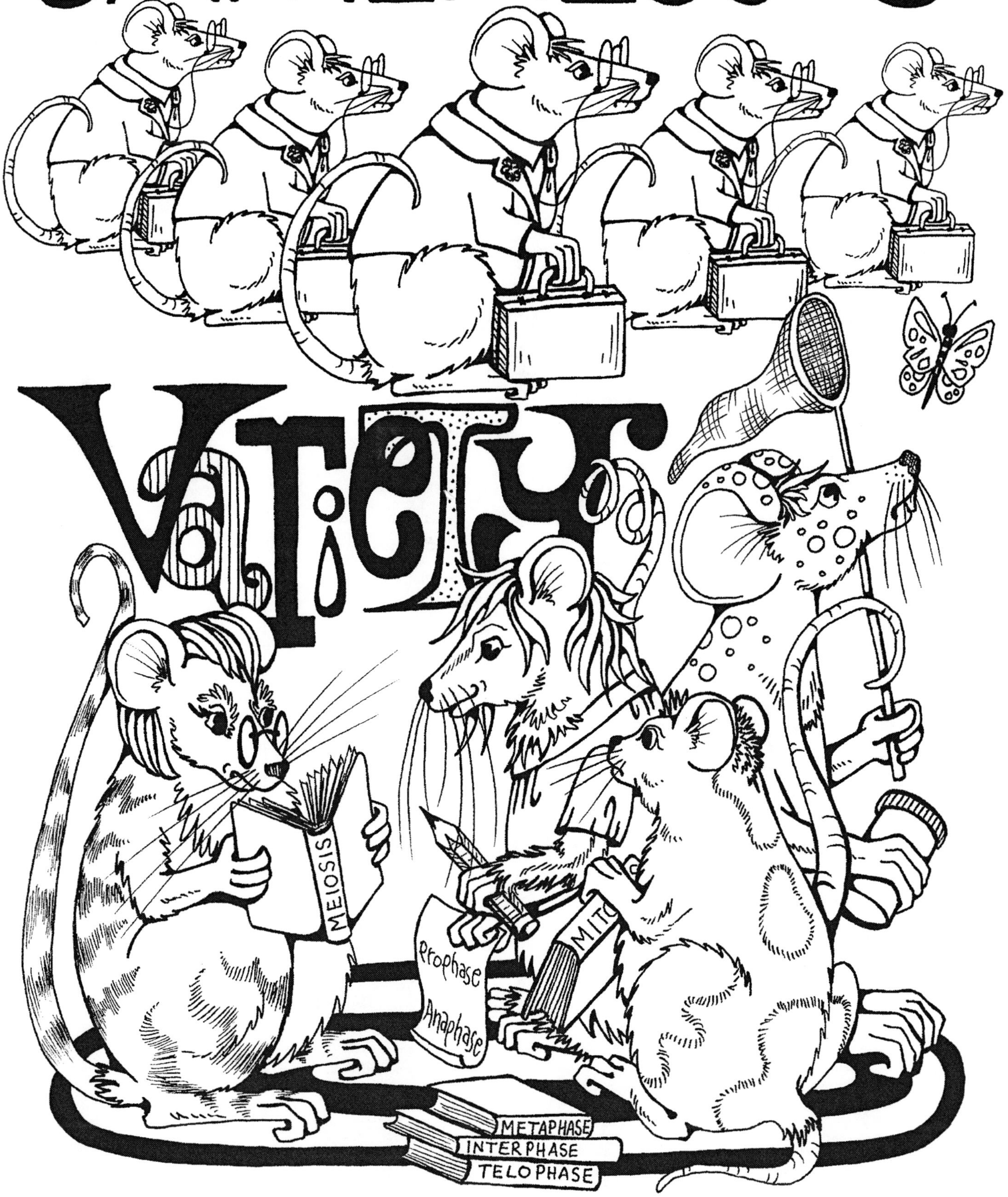

MEIOSIS

erophase

Anaphase

METAPHASE
INTERPHASE
TELOPHASE

Tetrahymena thermophila, a single-celled organism found in pond water, possesses seven (7) different genders. Such abundance of sexes leads to enhanced diversity.

—"Numbers: Sex" by Shannon Palus, *Discover Magazine,* June 2011, p. 12

Homosexuality in animal species has been documented in more than 500 species. Nearly half of bottle-nosed dolphins engage in same-sex relations; 31% of Hawaiian Laysan albatross pairings occur between females.

—"Numbers: Sex" by Shannon Palus, *Discover Magazine,* June 2011, p. 12

The number of chromosomes a species possesses has very little association with its size or complexity. The males of the ant species, *Myrmecia pilosula,* is haploid and has only one chromosome. The swamp wallaby has 10 (male) or 11 (female) chromosomes. The adder's tounge fern has the highest known chromosme number at 1260.

—http://www.ask.com/wiki/List_of_organisms_by_chromosome_count#cite_note-Simmonds-1

We share a significant percentage of DNA with other life-forms on Earth:

Life-form	Percent
E. coli	7%
yeast	23%
cabbage	40%
bananas	50%
fruit flies	51%
chickens	60%
slugs	71%
earthworms	74%
dogs	85%
mice	90%
chimpanzees	98%
other humans	99%
human relatives	99.5%

SAMENESS AND VARIETY

(MITOSIS AND MEIOSIS)

INTRODUCTION

Is it better to be the same as everyone else?
or
Is it better to be different?

We struggle with these questions in our personal lives. Would it surprise you to learn that all life, in terms of its reproductive strategy, has struggled with the same basic questions? It might also surprise you to learn that there is no *one* answer to reproduction, but *two* answers.

The strategy of producing offspring that are genetically the same as the parent is called **asexual reproduction,** and is accomplished through a cell division process termed **mitosis**. Asexual reproduction is the simplest and oldest form of reproduction, and it relies on a single parent.

The strategy of producing offspring that express genetic variety is termed **sexual reproduction**. It is accomplished through a cell division process called **meiosis** and a fusion process called **fertilization**. Sexual reproduction is complex and it usually relies on two parents.

Many organisms have lost the means to reproduce asexually except for cell replacement or growth. But some less specialized species use both modes, depending on the time of year. The one certainty is that organisms exist today only because they have incorporated both sameness and variety in their struggle to live and reproduce.

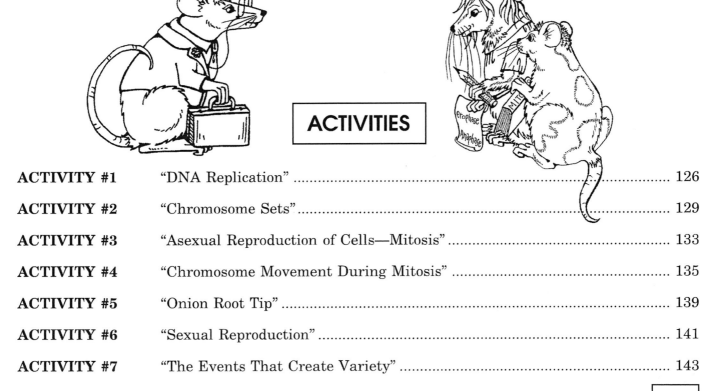

ACTIVITIES

ACTIVITY #1

"DNA REPLICATION"

Sixty years ago, the study of biochemistry revealed a fact that stunned the scientific establishment and transformed our approach to biology.

The fact is this: *A chemical called DNA reproduces—not the individual.*

Also, it was discovered that the sorting of DNA by the cell is what controls the sameness or variety of the next generation. This does not mean that the organism isn't important. The organism is made of cells that contain the DNA molecules. But the genetic unit that actually gets passed on to the next generation is the DNA. That's why the discussion of reproduction is centered around this unique molecule.

So, first let's take a look at the structure of DNA and how it reproduces itself. Then, we will see how DNA uses an organism to achieve sameness by asexual reproduction, or achieves variety by sexual reproduction.

DNA STRUCTURE

DNA is an extremely thin, long, ladder-like molecule that has two "rails" made of sugar and phosphate, and many "rungs" made of special complementary bases.

The DNA bases (rungs) are molecular units that combine only in two kinds of pairs.

The base *adenine* (A) is always paired with *thymine* (T), and *cytosine* (C) is always paired with *guanine* (G). Therefore, if you know *one* of the complementary bases, you can easily figure out the other.

The term *nucleotide* is used as a name for the repeating subunits in a DNA molecule. A nucleotide is actually a phosphate, a sugar, and a base hooked together as a basic building unit.

DNA Molecule

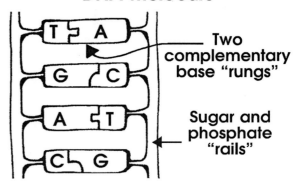

Two complementary base "rungs"

Sugar and phosphate "rails"

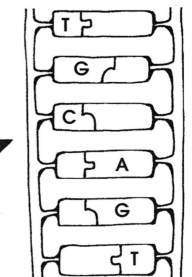

? QUESTION

1. Guanine always pairs with _____.

2. Thymine always pairs with _____.

3. Fill in the complementary nucleotides on this DNA ladder.

REPRODUCTION OF DNA

Before DNA can copy itself the cell must make lots of extra A, T, G, and C. Then the DNA unzips between the two bases and adds nucleotides to each side of the unzipped DNA molecule.

Original DNA ⟶ **Splits Open** ⟶ **Adds New Nucleotides**

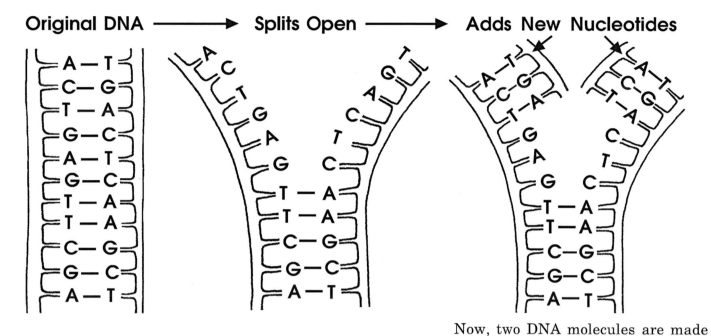

Now, two DNA molecules are made where there was only one before.

? QUESTION

1. Finish unzipping the DNA molecule pictured above, and draw the completed picture of the two "new" DNA molecules. Use the same DNA sequences as the example above.

2. What are the two "new" DNA molecules built from? Explain.

3. Are the two "new" DNA molecules absolutely identical to the "original" DNA molecule?

EXAMPLE

Expressed using apples, DNA replication looks like this:

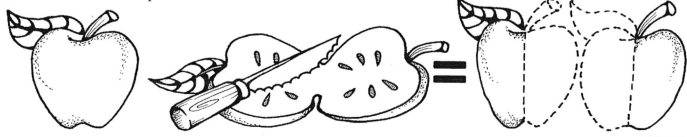

Look at the model of DNA on the demonstration table.

We have been presenting DNA as a straight ladder, but actually it is twisted on itself like a spiral staircase. This shape is called a *helix*.

THE CHROMOSOME

Normally DNA exists as loose strands (*chromatin*) in the nucleus of a cell. This nuclear DNA sends a message (RNA) to the ribosomes where protein and enzymes are synthesized.

When stretched out, the length of one DNA molecule in a human cell is almost 4 cm. However, the cell itself is but a tiny fraction of that size.

Problem: During cell reproduction the DNA must be able to move around. So it shortens its length by tightly coiling up. In doing so, the DNA strands become wider and are visible under a microscope. Visible DNA is called a *chromosome*.

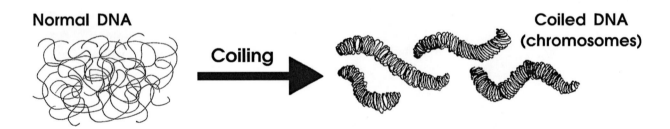

Normal DNA — Coiling → Coiled DNA (chromosomes)

? QUESTION

1. A chromosome is made up of tightly _____ DNA.

2. Explain the reason for this shape.

3. When not reproducing, DNA is found in the _____ of a cell and exists in the form called _____.

4. Visible DNA is called a _____.

ACTIVITY #2

"CHROMOSOME SETS"

The number of chromosomes in a cell varies from species to species, but it is exactly the same among individual members of the same species.

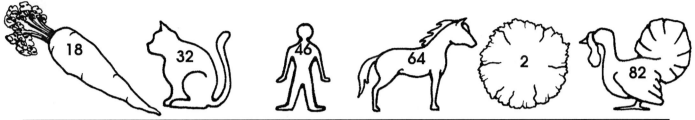

THE ONE-SET CONCEPT OF CHROMOSOMES: WHAT IS HAPLOID?

All species have one or more sets of chromosomes. This means that chromosomes come in *sets*, and the *number* of chromosomes in a set depends on the particular species.

A set of chromosomes includes *one copy* of all of the genes necessary to control the biochemical activities of a species. Most species have either one or two chromosome sets.

In genetics a single set of chromosomes is symbolized by the letter "**n**." Any cell that has only one set of chromosomes is termed **haploid**. Haploid means that the cell has *one* of each *kind* of chromosome.

? QUESTION

The set concept will be used throughout the rest of this lab, so the following questions were designed to aid you in understanding and recognizing sets. Remember that a set is a group of objects related in function and generally used together.

1. Pretend that the *fingers* of one hand represent chromosomes. (Count your thumb as a finger.) Hold up your hand.

    a. How many fingers (chromosomes) do you have on one hand? _____

    b. Do you have different kinds of fingers on one hand? _____

    c. Do you have more than one of each kind of finger on one hand? _____

    d. Judging by the definition of a set, you have _____ set(s) of fingers on one hand.

2. Pretend that all the numbers within the circle represent chromosomes.

    a. How many numbers are there? _____

    b. Are there different kinds of numbers? _____

    c. Is there more than one of each kind of number? _____

    d. Judging by the definition, you have _____ set(s) of numbers.

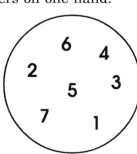

3. Pretend these lines represent chromosomes.

    a. How many lines are there? _____

    b. Are there different kinds of lines? _____

    c. Is there more than one of each kind of line? _____

    d. Judging by the set definition, you have _____ set(s) of lines.

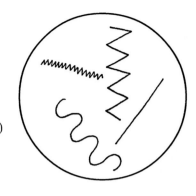

    Answers:

#1	#2	#3
a=5	a=7	a=4
b=yes	b=yes	b=yes
c=no	c=no	c=no
d=1	d=1	d=1

4. Explain the one-set concept of chromosomes.

THE TWO-SET CONCEPT OF CHROMOSOMES: WHAT IS DIPLOID?

Simple organisms and the gametes of complex organisms are haploid. That is, they have a single set of chromosomes. Complex organisms require *two sets* of chromosomes to survive. We will discuss the details of this two-set requirement in a later lab.

In genetics, the two-set condition is symbolized as "**2n**," and is called ***diploid***. Diploid means that the cell has *two* of each *kind* of chromosome.

? QUESTION

1. Pretend that the fingers of *both* of your hands represent chromosomes. Hold up your hands.

    a. How many fingers (chromosomes) do you have?

    _____

    b. Regarding both hands, do you have a *duplication* of each of the *kinds* of fingers? _____

    c. How many sets of fingers do you have? _____

    d. How many fingers are in a single set? _____

    e. Draw a simple sketch of a single set of fingers.

2. Pretend that all the numbers within the circle represent chromosomes.

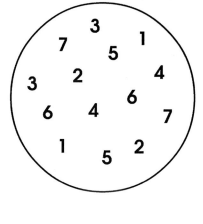

   a. How many total numbers are there? _____

   b. Is there a duplication of each kind of number? _____

   c. How many sets of numbers are there? _____

   d. How many numbers are in each set? _____

   e. Draw a sketch of a single set of numbers.

3. Pretend that the lines within the circle represent chromosomes.

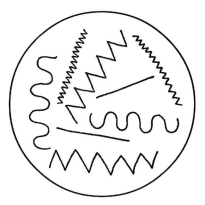

   a. How many lines are there? _____

   b. Is there a duplication of each kind of line? _____

   c. How many sets of lines are there? _____

   d. How many lines are there in each set? _____

   e. Draw a sketch of a single set of lines.

Answers:

#1	#2	#3
a=10	a=14	a=8
b=yes	b=yes	b=yes
c=2	c=2	c=2
d=5	d=7	d=4

4. Explain the two-set concept of chromosomes.

HOMOLOGOUS CHROMOSOMES

The word *homologous* means "the same," and the term ***homologous chromosomes*** refers to the pairs of chromosomes in a diploid cell that carry genes for the same traits. We will discuss more details about cell division in the following Activities, but for now, keep this note in mind: ***Each chromosome of a homologous pair comes from a different parent.*** Humans are diploid and have 46 chromosomes (two sets of 23). This means that we have 23 homologous chromosome pairs.

Although both chromosomes of a particular homologous pair carry the *same genes*, these genes may be slightly different *forms*. For example, one might be the "blue eye" form, and the other might be the "brown eye" form. (More about that later.)

? QUESTION

1. Pretend that the fingers of both of your hands are chromosomes. Hold up both your hands.

   a. How many individual fingers (chromosomes) do you have? _____

   b. How many homologous pairs are there? _____

   c. How many sets of fingers do you have? _____

   d. How many homologous pairs are in one set of fingers? _____

2. Pretend that the numbers in the circle are chromosomes.

   a. How many individual numbers are there? _____

   b. How many homologous pairs of numbers are there? _____

   c. How many sets of numbers are there? _____

   d. How many homologous pairs are in one set of numbers? _____

3. Pretend that all the lines within the circle are chromosomes.

   a. How many individual lines are there? _____

   b. How many homologous pairs of lines are there? _____

   c. How many sets of lines are there? _____

   d. How many homologous pairs of lines are in one set? _____

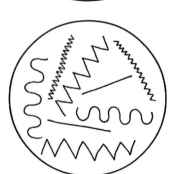

Answers:

#1	#2	#3
a=10	a=14	a=8
b=5	b=7	b=4
c=2	c=2	c=2
d=0	d=0	d=0

4. Explain in simple terms what homologous chromosomes are.

ACTIVITY #3

"ASEXUAL REPRODUCTION OF CELLS—MITOSIS"

Asexual reproduction of cells is called *mitosis*. Immediately before this cell division process begins, the DNA of a cell (either haploid or diploid) duplicates itself creating two identical copies of every DNA molecule (and chromosome). The DNA copies move to opposite ends of the cell. Then the cell partitions itself into two cells (each with *exactly* the same DNA as the original cell). The purpose of asexual reproduction by mitosis is to create new cells that are genetically *identical* to the original cell.

Haploid Mitosis

Haploid mitosis does happen in some organisms,
but will be covered in a more advanced biology course.

Diploid Mitosis

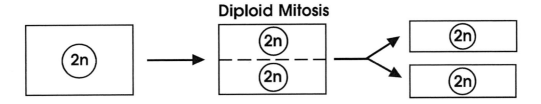

PROBLEM

1. Let's imagine what would happen to the amount of DNA material in a cell if, when it reproduced, it did not duplicate the DNA first. Complete this cell box.

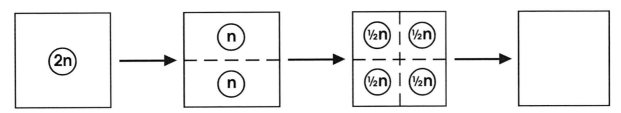

2. Explain what this mistake creates in the new cells.

FINALLY

For a dividing cell to maintain its original set # in the new cells, it must duplicate its genetic material prior to beginning mitosis. In addition, the genetic material must be divided in such a way that no new cell is missing any DNA, or has more DNA than the original cell.

*Whatever amount of DNA the original cell has prior to mitosis,
its offspring cells will have the same amount after the process is complete.*

1. When the process of mitosis is used for organism reproduction, are the new organisms exact genetic duplicates of the parent organism?

2. If organisms use mitosis for reproduction, would their offspring exhibit *sameness* or *variety*?

3. If asexual reproduction produces identical offspring, then how does such an organism "change" over time?

4. What would be the *advantage* of reproducing asexually?

5. What would be the *disadvantage* of reproducing asexually?

6. Starting with the *haploid* cell below, draw the next *three* generations of that cell as it reproduces.

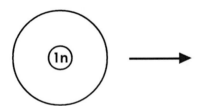

7. Starting with the *diploid* cell below, draw the next *three* generations of that cell as it reproduces.

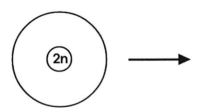

ACTIVITY #4

"CHROMOSOME MOVEMENT DURING MITOSIS"

Chromosomes move during mitosis. They replicate themselves (see Activity #1), and the copies separate, allowing two cells to be created from one. This movement of DNA material in the form of chromosomes (coiled DNA) has several "phases," which are described in this Activity.

| GO GET | 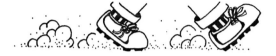 |

1. One red and one yellow crayon.

2. A package of chromosome beads. Each package should contain 8 chromosomes.

NOW

The human has 46 chromosomes (23 homologous pairs). We will follow the movements of 4 chromosomes (2 homologous pairs) as an example of what all the chromosomes are doing during mitosis.

Start with 4 of the chromosomes from your package. This is how a cell would look *prior* to duplicating its genetic material and undergoing the process of mitosis:

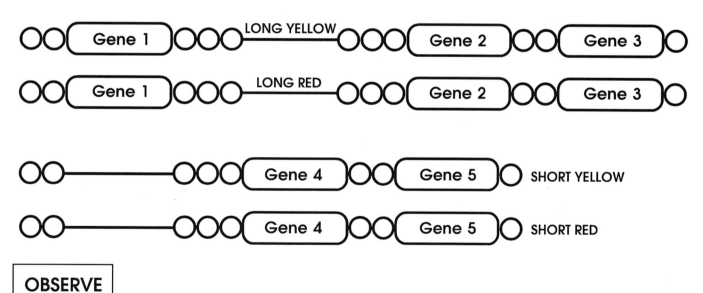

OBSERVE

1. The two short chromosomes represent *one* homologous pair, and the two long chromosomes represent *another* homologous pair. The *red* set represents the chromosomes from your mother, and the *yellow* set is the chromosomes from your father.

2. Color the chromosome beads above with your crayons, and as you go through this Activity, use the crayons to help you keep track of the chromosomes that came from your father and from your mother.

3. The bead chromsomes are labeled A[1], A[2], B[1], and B[2] in the next section.

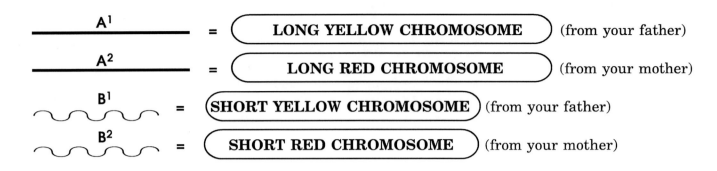

A[1]	= LONG YELLOW CHROMOSOME	(from your father)
A[2]	= LONG RED CHROMOSOME	(from your mother)
B[1]	= SHORT YELLOW CHROMOSOME	(from your father)
B[2]	= SHORT RED CHROMOSOME	(from your mother)

PHASES OF MITOSIS

Biologists sometimes describe mitosis as having several phases. Ask your instructor if you are required to memorize the names of the phases. If so, remember the phrase: **P**ay **M**e **A**ny **T**ime. This will help you to remember the sequence of phases in mitosis.

Pay attention to the different events as they occur in each phase, and mimic the phases by using your bead chromosomes. Interphase is usually considered to be the stage *before* mitosis actually begins. We include it as part of the mitosis discussion, but your textbook will say that mitosis begins with prophase.

1. **Early Interphase:** Although we have diagramed the DNA as long, thin chromosomes, in reality it is not coiled up yet, and is *not* visible as chromosomes until **prophase**. However, it is best to label the DNA at this stage so that we can remember what the parent cell starts with.

2. **Later Interphase:** Each DNA molecule has duplicated itself.

   We have diagramed these "doubled" DNA molecules as though we could see them. Actually, DNA is still in the long, thread-like form.

   Duplicate your beads now, using the other four bead chromosomes from the package.

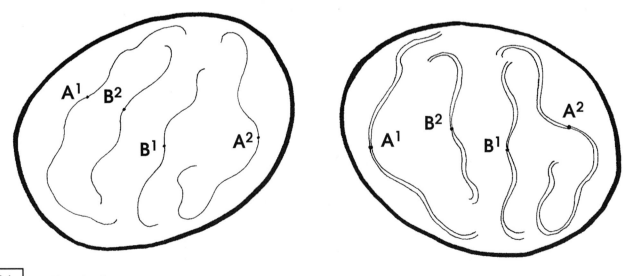

3. **Prophase:** This is when the DNA coils up and the chromosomes are now *visible* under the microscope.

   Each chromosome is now doubled, and consists of two absolutely *identical* "chromatids." (A **chromatid** is the name for one of the duplicated DNA molecules that has coiled itself into a chromosome form and is attached to the other chromatid.)

4. **Metaphase:** The chromosomes (each consisting of two chromatids) line up end to end, in random order, along the *midline* of the cell. Spindle fibers have formed and are attached to the chromosomes. You will have to imagine fine threads attached to your beads.

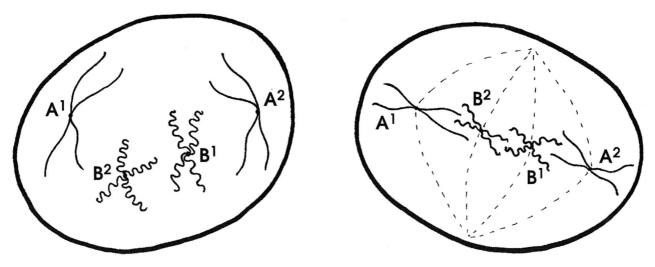

5. **Anaphase:** The spindle fibers pull the duplicated chromatids apart and move them to opposite ends (poles) of the cell.

6. **Telophase:** Chromosomes are at opposite ends of the cell, and the cell divides into two cells.

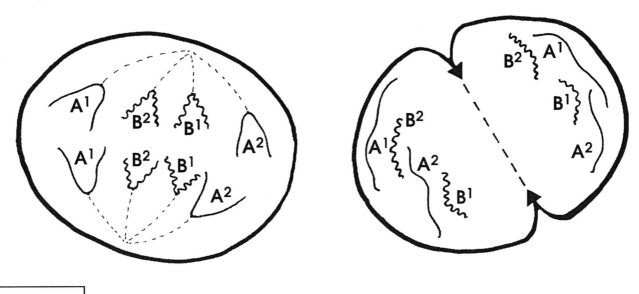

OBSERVE

Notice that you started with a cell having two sets of chromosomes, and you ended with two cells, each having two sets of chromosomes.

1. Are the two groups of chromosomes at *telophase* identical to the group of chromosomes you started with in *interphase* prior to DNA duplication?

2. Are the new cells identical to the original cells?

3. What is the name for this cell division process?

4. What kind of reproduction is it?

5. Is mitosis going on in your body right now?

    What kind of cells are you producing by this process?

6. Name two processes during which your body must reproduce cells by *mitosis*.

    a.

    b.

7. What do you think might be going on as you age (get wrinkles, grey hair, lose your hair, etc.)?

ACTIVITY #5

"ONION ROOT TIP"

It's time to review what you learned in Activity #4.

You will use a microscope to find the various phases of mitosis (cell division) in the root tip of an onion. Put on your investigator's hat and search for the "clues" that reveal each phase.

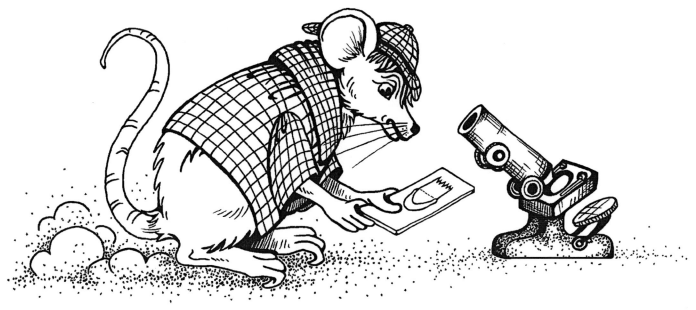

GO GET

1. A compound microscope.

2. A prepared slide of an onion root tip.

NOW

1. Under low power, notice that the root tip is covered by a root cap (like a thimble over your finger). Behind the root cap is an area of square-shaped cells that are undergoing cell division.

2. Look at this area under the high power (430x). If the cells are *rectangular,* then you are in the wrong place.

3. *Find every stage of mitosis.*

Onion Root Tip

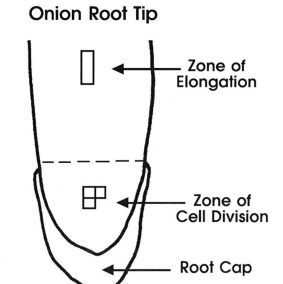

Zone of Elongation

Zone of Cell Division

Root Cap

4. Draw a simple sketch of what you see at each phase of mitosis.

Interphase*

Prophase

Metaphase

Anaphase

Telophase

* Interphase will look like a stained nucleus. You won't be able to see the DNA threads.

5. Optional: (Ask your instructor if you are to do this experiment.) There is a way that you can estimate the relative amount of time that a cell spends in each phase of the cell cycle. Count all of the cells in the zone of cell division and record how many of them are in each phase. Then figure what percent each stage is of the total. This is an indication of the relative time a cell spends in each stage of cell division. Does this make sense to you? Do it; it will.

Phase	# of Cells in Phase	% of Total Cells
Interphase		
Prophase		
Metaphase		
Anaphase		
Telephase		

ACTIVITY #6

"SEXUAL REPRODUCTION"

Sexual reproduction is the process of creating *variety* in the offspring of a species. It consists of two parts: *meiosis* and *fertilization*.

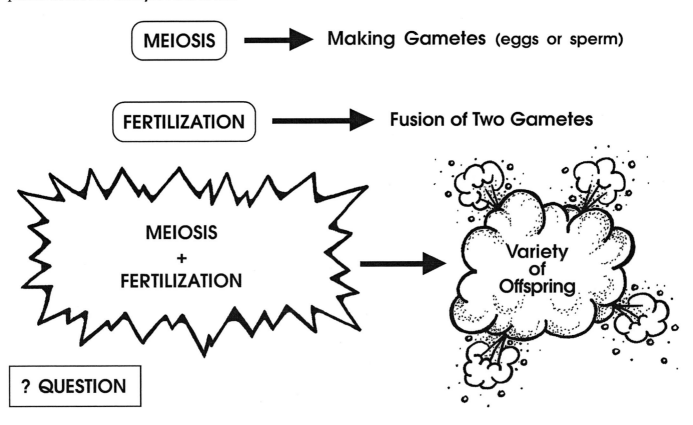

MEIOSIS ⟶ Making Gametes (eggs or sperm)

FERTILIZATION ⟶ Fusion of Two Gametes

MEIOSIS + FERTILIZATION ⟶ Variety of Offspring

? QUESTION

1. What is the advantage of producing variety in offspring?

2. What is the disadvantage of producing variety in offspring?

SET CHANGES DURING MEIOSIS AND FERTILIZATION

Review Activity #2 if you have forgotten what a "set" is.

MEIOSIS

Meiosis starts with a single *diploid* cell and ends with four *haploid* cells.

The original cell has two sets (2n) of DNA molecules which are then duplicated. After DNA duplication, the original cell divides *twice*, producing *four* cells—each with a *single* set (1n) of DNA molecules (chromosomes).

The four cells are haploid. Their chromosomes have been mixed in such a way as to produce *genetic variety*. We will present some of the details of that process in Activity #7.

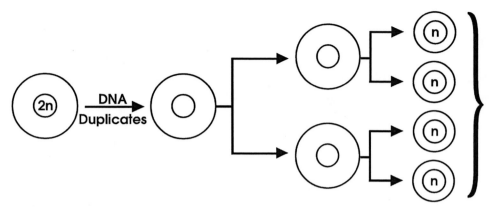

NOTE:

1. Reduction to one set.

2. Products are variable.

The product cells of meiosis are called **gametes**, and these can fuse with gametes from another organism of the same species to begin the next generation.

FERTILIZATION

Fertilization is the fusion of *two haploid gametes*. It results in the chromosome set number returning to 2n. This allows the next generation of the species to have the same "set" number of chromosomes as the parent generation.

Gametes:
the end
product of
meiosis

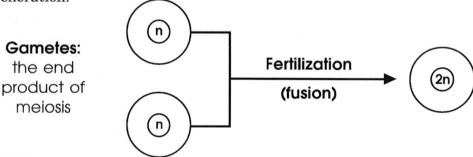

? QUESTION

1. What type of cell division reduces the set number? _____

2. What process takes this reduced set number and returns it to match the original set number of the parent cell? _____

3. How many *sets* of chromosomes are in a human sperm? _____

4. How many *chromosomes* are in a human sperm? _____

5. How many *sets* of chromosomes are in a human egg? _____

6. How many *chromosomes* are in a human egg? _____

7. When a human egg and sperm fuse, how many *sets* of chromosomes are there? _____

8. When a human egg and sperm fuse, how many *chromosomes* are there? _____

ACTIVITY #7

"THE EVENTS THAT CREATE VARIETY"

The essence of meiosis is the production of haploid cells from diploid cells. The essence of fertilization is the recombination of two haploid gametes to produce the next diploid generation. During meiosis and fertilization there are *three* events that create *genetic variety* in the next generation: ***crossing-over, independent assortment,*** and ***random fusion of gametes***.

None of these genetic variety events would be possible without a very special process during meiosis called ***synapsis***. This is the single most critical event that makes meiosis so different from mitosis.

SYNAPSIS

Synapsis is defined as the "pairing up" process of *homologous pairs* early in meiosis.

Let's illustrate the differences between mitosis and meiosis using the same chromosomes from our earlier mitosis diagrams.

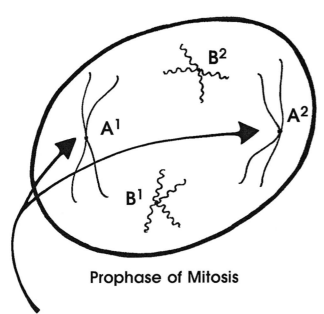

Prophase of Mitosis

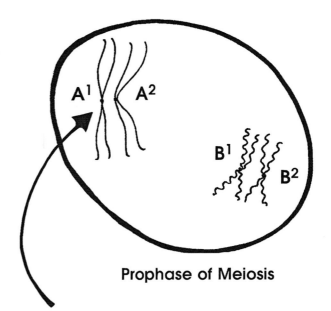

Prophase of Meiosis

Notice that the two members of the "A" homologous pair have duplicated themselves, and they will be moved around the cell *separately* from each other.

Notice that the two members of the "A" homologous pair have duplicated and they have "paired up" *(synapsis)*. This paired grouping is called a ***tetrad*** (meaning four chromatids) and they will be moved around the cell *together*.

1. The two "A" chromosomes are concerned with the same traits and are called _____ pairs.

2. Are the chromatids of the "A^1" chromosomes identical or different? _____

3. Are the chromosomes "A^1" and "A^2" absolutely identical? _____

4. Are the "A" and "B" chromosomes homologous pairs? _____

5. In meiosis, do the "A" and "B" chromosomes pair up with each other (synapse)? _____

CROSSING-OVER

Crossing-over is the exchange of DNA between the four chromosomes (chromatids) of a *tetrad*.

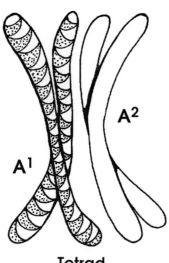

Tetrad

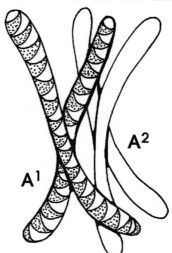

Tetrad Crossing-Over

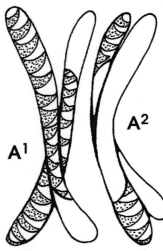

Exchanged DNA from Crossing-Over

If you consider that a single chromosome may carry a thousand or more genes, then these small cross-over exchanges are capable of creating hundreds of mixtures of chromosomes. Remember, you received one of the homologous chromosomes of a pair (A^2) from your mother and the other (A^1) from your father. The process of crossing-over makes "*new mixes*" of those chromosomes.

? QUESTION

1. What event during meiosis prophase (as opposed to mitosis prophase) makes it possible for crossing-over to occur?

2. As a result of crossing-over, will the "A" chromosome that you pass on to your children be your mother's, your father's, or will it be a mixture of your mother's and father's?

INDEPENDENT ASSORTMENT

During meiosis the tetrads formed by synapsis move around the cell and divide in different ways than we saw in mitosis.

The simplest description of the difference is:

1. the tetrads line up in the middle of the cell (during metaphase), and
2. the cell divides twice, separating the tetrads first into pairs of chromatids and then into single chromosomes, resulting in *four separate cells*.

Each of these cells contains only *one of each kind of chromosome*. They are haploid.

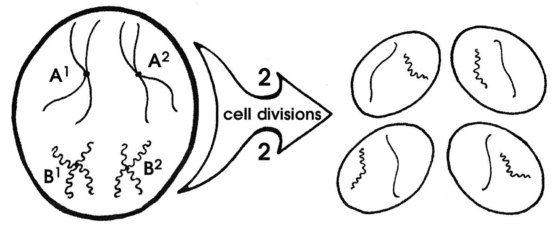

However, there is a very important detail called *independent assortment* that occurs during the chromosome separations of meiosis. Notice that the tetrads are drawn so that the A^1 and B^1 chromosomes are placed on the left side of the cell, and the A^2 and B^2 chromosomes are lined up on the right.

If the tetrads separated equally as drawn here you would see only two kinds of gametes from this process containing the following chromosomes:

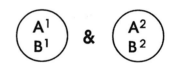

But, if the top tetrad had originally lined up during metaphase with the A^1 chromosomes on the right, then A^2 would have moved with B^1 into a gamete, and A^1 would have moved with B^2 into a gamete as pictured here:

This production of gametes containing different combinations of chromosomes is called ***independent assortment*** because one pair of homologous chromosomes is separated (segregated) into individual gametes independently of how another pair is separated. (A^1 and A^2 have been separated independently of how B^1 and B^2 have been separated.)

IMPORTANT MESSAGE

Remember: Every gamete gets a complete set of chromosomes with only one A chromosome and only one B chromosome.

1. How many *genetically different* gametes were produced in the independent assortment of these two homologous pairs?

2. The human contains 23 pairs of homologous chromosomes, all of which are independently assorted. What do you think the chance would be that one of your gametes would contain either all your mother's or all your father's chromosomes?

RANDOM FUSION OF GAMETES

Two mating individuals have the same kinds and same number of chromosomes, but those chromosomes are *not exactly* identical. Because individuals possess different variations of genes, the ***random fusion of gametes*** (fertilization) from any two individuals will result in more genetic variety in the offspring. Through fertilization the diploid set number is recreated with the offspring receiving one chromosome of a homologous pair from one parent, and the other chromosome of the pair from the other parent.

? QUESTION

To keep the example relatively simple, let's consider only one of the homologous pairs of the human—the A chromosome. (Actually, human chromosomes are referred to by numbers from 1 to 23.)

1. Where did chromosome A^2 come from?

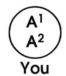

A^1 came from your father

You

2. Where did chromosome A^4 come from?

3. What are your possible gametes?

A^3 came from your mate's father

Your Mate

4. What are your mate's possible gametes?

5. Determine the four possible combinations of your gametes with your mate's gametes. In other words, what genetic variety can we expect in your offspring?

6. Are any of the offspring identical to either parent?

7. What are the three events during *sexual reproduction* that prevent identical children?

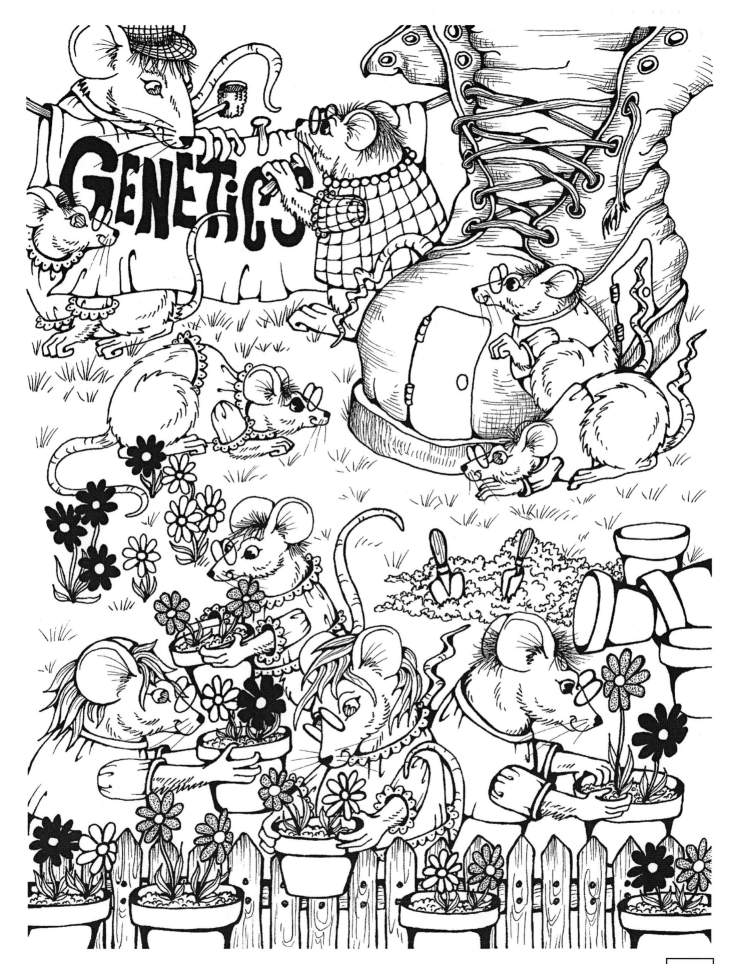

DYNAMIC DEVELOPMENTS
AND
FASCINATING FACTS
IN BIOLOGY

In a single human cell there are between 10,000 and 100,000 genes. If all the instructions contained in all these genes were written down as words, they would fill the equivalent of 10,000 volumes of the Encyclopaedia Britannica.

—HTTP://WWW.SKYGAZE.COM/CONTENT/FACTS/BIOLOGY.SHTML

It is possible to be your own twin. Human *chimeras* have two genetically distinct types of cells. Most are "blood chimeras"—non-identical twins who shared a blood supply in the uterus. Those who are not twins have blood cells from a twin that died early in gestation. About 8% of non-identical twin pairs are chimeras. Many more people are *microchimeras* and carry smaller numbers of foreign blood cells that may have passed from mother across the placenta, or persist from a blood transfusion.

—HTTP://WWW.VIVO.COLOSTATE.EDU/HBOOKS/GENETICS/MEDGEN/CHROMO/MOSAICS.HTML
—HTTP://WWW.MEDTERMS.COM/SCRIPT/MAIN/ART.ASP?ARTICLEKEY=8905

Once considered to be the exclusive carrier of heredity, DNA is influenced by life experiences. *Epigenetics* is the study of environmental influences on gene expression. Events like smoking before puberty, alcoholism, malnutrition, and a high-stress pregnancy can trigger cellular changes that transmit to future generations.

—*EPIGENETICS: THE ULTIMATE MYSTERY OF INHERITANCE* BY RICHARD C. FRANCIS

Sequences of DNA at the ends of chromosomes called *telomeres* get shorter every time the cell divides. When the telomeres get too short, the cell dies. Research in longevity has discovered that adding *telomerase*—an enzyme that appends DNA to telomeres—prolongs cell life, and therefore the lifespan of the animal. One drawback to be worked out: Cancer cells have an enhanced affinity for telomerase and multiply with abandon in its presence.

—ARMANIOS, MARY, ET AL, "SHORT TELOMERES ARE SUFFICIENT TO CAUSE
THE DEGENERATIVE DEFECTS ASSOCIATED WITH AGING,"
AMERICAN JOURNAL OF HUMAN GENETICS,
DECEMBER 11, 2009; 85(6):823832

GENETICS

INTRODUCTION

More than a hundred years ago Gregor Mendel discovered that hereditary particles are passed from parent to offspring during the reproductive process. These particles were later named *genes,* and the science of studying inheritance was called *genetics*.

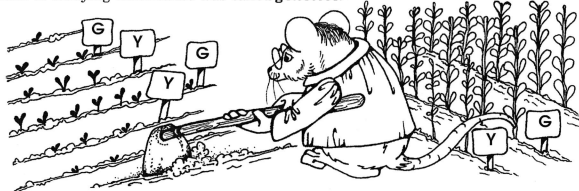

Genes can be traced backwards to the very origin of life about 4 billion years ago. When we do so, we find that all traits were new at some point in time, and that a gene's success is determined by natural selection. However, genes do not last forever. And most have already gone extinct.

The investigation into the mechanics of inheritance—the mixing, the passing on, and the function of genes—is one of the greatest scientific puzzles of the 21st century. Understanding genetics has led to the prevention and curing of numerous hereditary diseases. It has substantiated the principle of evolution by natural selection, and has helped human beings to realize their place in Nature's Family Tree.

As a contemporary student, you should note that your individuality is not the result of possessing a trait that no other individual has, but is a result of a particular *combination* of genes. These genes came from your parents and their ancestors before them.

This lab will explore some of the basic principles of genetics, introduce you to basic terminology, and help you apply genetic rules to some hypothetical problems.

ACTIVITIES

ACTIVITY #1

"BASIC TERMINOLOGY"

In order to understand the mechanics of inheritance, we must understand the terminology used to describe this very complex process.

GENES AND CHROMOSOMES

A *gene* is a segment of the DNA molecule and is responsible for manufacturing a protein that either becomes part of the organism's structure or becomes an enzyme that controls biochemical events.

Every organism has a certain number of chromosomes—the exact number depends on the species— and each chromosome is made of many genes. DNA coils up into the form of a chromosome during cell division, and a gene becomes a distinct particle on that chromosome. *Remember:* Chromosomes and DNA molecules are basically the same thing.

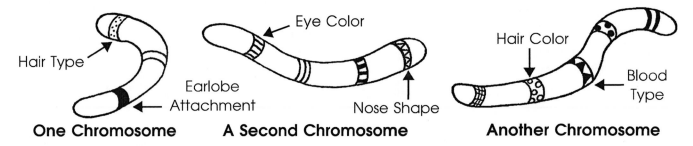

| One Chromosome | A Second Chromosome | Another Chromosome |

Genes can be described by their exact location on a chromosome. The process of locating genes is called *mapping.* The location of a gene is its *locus,* and geneticists go through great efforts to pinpoint these locations. Knowing where a gene is found on the chromosome is what allows scientists to do genetic research.

? QUESTION

1. The particles that control inherited traits are called _____.

2. These particles are segments of _____ , and are responsible for manufacturing a _____ that becomes either _____ or _____.

3. Every living thing on the planet has the same number of chromosomes. _____ (T or F) Explain your answer.

4. Every chromosome has the same identical genes as every other chromosome. _____ (T or F) Explain your answer.

5. The place where you find a particular gene on a chromosome is called the _____.

HOMOLOGOUS CHROMOSOMES

We have discussed homologous chromosomes before. This idea is essential to the understanding of genetics, so we will review it again.

INFORMATION

1. Very simple organisms have only one set of chromosomes and they are *haploid*.

2. More complex organisms have two sets of chromosomes and are *diploid*.

3. Haploid organisms have one of each kind of chromosome and one of every kind of gene.

4. Diploid organisms have two of each kind of chromosome and two of every kind of gene.

5. The two chromosomes of each kind are called **homologous chromosomes** because they are carrying the same kind of traits (genes). *Homo* means "same."

6. A human has 23 different kinds of chromosomes that are given numbers from 1 to 23. Because we are diploid organisms we have two of each of the different kinds. So, we have 46 chromosomes in all, made up of 23 *homologous pairs*.

? QUESTION

1. How many sets of DNA molecules or chromosomes does a diploid organism have? _____

2. How many sets of DNA molecules or chromosomes does a haploid organism have? _____

3. Humans are _____. (haploid or diploid)

4. How many homologous pairs of chromosomes does a human have? _____

5. Because chromosomes occur in pairs in a diploid organism, how many genes for one trait would a diploid organism possess? _____

6. How many genes for a trait would a haploid organism possess? _____ Why?

ALLELES: THE VARIOUS FORMS OF A GENE

Humans are diploid, and they have two copies of every kind of gene. One of the purposes of genetics is to figure out which form (variation) of these two genes you have, and what expression of those genes you can expect.

The *alternate forms* of a particular gene are called **alleles**. For example, there are three alternate forms—three alleles—for blood type: A, B, and O.

The reason all species have various alleles (forms of genes) is that *mutation* events change the structure of genes.

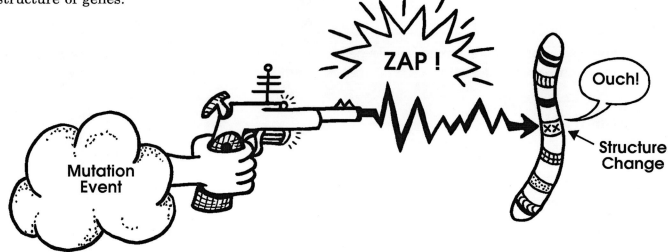

A gene can be mutated (changed) by radiation, chemicals in the environment, or other spontaneous events that are surprisingly common on this planet. There may have been a time when all the genes for eye color were identical and resulted in brown eyes. But over time, mutations occurred and changed the DNA of this eye color gene, creating a new "allele" (variation) for the eye color trait. Perhaps this new allele was for blue eyes.

Alleles are always for the same trait, and are located at the exact *same* spot on homologous chromosomes. (This is how we know that they are truly alleles of each other, and not different genes.) *Remember:* Alleles are variations of the same gene!

? QUESTION

1. What is an allele?

2. Where are alleles located?

3. What process creates the various alleles in a species? Explain how.

4. Which of the following genes (1 through 9) are alleles?

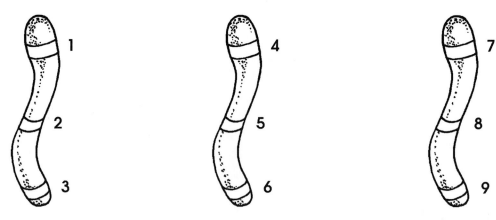

Chromosome #3   Chromosome #7   Another Chromosome #3

GENOTYPE

A *genotype* is the description of the alleles an individual possesses for a particular trait. Observe the following situation where there are two different alleles for a particular trait.

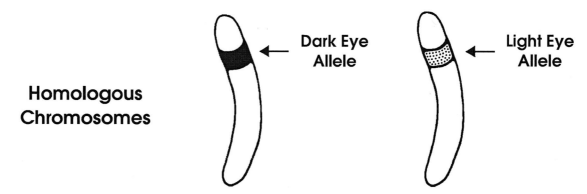

Homologous Chromosomes

Dark Eye Allele

Light Eye Allele

Note: Even though the two genes look different, they are alleles because they are at the *same locus* on homologous chromosomes.

NOW

1. Study the chromosomes above. Draw and label the three combinations of eye color alleles that are possible in individuals of the same species.

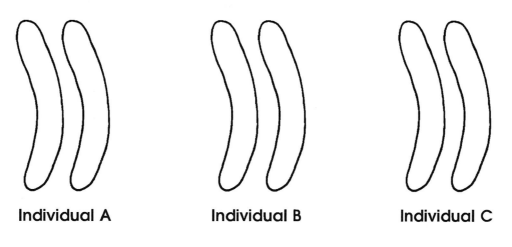

Individual A   Individual B   Individual C

_____   _____   _____

2. If an organism has *two identical alleles*, we say that it is *homozygous* for that trait (meaning the "same" two alleles).

3. If an organism has *two different alleles*, we say that it is *heterozygous* for that trait (meaning "different" alleles).

4. Go back to the diagram of the three individuals above and label each as to whether it is *homozygous* or *heterozygous*.

PHENOTYPE

The physical expression of the alleles—what an organism looks like—is termed the *phenotype*. Because there are different possible combinations of alleles (genotypes), there are alternative possible phenotypes for a trait that can be expressed in a population.

NOW

Draw this survey chart on the chalkboard, and record your phenotype for each of the six traits. After everyone in the class has recorded their phenotypes, write the class totals on the chart below. Your instructor will tell you the genotypes of these traits at the end of the next Activity.

Trait	Class Phenotype Totals		
Eye Color	*Dark # _____		Light # _____
Earlobes	Attached # _____		Unattached # _____
PTC Paper	Can taste # _____		Cannot taste # _____
Hairline	Widow's peak # _____		Straight across forehead # _____
Hair Type	Straight # _____	Wavy # _____	Curly # _____
Fingers	Five # _____		Six # _____
Little Finger	Bent # _____		Straight # _____
Tongue	Roller # _____		Non-Roller # _____
Long Palmer Muscle	Present # _____		Absent # _____

* Dark is considered to be black, brown, hazel, green, or grey.

INFORMATION

1. The phenotype is the description of the physical expression of a trait (brown eyes), whereas the genotype is the description of the exact combination of alleles (for example, 1 allele for brown eyes + 1 allele for blue eyes).

2. The genotype results from the combination of genes you inherited from your parents.

3. The phenotype results from the physical expression of the genes in the genotype, and also may be influenced by the organism's environment. In some cases there may be only two phenotypes for a trait, and in other cases there are *more than two* phenotypes for a trait.

ACTIVITY #2

"SOME RULES OF GENETICS"

*Nine times out of ten, in the arts as in life,
there is actually nothing to be discovered;
there is only error to be exposed.*

—H. L. Mencken
American editor and critic (1880–1956)

RULE OF THE GENE

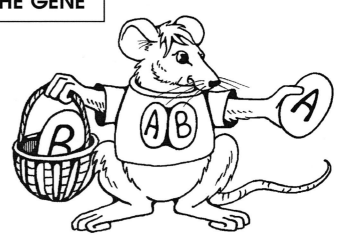

The parent must possess the gene in order to pass it on.

The source of all genes in the offspring is the parents. Always look to the parents to figure out what genes the sperm or egg can possibly carry, and remember that a parent does not possess all of the genes found within a reproducing population of a species.

? QUESTION

1. How many different *alleles* for a single trait can a homozygous parent pass on? _____

2. How many different *alleles* for a single trait can a heterozygous parent pass on? _____

RULE OF SEGREGATION

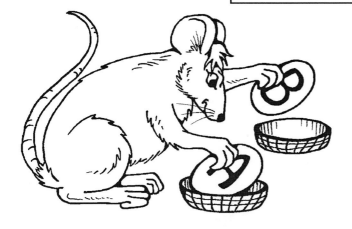

Only one gene of the two alleles that you have is put into each gamete that you make.

Alleles are located on homologous chromosomes, and since homologous chromosomes are segregated during meiosis, the genes are also segregated.

Numerous gametes are formed during gamete production, and if the alleles are different (heterozygous), 50% of the gametes will carry one gene and 50% of the gametes will carry the other.

When alleles are the same (homozygous), 100% of the gametes will carry the same allele.

1. A parent possesses two copies of each gene. When this parent passes on its alleles for a gene, how many does it contribute to each of the offspring? _____

2. How many copies of a gene does the other parent contribute to each offspring? _____

3. How many copies of each gene for the trait does each offspring receive? _____

RULE OF DOMINANT AND RECESSIVE ALLELES

Some alleles control the phenotype even if they are paired with a different allele.

An obvious example is the dark eye allele that will create the dark eye phenotype in an individual even if the allele for light eyes is present.

If two different alleles are together in an organism, and only one phenotype is expressed, then the allele that is expressed is called *dominant*.

The other allele that is "hidden" is called *recessive*.

? QUESTION

1. Can the individual carry an allele that is not expressed? Explain.

2. What word is used to describe the *genotype* condition where there are two different alleles together in the same organism? _____

3. What word is used to describe the *genotype* condition where there are two of the same alleles together in the same organism? _____

INFORMATION

Since dominance and recessiveness have intricate biochemical explanations, the only way of determining dominance is to cross two individuals that are homozygous (pure) for the two different phenotypes. This produces the heterozygous condition. Whichever phenotype is exclusively expressed is said to be the *dominant phenotype*.

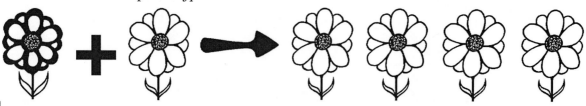

1. A homozygous blue-eyed mouse with short whiskers mates with a homozygous brown-eyed mouse with long whiskers. All of their offspring have brown eyes and short whiskers. Which alleles are dominant?

2. A homozygous five-clawed cat is crossed with a homozygous six-clawed cat and all of the kittens have six claws. Which allele is dominant?

3. In humans, the five-fingered condition is *recessive* to the six-fingered condition. Yet, most people have five fingers. Explain how this can happen.

IMPORTANT MESSAGE

Ask your instructor which alleles are dominant in the class Phenotype Chart. It is a common *mistake* to assume that the allele found most frequently is always the dominant allele. *Natural selection* determines the success of an allele.

RULE OF INCOMPLETE DOMINANCE

When two different pure-breeding strains are crossed, and their offspring show a blending of phenotypes, then neither allele is dominant.

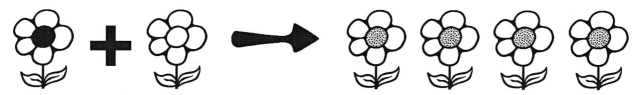

This is easily recognized when the phenotype is somewhere between two extremes. Counting the parents, there are *three* phenotypes (*black, white, grey*) being expressed in these flowers instead of only two, and that third phenotype is *intermediate* between the other two. This heterozygous condition is called *incomplete dominance*.

? QUESTION

1. On the chart you did earlier, which of the three hair types (wavy, curly, or straight) represents incomplete dominance—the *blended* heterozygous condition? _____

2. You cross a herd of red cattle with white cattle and all of the calves appear to be roan (reddish white). Is this an example of incomplete dominance? _____ How do you know?

3. You cross a blue flowering pea plant with a white flowering pea plant and all of the offspring are blue flowered. Is this an example of incomplete dominance? _____ How do you know?

ACTIVITY #3

"HOW TO SOLVE GENETIC PROBLEMS"

USING LETTERS FOR ALLELES

For convenience, the genes of an allele pair are usually symbolized by a letter from the alphabet. A *large* letter is used for the dominant trait and a *small* letter for the recessive trait. When we want to describe the *genotype* of an organism, we use both letters to represent the alleles inherited from the parents.

For example, free earlobes is a dominant allele and attached earlobes is recessive. You would use a capital "**F**" to indicate the dominant allele and a small "**f**" to indicate the recessive allele in describing an individual.

? QUESTION

1. Write the three genotypes for earlobe attachment as it applies to the following individuals.

    a. Heterozygous _____ _____

    b. Homozygous Dominant _____ _____

    c. Homozygous Recessive _____ _____

2. When it comes to symbolizing incomplete dominance with letters, it is best to use the letter "**C**" for one allele and "**C'**" for the other allele.

    List the three possible genotypes for hair type.

    a. Curly _____ _____

    b. Wavy _____ _____   Why not use a small letter "**c**" for the heterozygous genotype?

    c. Straight _____ _____

USING THE PUNNETT SQUARE

The ***Punnett Square*** is a method of predicting the probable outcome of genetic crosses.

| STEP 1 | Draw a square like this:

Put the gametes of one parent here.

Put the gametes of the other parent here.

STEP 2 | Determine what kinds of gametes are made by each parent in the cross, and put those gametes into the boxes of the Punnett Square.

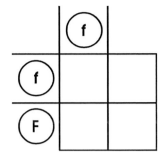

If your mate is heterozygous (Ff), then those gametes are (F) and (f).

For example, if you are homozygous recessive for attached earlobes (ff), then all of your gametes are (f).

STEP 3 | Fill in the offspring boxes of the Punnett Square.

In this example there are only two possible offspring genotypes. The Punnett Square tells us to expect about 50% ff and 50% Ff.

Sometimes the Punnett Square is more complex than this and you must figure out more than one trait at a time. Nevertheless, you use the same basic method.

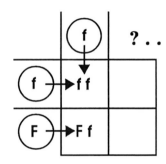

? . . . Why is it unnecessary to fill in this box with another small (f)?

NOW

Make up your own genotype example and work out the crosses.

1. Traits:

2. Symbols:

3. Male Genotype:

4. Female Genotype:

5. Offspring Genotypes:

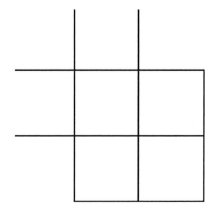

Punnett Square

ACTITITY #4

"GENETIC PROBLEMS"

CASES OF COMPLETE DOMINANCE

1. Gregor Mendel grew different varieties of pea plants in his garden. When he crossed yellow-seed plants with green-seed plants, he always got yellow pea seeds.

   a. What is the dominant allele?

   b. What is the genotype of all green-seed plants?

   c. Use the Punnett Square to show Mendel's cross.

   d. Do the parent yellow-seed plants have the same genotype as the offspring yellow-seed pea plant?

   Parent: _____ Offspring: _____

   e. What genetic fact do you know about any yellow-seed pea plant?

   f. If yellow-seed pea plants are dominant to green-seed pea plants, why are there mostly green pea seeds in nature?

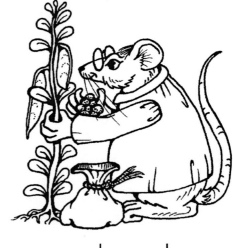

2. A dark-eyed man mates with a light-eyed woman and they have ten dark-eyed children.

   a. What is the dominant allele?

   b. What is the genotype of all light-eyed people?

   _____

   c. What are the genotypes of the two parents?

   _____ and _____

   d. What is the genotype difference between the dark-eyed parent and the dark-eyed offspring?

   Parent: _____ Offspring: _____

   e. When two heterozygous dark-eyed people (Dd) are crossed, what is the *phenotype* ratio of dark-eyed offspring to light-eyed offspring? (Use the Punnett Square to get your answer.)

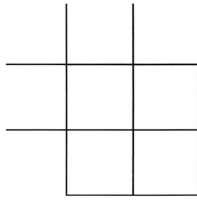

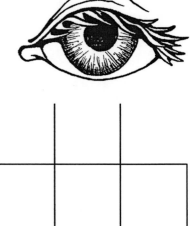

A SPECIAL NOTE ON EYE COLOR

Eye color is probably due to multiple alleles and more than one gene pair. The numerous phenotypes are determined by genes that control both the *amount* and the *distribution* of a dark pigment called *melanin*. Except for albinos, everyone has some eye pigmentation.

Eye color is determined mainly by the location of melanin in the iris of the eye. Concentrated melanin particles appear as brown; dilute melanin particles appear as yellow or yellow-brown.

VARIOUS EYE COLORS

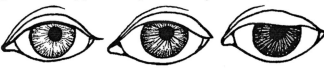

Blue: no melanin in the front part of the iris. The color is due to minimal amounts of melanin in the rear of the iris with the clear front portion scattering the light reflected off the melanin. This scattering is greatest in the blue spectrum giving the iris its blue color.

Grey: the same as blue, but with a slight amount of melanin in the front of the iris which tones down, or greys, the blue reflected from behind.

Green: a bit more melanin particles scattered in the front part of the iris create yellow. Blended with the light blue from the rear of the iris, it produces an overall green color.

Hazel: even more melanin particles in the front of the iris give a slight brown color, and dilute melanin particles scattered throughout the iris add some yellow.

Brown: melanin particles in the front part of the iris and throughout the iris. The amount of melanin varies, leading to gradations of brown color in the eye.

Black: large amounts of melanin in the front and throughout the iris.

TEST CROSS TO CHECK GENOTYPE

If an organism shows the dominant phenotype, then one of its genes has to be the dominant allele, but you cannot be sure of the identity of the other allele unless you do a **test cross** to see if the dominant parent breeds pure. Let's pretend that you are in the dog-breeding business. You know that long hair on a "pooch hound" is a dominant allele and short hair is recessive. You purchase a male long-haired "pooch hound." How do you figure out if your male "pooch hound" is homozygous or heterozygous for long hair? Which genotype of female should you breed him to?

If a proper test cross is used, what phenotypes of puppies would you see if your male dog is heterozygous dominant? _____

What puppy phenotypes would you see if your male dog is homozygous dominant? _____ Complete the Punnett Square to show the test cross that would convince someone that your "pooch hound" is homozygous for long hair.

Male Genotype: _____ Female Genotype: _____

CASES OF INCOMPLETE DOMINANCE

1. When a straight-haired mouse is crossed with a curly-haired mouse, the result is always wavy hair. Two wavy-haired mice cross.

   a. What are the genotypes of the two wavy-haired mice? _____

   b. Draw the Punnett Square of a cross between two wavy-haired mice, and show the probable genotypes of their offspring.

   c. What is the expected *phenotype* ratio of the offspring?

   _____ %   _____ %   _____ %

   d. What is the expected *genotype* ratio of the offspring?

2. Red orchids with straight petals are crossed with white orchids with curly petals. The results are pink orchids with wavy petals.

   a. What are the genotypes of the two parent orchid plants? *Remember:* You are dealing with *two different* traits.

      First parent: ___ ___   ___ ___
                    (color)   (shape)

      Second parent: ___ ___   ___ ___

   b. What is the genotype of the offspring orchids?

      Offspring: ___ ___   ___ ___

ACTIVITY #5

"SEX-LINKED TRAITS"

SEX DETERMINATION

Humans have 23 homologous pairs of chromosomes. Twenty-two of these pairs are named using the numbers 1 through 22. The 23rd pair is individually labeled with the letters "*X*" and "*Y*" for males, and "*X*" and "*X*" for females. These labels distinguish them as the *sex chromosomes*.

During meiosis in the male two types of sperm are produced: those carrying the X and those carrying the Y chromosome. Females produce eggs carrying only the X chromosome.

If a Y chromosome is present in the cells of an embryo, then the child becomes a male. If the Y is not present, the child becomes a female. It is the presence or absence of the Y chromosome that determines the sex of a child!

This means that a male child receives a Y chromosome from his father and an X chromosome from his mother. A female child receives an X chromosome from her father and the other X chromosome from her mother.

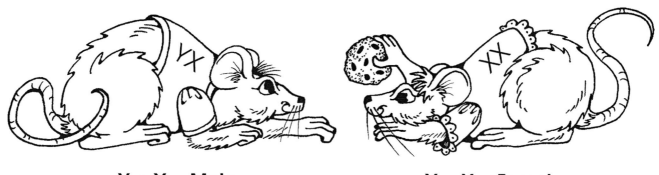

Y + X = Male   X + X = Female

? QUESTION

Draw a Punnett Square to show a cross of X and Y chromosomes in the fertilization of male and female gametes.

The offspring boxes should reveal why we have about a 50% male to 50% female ratio within the human population.

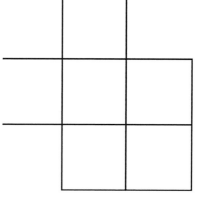

SEX-LINKAGE

The X and Y chromosomes are not exactly identical, and we should expect that there would be differences in how each of them carries genes. These differences are expressed in the unequal frequencies of phenotypes in the male and female offspring.

If any phenotype is distributed *unequally* between male and female offspring, and those differences are due to X and Y chromosome differences, then we call those traits *sex-linked*. Actually, "sex-linked" means that the gene is carried on the X chromosome and not on the Y chromosome. We call these genes *X-linked*. It is easier to understand sex-linkage by looking at the sex chromosomes.

The 23rd Pair of Chromosomes

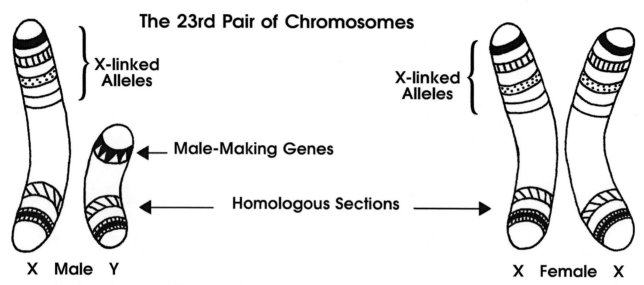

Two genetic situations are illustrated above.

First: There is a homologous section of the X and Y chromosomes that is the same, and there will be no differences in phenotype between male and female children.

Second: Notice that the Y chromosome is very short. We would expect it to lack some of the genes that are carried on the X chromosome. There is an X-linked section on the X chromosome that carries genes that are *missing* from the Y chromosome.

? QUESTION

1. How many copies of an X-linked gene does a male have? _____

2. Will a male be able to give X-linked genes to his daughter? _____ Explain.

3. Will a male be able to give his X-linked genes to his son? _____ Why or Why not?

4. How many copies of an X-linked gene does a female have? _____

5. A male child gets X-linked genes from which of his parents? _____

6. A female child gets X-linked genes from which of her parents? _____

7. If a father is carrying an X-linked allele, then how many of his sons will get that allele? _____

   How many of his daughters will get that allele? _____

8. If a mother has a defective X-linked allele on one of her chromosomes and the other chromosome is normal, then how many of her sons will get that defective allele? _____

   Will any of her daughters get the defective allele? _____ How many? _____

9. If we found that none of the daughters actually showed the defective phenotype, then how could we explain it?

TIPS FOR SOLVING SEX-LINKED GENETIC PROBLEMS

There is a sex-linked gene on the X chromosome that causes a disorder called *hemophilia,* where the blood fails to clot properly when a person is injured. This disorder is recessive and can be symbolized by the small letter "n." Normal blood clotting is dominant and can be symbolized by the capital letter "N."

▶ In sex-linked cases we not only use letters to symbolize the genes, but also include the X or Y chromosome to indicate gender and to follow the sex chromosomes into the next generation.

▶ Using these symbols we can indicate a female who is heterozygous for clotting as $X^N X^n$.

▶ A homozygous female for normal clotting would be $X^N X^N$.

▶ A hemophilic male would be $X^n Y$.

We would diagram a Punnett Square of a cross between a heterozygous female and a normal clotting male like this:

Complete the Punnett Square showing the offspring.

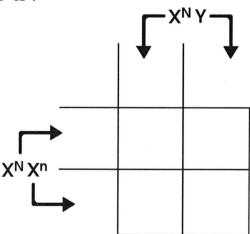

1. Looking at the Punnett Square you just completed, answer the following questions.

    a. What is the genotype for the female parent? _____

    b. What is the genotype for the male parent? _____

    c. What are the genotypes for their offspring? _____

    d. What are the chances that any child will be a hemophiliac? _____

    e. Is it the father or the mother that passes the hemophilia gene to the male child?
    _____

2. Failure to distinguish between red and green colors is caused by a recessive allele and is a sex-linked gene carried on the X chromosome.

    A red-green color-blind male marries a normal female. Of their six children (four boys and two girls), all have normal vision.

    a. What is the most probable genotype of the mother? _____

    b. Will any of their four male children pass this disorder on? _____ Explain.

    c. Draw a Punnett Square of this cross to prove your answers.

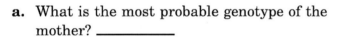

3. A normal-visioned female gave birth to a color-blind daughter. Her husband has normal vision. He claims that the child is not his. Does the genetic information suggest that someone else is the child's father?

Explain and prove your answer using a Punnett Square.

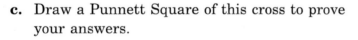

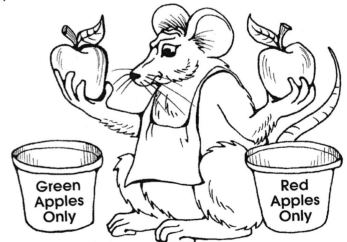

Green Apples Only

Red Apples Only

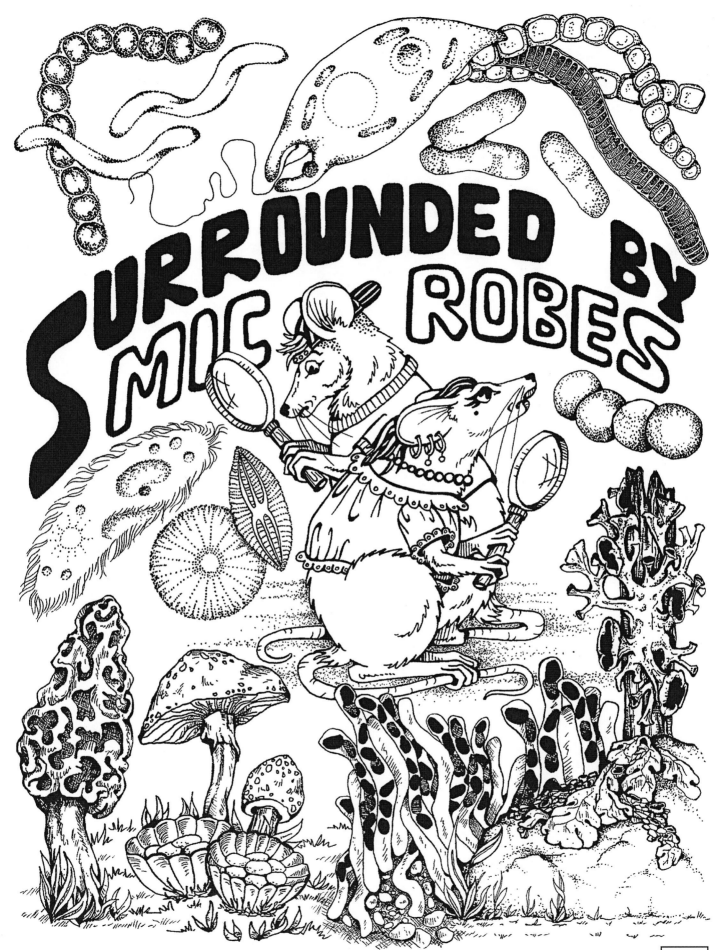

SURROUNDED BY MICROBES

┌─────────────────────────────┐
│ **DYNAMIC DEVELOPMENTS**   │
│   **AND**   │
│ **FASCINATING FACTS**   │
│   **IN BIOLOGY**   │
└─────────────────────────────┘

Humans are more than just human: We coexist with over 500 trillion microbes in and on us—a *microbiome.* In fact, we harbor 10 microbes for every human cell—which make us 90% *not us.* Without microbes, we would be unable to digest our food, suffer from multiple vitamin deficiencies (bacteria synthesize many vitamins, including niacin, biotin, and vitamin K), have weak and ineffective immune response (innocuous bacteria "train" our immune systems), and be vulnerable to detrimental microbial attack through our skin (protective bacterial colonies on our skin defend us from infection by harmful bacteria).

—HTTP://DISCOVERMAGAZINE.COM/2011/MAR/04-TRILLIONS-MICROBES-CALL-US-HOME-HELP-KEEP-
HEALTHY?SEARCHTERM=BACTERIA%20IN%20HUMAN%20GENOME

SURROUNDED BY MICROBES

INTRODUCTION

Small unicellular organisms developed on Earth sometime before 3.5 billion years ago. The vast majority did not fossilize, so we don't have a clear picture of what happened during early evolution. Therefore, we must depend on the few fossils that have been found and the characteristics of modern-day organisms to reconstruct life's story. That story begins with the simplest cell type called *prokaryote* ("before the nucleus"). Prokaryotic cells are very small and do not have a nucleus or other cell organelles. Those traits took another 2 billion years to evolve and produce the second type of cell called *eukaryote* ("new nucleus"). Eukaryotic cells are larger, and have a nucleus and other specialized cell organelles. (See Figure 1.)

THE THREE DOMAINS

Taxonomists use the similarities and differences among organisms to hypothesize probable evolutionary relationships. They create categories to sort organisms based on those relationships. (More details about organism taxonomy are discussed in the "Survey of Animals" lab.) The most general categories are called **Domains**. The subgroups of domains are called **Kingdoms** and the divisions of Kingdoms are called **Phyla**. Current taxonomic models start by dividing organisms by their cell types, either prokaryotes or eukaryotes.

Biochemical evidence suggests that there were profound evolutionary changes within the prokaryotic organisms, and two subgroups have been proposed. One group is called **Domain Archaebacteria** ("ancient bacteria") and the other group is called **Domain Eubacteria** ("new bacteria"). The specific differences between Archaebacteria and Eubacteria are described in your textbook. Domain Archaebacteria includes bacteria that live in very exotic environments like hot springs and thermal vents in the deep ocean along with some other marine bacteria. Domain Eubacteria includes the "common bacteria" we encounter in our daily lives.

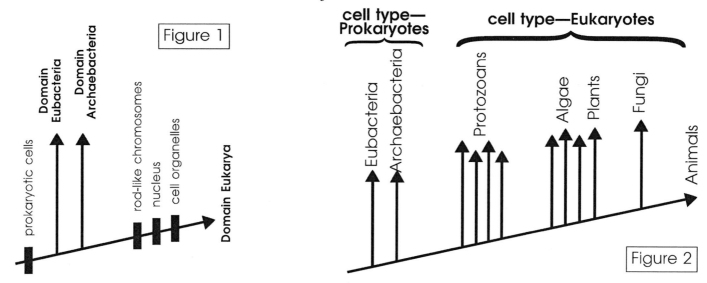

The third domain is **Eukarya** (the eukaryotes), and it includes all other organisms. It may seem surprising that eukaryotes are put into a single domain, but the uniting feature is the similar structure of their cells. Therefore, protozoans, algae, plants, fungi, and animals are all considered subgroups under the Domain Eukarya. (See Figure 2.)

ACTIVITIES

ACTIVITY #1

"BACTERIA IN OUR ENVIRONMENT"

This Activity must be completed during the week prior to the "Surrounded by Microbes" Lab so that there will be enough time for the bacterial colonies to grow and be seen.

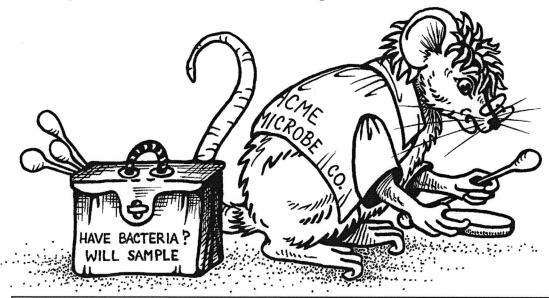

WHERE ARE THE BACTERIA IN OUR ENVIRONMENT
AND HOW MANY ARE THERE?

Today your class will pose one or two questions related to bacteria that live with you on this campus. Then you will design a sampling procedure that answers your questions.

NOW

1. Divide the class into three large groups.

2. Each group has 5 minutes to discuss interesting bacteria questions that you think are possible to answer by sampling with agar plates.

3. Decide which question is the most interesting to your group.

THEN

1. Each group will present its favorite question to the entire lab class.

2. As a class you will decide the final experimental questions.

3. You will have sterile agar plates for growing bacteria.

4. As a class, decide how you will use these plates in your experimental design.

AGAR PLATES

The special glassware used for agar sampling are called Petri dishes. The top of the Petri dish loosely covers the bottom. This permits oxygen gas in the air to enter the plate without allowing contamination by spores and other microbes in the environment.

Agar has been poured into the bottom half of a Petri dish. Agar is a derivative of a red algae called *agar-agar*. It is a solidifying agent. The true nourishment is added to the agar, and consists of partially digested protein, carbohydrates, minerals, and other nutrients.

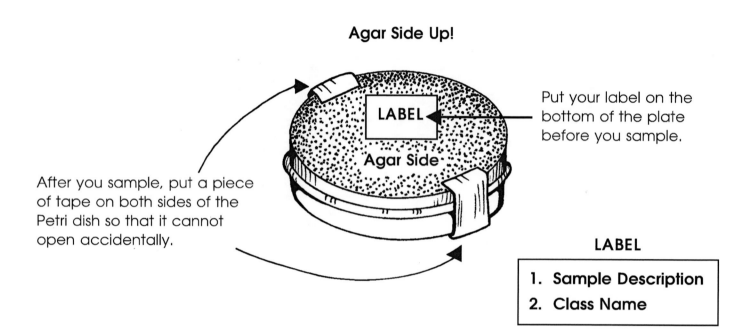

Agar Side Up!

LABEL

Agar Side

Put your label on the bottom of the plate before you sample.

After you sample, put a piece of tape on both sides of the Petri dish so that it cannot open accidentally.

LABEL

1. Sample Description
2. Class Name

IMPORTANT

It is important that the label be placed on the bottom of the Petri dish (the one containing the nutrient agar).

The Petri dishes will be incubated in an inverted (bottoms up) position.

When the label is placed on the bottom half of the dish, it will be easily identified and will be on the same side as the bacteria.

Another reason that the Petri dish is inverted during incubation is to prevent drops of moisture from collecting on the agar and permitting the bacteria to swim out into your environment.

SAMPLING FOR BACTERIA

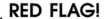

RED FLAG!   WARNING!   WARNING!

Do not obtain sampling specimens from your mouth, throat, groin, nose, or any area of your body except for healthy skin.

Be very careful when carrying out this experiment. The environment contains a large variety of different microbes (bacteria and fungi). Some of these microbes may be ***pathogenic*** (disease causing).

NOW

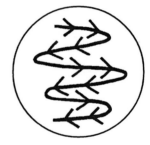

1. You have labeled your dishes before sampling. Check your label for complete information. Print your Sample Description and your Class Name.

2. A sterile moistened swab will be used to sample the environment and then to inoculate the sterile agar in the Petri dish.

3. *Swab the plate in this fashion:*

    Gently roll the swab across the surface of the agar. *Do not dig!*

    Skimming the surface as you roll the swab back and forth will do the trick.

4. Tape the two sides of the Petri dish together.

5. Put a piece of tape around the entire class's agar plates so they don't get mixed up with those from other lab classes.

6. Place the *inverted plates* in the tub labeled "To Be Incubated."   Be sure that your plates are all inverted in the same direction (agar side up).   The Petri dishes will be incubated during the next week.

IMPORTANT

After you obtain your sample and inoculate your agar plate, discard the used swabs in the test tube or envelope provided.

Then place the test tube or envelope in the laboratory area marked:

Danger—Contaminated Materials to be Autoclaved

A special machine called an *autoclave* will be used to decontaminate these materials by using a process that involves steam sterilization under pressure.

ACTIVITY #2

"WHAT ARE SOME BASIC CHARACTERISTICS OF ORGANISMS?"

By the end of this lab you will know three very basic characteristics for the majority of organisms in each of two domains — *Eubacteria*, and *Eukarya*.

FIRST CHARACTERISTIC

All cells can be divided into one of two types.

Prokaryotic
vs.
Eukaryotic
} **How do you tell?**

- A prokaryotic cell is very small compared to a eukaryotic cell.
- A prokaryotic cell does not have a nucleus.
- A prokaryotic cell does not have any chloroplasts. If the cell does photosynthesis, then the light-catching pigments are spread throughout the cell water and not in plastids.
- A eukaryotic cell has many organelles (including a nucleus, chloroplasts, mitochondria, and others).
- A eukaryotic cell is big compared to a prokaryotic cell.
- By the way, the word *prokaryotic* means "before nucleus," and the word *eukaryotic* means "true nucleus."

? QUESTION

1. Remember the onion cells that you saw in an earlier lab? What kind of cells were they—prokaryotic or eukaryotic? _____

2. How do you know?

SECOND CHARACTERISTIC

All living organisms are composed of one or more cells.

Unicellular
vs.
Multicellular
} **How do you tell?**

- *Unicellular* means that the organism is a single cell, or it is a small chain or cluster of identical cells.
- *Multicellular* means that the organism is made of more than one kind of cell type.

? QUESTION

1. The plant leaves that you saw in an earlier lab are part of what type of living organism—unicellular or multicellular?

2. How do you know?

THIRD CHARACTERISTIC

All living organisms get their energy for their life processes from a specific source.

Phototrophic
vs.
Heterotrophic
} **How do you tell?**

- The word *phototrophic* means "light-eater," and the word *heterotrophic* means "other-eater."

- A phototrophic organism will either have chloroplasts or photosynthetic pigments spread throughout the cytoplasm of the cell. These organisms require light for their survival.

- A heterotrophic organism does not have photosynthetic pigments or chloroplasts. It cannot do photosynthesis.

  This type of organism must eat some other organism or the by-products of that organism to get its energy. Sometimes, this category of organism is called a *chemotroph* because it gets its energy from chemicals. If you go on to advanced biology classes, then you will study a more detailed distinction in energy categories. For this class, we will combine all non-phototrophs under the one word *heterotroph*.

ACTIVITY #3

"BACTERIA"

Bacteria are the most numerous organisms on this planet. They exhibit more variety in the way they get their energy than any other group. They are an essential organism for the recycling of dead plants and animals.

Last week, various parts of the environment were sampled for different kinds of bacteria, and Petri dishes were inoculated. Now . . .

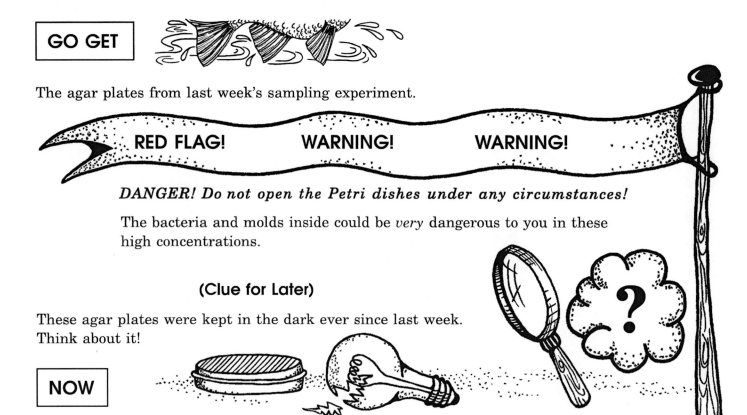

GO GET

The agar plates from last week's sampling experiment.

RED FLAG!   WARNING!   WARNING!

DANGER! Do not open the Petri dishes under any circumstances!

The bacteria and molds inside could be *very* dangerous to you in these high concentrations.

(Clue for Later)

These agar plates were kept in the dark ever since last week. Think about it!

NOW

1. Determine the answer to your experimental question.

2. You should be able to tell the difference between bacterial colonies and fungus colonies. (Fungus looks "fuzzy" and bacteria usually don't.)

3. Look at your bacterial colonies and describe their growth (color and shape).

4. When you are finished, *put all the agar plates in the container labeled* "To Be Sterilized."

5. *Wash your hands!*

GO GET	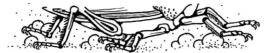

1. A compound microscope.

2. A prepared microscope slide of bacterial shapes.

NOW

1. Examine the three different samples on this slide and determine the three basic shapes of bacteria. (The bacteria may be grouped together, so look at the individual cells.)

2. The 3 shapes of bacteria are:

   _____

   _____

   _____

3. *Return the slide when you are finished.*

FINALLY

You should have enough information to determine the three basic characteristics of bacteria. (circle your choices)

Prokaryotic	Unicellular	Phototrophic
vs.	vs.	vs.
Eukaryotic	Multicellular	Heterotrophic

ACTIVITY #4

"CYANOBACTERIA AND THE TRUE ALGAE"

The *cyanobacteria* and the *true algae* are very different kinds of organisms, but *both* of them do photosynthesis.

The objective of this Activity is to determine the difference between the algae and the cyanobacteria.

You will need to work with another microscope group in order to make comparisons of the two kinds of organisms.

 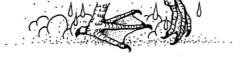

1. One microscope group is to get a prepared microscope slide of *Spirogyra*.

2. The other group is to get a prepared microscope slide of *Nostoc*.

NOW

1. Work as a team with another group at your table. Each microscope group is to find their organism, and put it under the *same* high magnification.

2. These two organisms grow in chains of identical cells.

3. Look back and forth between the microscope views until the most basic differences become obvious. (Ignore the color of the stain.)

4. *Nostoc* is a cyanobacteria and *Spirogyra* is a true algae.

5. *Remember:* You are going to have to answer the three basic characteristics questions about both of these organisms. Make some quick notes and a sketch of both organisms.

Nostoc	*Spirogyra*

Ask your instructor about the ribbon-shaped structure inside the *Spirogyra* cells.

6. *Return the slides to where you found them.*

BASIC CHARACTERISTICS

Talk it over with your group and decide which features represent each group. (circle your choices)

CYANOBACTERIA

Prokaryotic	Unicellular	Phototrophic
vs.	vs.	vs.
Eukaryotic	Multicellular	Heterotrophic

TRUE ALGAE*

Prokaryotic	Unicellular	Phototrophic
vs.	vs.	vs.
Eukaryotic	Multicellular	Heterotrophic

* We have examined only unicellular algae. There are also multicellular forms, but they are studied in advanced botany courses.

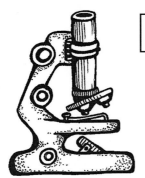

TESTING . . . TESTING

Now for a test of your skills!

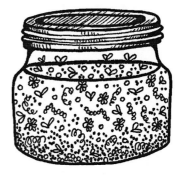

GO GET

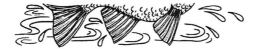

1. Use your compound microscope.

2. Make a slide using a sample from the "Live Mixed Algae" jar. (One drop of the green stuff will do it.)

NOW

1. Find two different cyanobacteria in the sample.
   Show them to your instructor. What characteristics tell you that they are cyanobacteria?

2. Find two different true algae in the sample.
   Show them to your instructor. What characteristics tell you that they are true algae?

ACTIVITY #5

"PROTOZOANS"

We've seen the Protozoans before in previous labs. Now, it's time for you to determine their basic characteristics.

 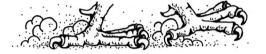

Make a slide using a sample from the "Live Mixed Protozoa" jar. (One drop from the bottom of the jar.)

NOW

1. Find at least two different kinds of Protozoans.

2. *Show them to your instructor.*

3. You may need to use Protoslo® to slow the swimming organisms enough to follow them with your microscope. Ask your instructor how to use Protoslo®.

4. You may also find some attached Protozoans in the sample.

5. We have a booklet that will give you the names of some Protozoans you are seeing. Try to identify your Protozoans.

BASIC CHARACTERISTICS

Talk it over with your group and decide which features represent Protozoans. (circle your choices)

Prokaryotic	Unicellular	Phototrophic
vs.	vs.	vs.
Eukaryotic	Multicellular	Heterotrophic

ACTIVITY #6

"BREAD MOLD AND MUSHROOMS"

Bread mold and mushrooms are strange beasts indeed!

During this Activity you will continue with your determination of basic characteristics, and you will discover some interesting structural features of this group, along with one of its strange methods of reproduction.

SPORE REPRODUCTION

Some organisms have a special type of reproduction to get through very tough times in their environment.

These organisms produce **spores**, which are small cells with a very thick protective coating. (They look like little balls.) When the environment changes, these spores will grow into the next stage in the life cycle of these organisms.

BREAD MOLD

NOW

1. Look at the bread mold samples growing on the bread.

2. Make observations about how you think it is "making a living" and talk this over with your group. What are your conclusions?

GO GET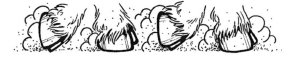

Go to the bread mold cultures growing on agar plates, and cut out a small part ($\frac{1}{4}$" x $\frac{1}{4}$") of the organism, and put it on a slide (no coverslip).

NOW

Bread Mold

1. Examine this organism with the *dissecting microscope* and make observations about its basic characteristics.

2. Find those "little balls" called *spores.*

3. Draw a simple sketch of the structure of the bread mold.

THEN

Filaments and Spores

1. Make a wet mount slide of the balls and a few of the filaments. Use a compound microscope, and examine under higher magnification.

2. Make a simple sketch of what you see. (The filaments are used for feeding, and the very little balls are spores.)

MUSHROOMS

GO GET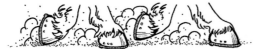

Remove a small piece of the brown-colored tissue from under the mushroom cap.

NOW

Mushroom

1. Make a slide of the mushroom tissue and determine what that brown-colored tissue is.

2. Make a simple sketch of what you see.

? QUESTION

1. How do you think that this mushroom organism gets its energy for life? Talk it over with your group. What are your conclusions?

2. Do you think that this organism does photosynthesis?
   Why or why not?

FINALLY

Talk with your group and decide what features represent the *bread mold* and *mushroom* organisms. (circle your choices)

Prokaryotic	Unicellular	Phototrophic
vs.	vs.	vs.
Eukaryotic	Multicellular	Heterotrophic

182   Chapter 11

ACTIVITY #7

"BASIC CHARACTERISTICS OF EUBACTERIA AND EUKARYA"

We designed this lab to include organisms that would define the basic characteristics of each of *two domains — Eubacteria and Eukarya.*

You have answered the three characteristics questions about each of the groups presented.

? QUESTION

1. Which **cell type** do you think is the most complex? (circle your choice)

    Prokaryotic   or   Eukaryotic

2. Which **cell arrangement** do you think is the most complex? (circle your choice)

    Unicellular   or   Multicellular

NOW

1. Using your answers to the above questions, list the four possible combinations of cell type and cell arrangement, placing them in order from *simple* to *more complex*. (Fill in the domain names after reading statement #3 below.)

Simple	Cell Type	Cell Arrangement	Domain
↓	_____ & _____	_____
	_____ & _____	_____
	_____ & _____	_____
More Complex	_____ & _____	_____

2. Refer to the descriptions of basic characteristics that you chose in earlier Activities for each of the subgroups examined in this lab. You should see that only one of the four possible combinations above is not represented.

    Cross out that combination of traits—it doesn't exist!

3. You are left with three combinations. The first combination is Domain Eubacteria. The second two combinations are Domain Eukarya.

    Put those domain names on the correct lines above.

4. Place each of the following five subgroups into the correct domain in the table below, and list whether that subgroup is a *heterotroph* or a *phototroph*.

Bacteria

Cyanobacteria

True Algae

Protozoans

Bread Mold and Mushrooms

Domain	Subgroup	Method of Energy
Archaebacteria (not examined in today's lab)	Thermal Vent and Hot Spring bacteria	Oxidation of various minerals
Eubacteria		
Eukarya		

FINALLY

You should be able to name the subgroups in each domain that you studied, and list the three basic characteristics of each.

Your textbook or lecture class may define the basic characteristics of the domains in more detail than this lab did. Also, your textbook or lecture class may point out some of the exceptions to the generalizations presented in this lab.

ACTIVITY #8

"LICHENS"

A little more than 100 years ago, botanists discovered that *lichens*, strange plant-like organisms, are actually a cooperative relationship between *two* very different organisms. One of the organisms provides the basic structural framework of the lichen, and the other organism does the energy collecting (photosynthesis). Lichens are often found growing on rocks, tree trunks, or fallen branches on the forest floor.

The metabolic lives of these two very distantly related species may be intimately intertwined in many different ways. Lichens exhibit a high resistance to unfavorable environments including the cold polar regions, barren mountain rocks far above the timberline, and fully exposed rocks in the hottest of desert areas.

INFORMATION

There are several different forms of lichens, and we have some in the lab today:

1. A crust-like form growing very close to the rock's surface,

2. A leaf-like form, and

3. A shrub-like or hair-like form.

GO GET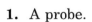

1. A probe.

2. A small sample of lichen from the station marked "Lichen Sample."

NOW

1. Crush a small amount of lichen with a probe in a drop of water on the slide. Cover and examine it with your compound microscope.

2. Search the slide for evidence of two very different kinds of organisms. *Show your instructor* the two organisms, and answer the next six questions based on your sample.

1. Which organism does the photosynthesis?

2. Draw a quick sketch of the organism.

3. What is your evidence that this organism does the photosynthesis?

4. Which organism makes up most of the body structure of this lichen?

5. Draw a quick sketch of this organism.

6. What is your evidence that this organism does *not* do photosynthesis?

Photosynthetic Part

Structural Part

FINISHED

We hope you've enjoyed discovering some of the many organisms that inhabit the domains of Eubacteria and Eukarya. The study of these organisms is what *microbiology* is all about.

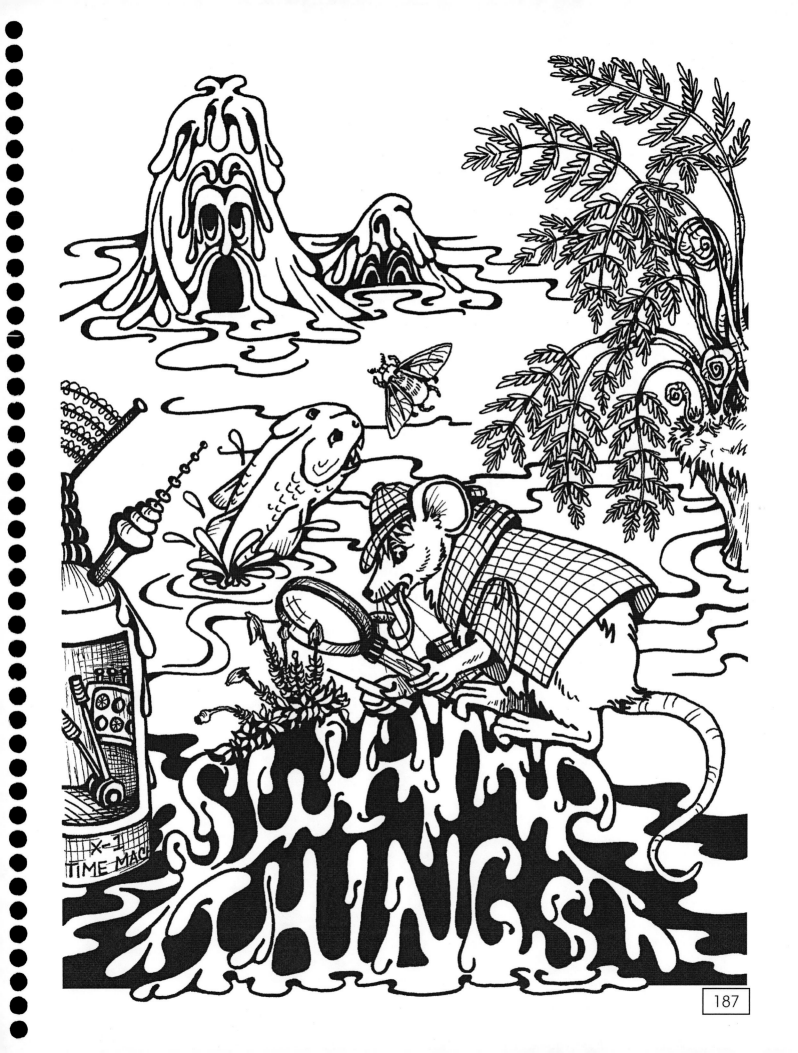

SWAMP THINGS

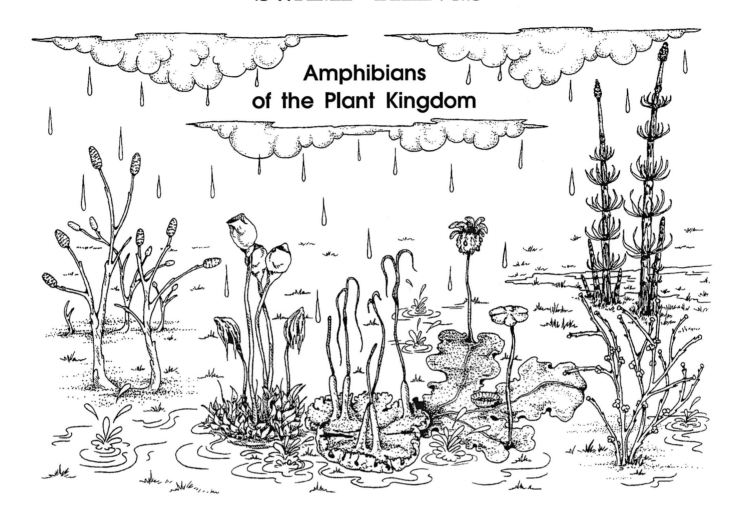

Amphibians
of the Plant Kingdom

INTRODUCTION

It was the time of the Rhyniophytes and whisk ferns, club mosses and horsetails. And the world was a swampy place. A botanist would trade a Porsche for a stroll in those Paleozoic times.

Ah, those were the days!

ACTIVITIES

ACTIVITY #1

"PLANT LIFE CYCLES"

This week's lab is a continuation of the evolutionary story of the plants on this planet. Last week we looked at algae, and saw that they started as one-celled organisms and developed into more complex algae. The advanced types of algae were the most probable ancestors of land plants.

Because there was a lot of swampy land about 400 million years ago, natural selection picked traits that allowed aquatic plants to move into that environment. Land would have been an excellent new opportunity for any plant. It provided "unlimited access" to sunlight for photosynthesis.

The two basic questions to understanding this evolutionary event are:

1. *What are the traits that would be needed by land plants?* and

2. *What traits did the algae already have before the land invasion?*

We will consider the traits needed on land as we look at **mosses** and **ferns** later in the lab. But, now we will begin with a basic understanding of the algae life cycle on which all land plant reproduction is based.

ALGAE LIFE CYCLE

Before plants were capable of invading land, the algae had already evolved a unique life cycle called **alternation of generations**. During this cycle, the algae alternated between a stage called **gametophyte** (which means "gamete plant") and a stage called **sporophyte** (which means "spore plant"). These two stages repeated one after the other, generation after generation.

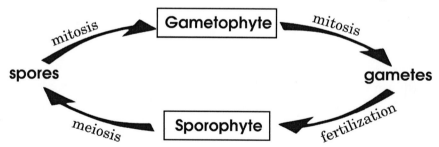

In early plants like the mosses and ferns the gametophyte is a small plant that produces gametes (eggs and sperm). Only, it turns out that the gametophyte is already haploid when it does so. The diploid sporophyte grows from the embryo created by the union of an egg and sperm. It is actually the sporophyte that performs meiosis when it makes spores. (In contrast, animals produce eggs and sperm directly by meiosis.)

1. The *alternation of generations* allowed plants to reproduce and multiply by using two different methods—*spores* and *gametes*.

2. As algae gave rise to land plants evolution changed the physical appearance of both the gametophyte and sporophyte generations.

Remember: We are talking about algae that lived in the water.

To be sure you understand these life cycles, and for practice:

1. Put the names of the correct stage inside the *Life Cycle* boxes below.

2. In which generation does meiosis occur (sporophyte or gametophyte)? _____.
   Put that generation name into each of the appropriate boxes in the Alternation of Generations
   Cycle. Put the other generation name into the other boxes.

3. Don't worry about the lines underneath the boxes; they'll come later.

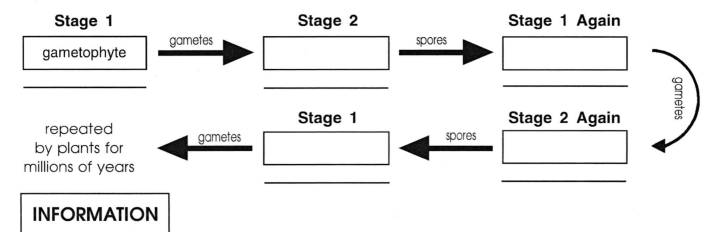

INFORMATION

1. The gametophyte stage is *haploid*. This means that the cells have only *one* set of chromosomes.

2. The sporophyte stage is *diploid*. This means that the cells have *two* sets of chromosomes.

? QUESTION

1. Which stage in the algae life cycle produces eggs and sperm? _____

2. How many sets of chromosomes does an egg have? _____

3. How many sets of chromosomes does a sperm have? _____

4. When the egg and sperm unite, we are back to . . . (circle your answer)

   a. one set of chromosomes
   b. two sets of chromosomes

5. The fertilized egg will grow into one . . . (circle your answer)

   a. gametophyte plant
   b. sporophyte plant

NOW

Go back to your *Life Cycle* diagram, and write the words *"diploid"* and *"haploid"* on the line under the appropriate stages (boxes).

SUMMARY

We have seen that the algae have two stages in their life cycle—the gametophyte stage and the sporophyte stage.

One of these stages is haploid and the other stage is diploid.

The algae used these two stages for different environmental and reproductive purposes.

Now, the question is: ***Which of these two stages would prove to be best able to adapt to a dry land environment?***

Any thoughts? Well, let's proceed to Activity #2.

ACTIVITY #2

"WHICH WORKS BETTER ON LAND—HAPLOID OR DIPLOID?"

| INFORMATION | GENES AND MUTATIONS |

Plants have many genes, and these genes are carried on the chromosomes.

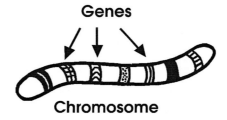

Each gene is involved with the making of a specific protein.

Each protein is used in one of two ways:

• A protein might be part of a plant structure.

• A protein might be an enzyme.

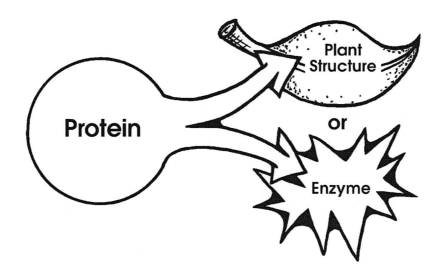

| ? QUESTION |

What will be lost if a gene is destroyed? _____ or _____

A *mutation* usually results in a destroyed gene. A gene can be destroyed by radiation, chemicals in the environment, or other spontaneous events involving the DNA of a cell.

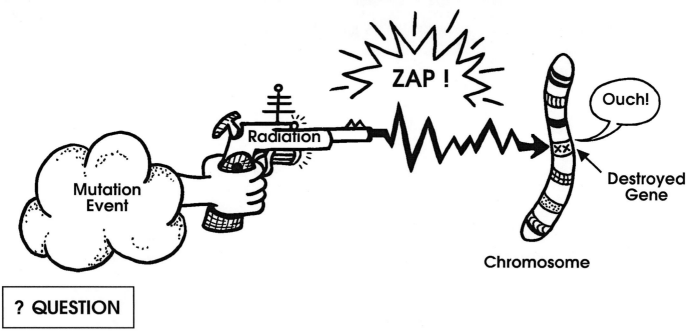

? QUESTION

Are mutations almost always a good thing, or a bad thing? _____
Explain your answer.

INFORMATION

A plant has a certain number of chromosomes (the number depends on the species) and each chromosome has many genes. Each gene produces a plant trait. The more genes that a plant has, the more traits it has. Presumably, more traits give the plant a better chance to adapt to dry land conditions.

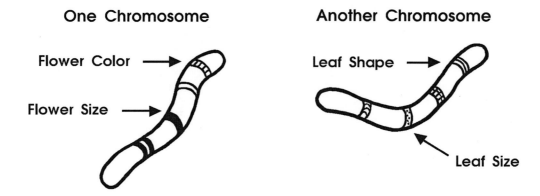

You are ready for the next two puzzles.

Put on your investigator's hat, get your magnifying glass, and try to solve *"The Mystery of the Helpless Haploid"* and *"The Mystery of the Dependable Diploid."*

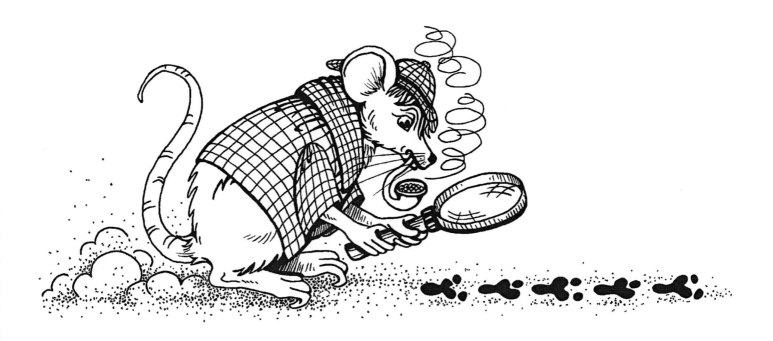

CASE 1

"THE MYSTERY OF THE HELPLESS HAPLOID"

1. Imagine that you are a plant.

2. You have a single set of chromosomes. (That is, you are *haploid*. **Remember:** Haploid means that you have only *one copy* of each different chromosome in your species.)

3. Assume that mutation events occur at a rate of one mutation for every 1000 genes. The probability of a mutation is, therefore, $\frac{1}{1000}$. (The actual probability of mutations is dependent on many factors, and the value of $\frac{1}{1000}$ has been chosen so that you can make comparison calculations during this lab.)

4. Assume that every gene (every trait) that you have is necessary for your survival as a plant.

5. Assume it takes *more than* 10,000 genes to be a *complex* plant with lots of structures and enzymes.

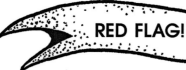

1. Assuming the previous information, what would be the safest number of genes for you if you lived as a haploid plant? (circle your choice)

    a. 1000

    b. more than 1000

    c. less than 1000

RED FLAG!   WARNING!   WARNING!

Check your answer to question #1 with your instructor before going on. This "clue" must be properly understood or you will spend the rest of this case chasing a "red herring"!

2. Describe your basic structure as a haploid plant using the conclusion in question #1. (circle your choice)

    a. You are a complex plant (lots of structures).

    b. You are a simple plant (fewer structures).

3. If you were an algae plant that was starting to move onto land through the process of evolution, then what would be the most likely requirement to ensure your survival in a land environment? (circle your choice)

    a. Don't change any genes.

    b. Add more genes (new traits).

4. You should have decided that more genes enable you to develop more traits to help you survive on land. But, you are still *haploid!* What risk would you be taking if you were to add many more genes?

5. Some of the algae plants that evolved onto land developed an emphasis on the haploid stage. These plants could not add very many more genes without risking extinction. Therefore, the algae plants that used this strategy were restricted to being . . . (circle your choice)

    a. simple plants (few structures).

    b. complex plants (many structures).

FINALLY

Some plants did move onto land with an emphasis on their haploid *gametophyte* stage. From what you have discovered, you should be able to deduce that their structure would be very simple.

It's elementary, my dear Watson!

Now you know why we call this problem, "The Case of the Helpless Haploid."

CASE 2

"THE MYSTERY OF THE DEPENDABLE DIPLOID"

All of the assumptions of Case 1 are also true for Case 2 *except* that now: You are a plant with a double set of chromosomes. (That is, you are *diploid*.) Diploid means you have *two copies* of each different chromosome in your species. You have two of every gene.

? QUESTION

1. Consider what would happen to a diploid plant when genes are destroyed by mutation. How many genes have to be destroyed in a diploid plant for one trait to be lost? _____

2. Case 1 assumed that the probability of a gene mutation was one chance for every 1000 genes. A rule in statistics states that: "If you want to know the probability of two events happening together, then *multiply* their separate probabilities."

   Based on your answer to the previous question, as a diploid plant, what is the probability of your losing both genes for the same trait because of destruction through mutation? _____

3. Consider your answer to question #2, and that mutation does destroy genes. How many genes can a diploid plant "safely" have? (circle your choice)
   a. about the same number as a haploid plant
   b. fewer genes than a haploid plant
   c. many more genes than a haploid plant

4. Based on your conclusions above, describe yourself as a diploid plant. (circle your choice)
   a. You are a complex plant (lots of structures).
   b. You are a simple plant (fewer structures).

5. How does your description above relate to your chances for doing well in a land environment? Explain.

FINALLY

Some plants did move onto land with an emphasis on their *sporophyte* stage. You should be able to deduce whether their structure would be simple or complex.

Now you know why we call this problem "The Mystery of the Dependable Diploid."

The time has come to test your detective skill in Activities #3 and #4 with the moss plant and the fern plant.

The game is afoot, Watson!

ACTIVITY #3

"THE MOSS PLANT"

During this Activity you will figure out the life cycle of the moss plant, and you will identify some distinguishing adaptations and limitations of the moss plant.

WHEN YOU SEE A MOSS PLANT

When you see green moss growing on a river bank or on a fallen tree, you are actually seeing only one of the two alternating generations in its life cycle. You must look closely at this generation to determine which it is—*gametophyte* or *sporophyte*.

 GO GET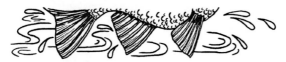

1. A dissecting microscope.
2. A moss plant.

OBSERVATIONS

---

1. Look at the green parts of the moss plant under the dissecting microscope. Moss leaves don't have veins for transporting nutrients or stomata for regulating air flow like typical plants. Does this suggest that moss leaves are as complex as tree leaves? _____ Leaf veins and stomata are land traits, and require many genes to create them. How many "leaf genes" would the moss have compared to a typical tree (many or few)? _____

2. Does the moss plant have much root? _____ Assuming that large complex roots require more genes than small simple roots, how many "root genes" would the moss have (many or few)? _____

3. In general, being bigger requires more genes than staying small. How many "size related genes" would the moss have (many or few)? _____

4. By looking at the general features of the moss plant you should be able to conclude that it has (many or few) _____ genes for land traits.

Remember: In Activity #2 you concluded that being haploid restricts the plant to being simple, whereas being diploid allows for much more complex structures. Now you are ready to identify which generation in the moss life cycle you are looking at.

? QUESTION

---

1. Is this stage of your moss plant . . . (circle your choice)

    a. a complex plant   or   **b.** a simple plant

2. Therefore, this stage of the moss plant is probably . . . (circle your choice)

    a. haploid   or   **b.** diploid

3. This means that you are looking at the (circle your choice)

a. *sporophyte*   or   **b.** *gametophyte*
generation   generation

4. Which means that this stage produces (circle your choice)

a. *gametes* (eggs and sperm)   or   **b.** *spores*

5. Draw a quick sketch of your moss plant.

6. *Save your moss plant.* You'll be needing it later.

Moss Plant

MOSS SEX ORGANS

It is not possible to see the details of the moss sex organs in a living plant, so . . .

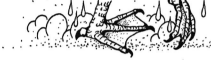 **GO GET**

1. A compound microscope.

2. A microscope slide marked "Moss Archegonia."

3. A microscope slide marked "Moss Antheridia."

NOW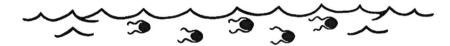

1. Don't worry about the fancy names of these sex organs. You will discover which one is male and which one is female as you continue.

2. Female organs usually have one large **egg** cell in the middle of a vase-like structure.

3. Male organs are usually round or oval in shape and have a dozen or more small round cells inside called **sperm**. *After a rain the moss sperm must swim to the egg for fertilization.* This means that moss reproduction depends on a *wet* environment.

4. Work with a partner so that one of you has the "Antheridia" slide, and the other has the "Archegonia" slide. You are viewing moss stem tips which look something like an artichoke sliced in half. The leaves at the stem tips surround the sex organs.

5. Finding the female organ is a bit difficult. The female sex organ looks like a vase or a bowling pin, depending on the species. If you are lucky, the thin section of the moss plant will cut exactly through the middle. Or, you may find odd-shaped sections. A large egg cell is a clue. Looking back and forth between both slides, as well as the slides of other students, may help. Find a female organ, and show it to your instructor! Draw a quick sketch of what you see.

Female

Male

6. Search the other slide and find a male organ. Show your instructor! Draw a quick sketch of what you see.

FUNNY-LOOKING STALK

The sex organs of mosses are considered to be very simple. These organs are part of the gametophyte which is haploid, and haploid forces a simple design (fewer genes). You can't make a fancy sex organ unless you are diploid. Now, we will examine the diploid reproductive stage of the mosses.

 GO GET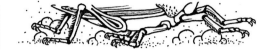

A fine-pointed probe and small tweezers.

NOW

1. Using your dissecting microscope, search for a funny-looking stalk coming out of the top of the moss plant you saved.

2. Look at the top of the stalk. You should see a small capsule. The stalk with its capsule is actually the next generation stage in the life cycle of the moss.

This next stage grows out of the female sex organ of the previous gametophyte stage. It grows from a fertilized egg.

Draw a simple sketch of what you see.

3. If there is a cap on the capsule, pry it off and look at what is inside.

4. Make a wet mount of the small balls, and look at them with your compound microscope.

5. Draw a simple sketch of the balls.

Dissecting Scope View of the stalk and capsule	Compound Scope View of the little round balls

? QUESTION

1. What are the little round balls? _____
   Hint: If you have trouble figuring out the answer, then look back at the *Life Cycle* in Activity #1.

2. Now that you know what the little balls are, you also know that the "funny looking stalk" is actually the . . . (circle your choice)

   a. *gametophyte* stage   **b.** *sporophyte* stage

MOSS ANCESTOR

We know that the spore grows into the gametophyte generation. Botanists tell us that the moss gametophyte developed from evolutionary changes in the growing spore of an algae. If this is true, then land traits were added to the algae gametophyte producing what we see today as the moss gametophyte. A logical implication of this theory is that the early growing moss spore should show some ancestral resemblance to the algae.

Protonema

 GO GET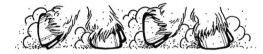

A microscope slide marked "Moss Protonema."

NOW

1. Using your compound microscope, search the slide for some branching filaments. The very first product of a growing *spore* is a branching chain of cells called the ***protonema***. Normally, spores are produced by mosses at the end of the wet season. With the next rains these spores grow into the protonema, which eventually matures into the new generation of gametophytes.

2. Draw a quick sketch of the protonema.

3. Compare the protonema structure to that of the filament algae (like *Spirogyra*) you saw in last week's lab. Explain how this is evidence that mosses may have evolved from the algae.

LIFE CYCLE

Diagram the *Life Cycle* of the moss plant below. Include: spores, gametes, sporophyte, and gametophyte. Draw a simple sketch of each generation as a visual reminder.

ACTIVITY #4

"THE FERN PLANT"

During this Activity you will figure out the life cycle of the fern plant, and you will identify some distinguishing adaptations and limitations of the fern.

WHEN YOU SEE A FERN PLANT

When you look at a fern plant growing in a forest or in your yard, you are seeing only one of the generations in the fern life cycle.

You must look closely at this generation to determine which it is—*gametophyte* or *sporophyte*.

 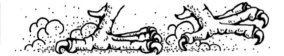

A fern plant.

NOW

1. Remember the logic steps we used in Activity #3. Look at the fern plant very carefully.

2. Decide whether it is simple or complex. _____ Therefore, whether it is haploid or diploid. _____ And conclude which generation it is (gametophyte or sporophyte). _____

3. Finally, what will it produce in this stage—spores or gametes? _____

GO GET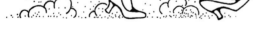

A microscope slide of a cross-section of a "Fern Stem."

NOW

Find vascular tissue in the fern stem using your compound microscope.

Vascular tissue is like the circulatory system in animals. It moves food and water up and down the plant through specialized tubes. The cells of these tubes will have *thicker cell walls* than other stem cells. The vascular tubes may be grouped in clusters that show a cylinder or a horseshoe-shaped arrangement in the cross-section of the stem. Ferns do not have well developed vascular tissue in their roots, so they don't thrive as well in dry environments compared to cone and flowering plants (see next lab). In contrast, moss plants have no vascular tissue at all.

or

Look for the vascular tissue cells in the stem and notice their thick cell walls compared to the other stem cells. Show your instructor!

Return the slide to where you got it!

CONCLUSIONS

1. The fern plant that you normally see is . . . (circle your choices)

Simple	Diploid	Sporophyte
or	or	or
Complex	Haploid	Gametophyte

2. Go back to the demonstration table and examine the fern plant. Based on your conclusions, what does this stage in the life cycle of a fern plant produce?

3. Look for them on the underside of leaves. Make a slide, snd show them to your instructor.

4. Draw these structures and the part of the fern plant that produces them. What are the small balls called? _____

5. What do these structures grow into?
   _____

FERN SEX ORGANS

We will have to depend on slides and preserved specimens for the next stage in the life cycle of ferns.

 GO GET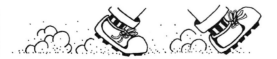

A prepared microscope slide of "Fern Prothallium" (Antheridia and Archegonia).

1. Use your compound microscope to examine the general structure of this stage of the fern plant life cycle. It grows from a spore that fell from the underside of a mature fern plant leaf. This very simple fern generation called the *prothallium* is normally found living on the forest floor, and may be only 1 or 2 centimeters in size. You should be able to conclude which stage you are looking at. Is it the sporophyte or the gametophyte? _____

   As a reminder, write your answer next to the word "prothallium."

2. Find the male and female organs. Show your instructor!

3. Draw the prothallium showing the male and female organs.

4. The egg and sperm unite to form the beginning of the next stage in the life cycle. (You already learned that stage as the fern plant you normally see.)

   Important! The ferns have swimming sperm just like the mosses. This means that fern reproduction is also dependent on a wet environment.

Prothallium _____

LIFE CYCLE

Diagram the *Life Cycle* of the fern plant below. Include spores, gametes, sporophyte, and gametophyte. Draw a simple sketch of each generation as a visual reminder.

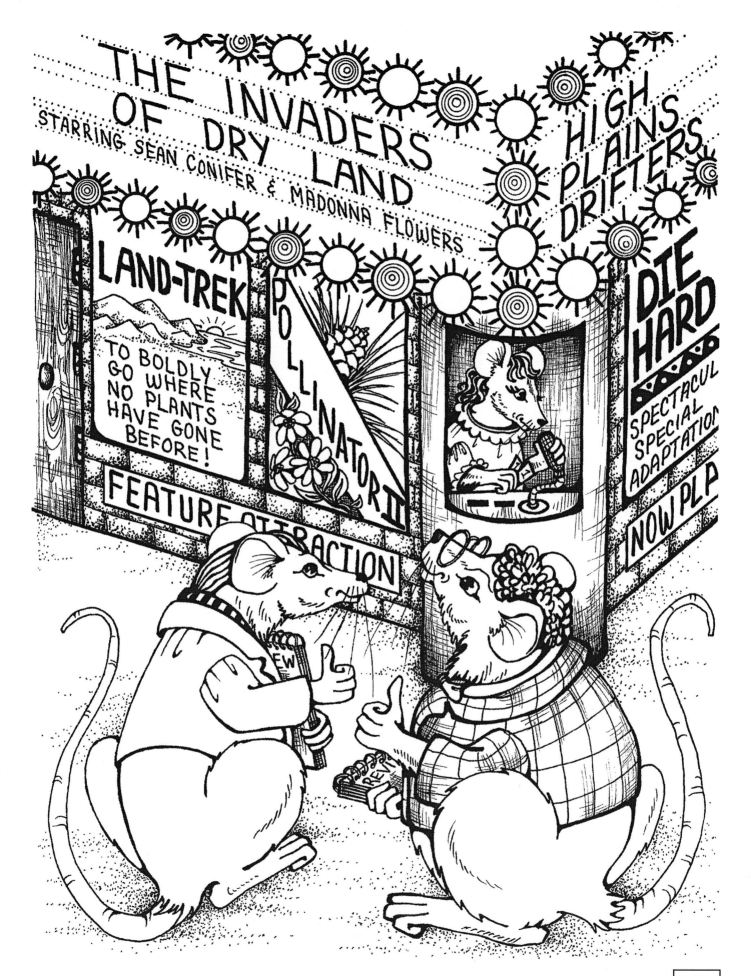

DYNAMIC DEVELOPMENTS AND FASCINATING FACTS IN BIOLOGY

The oldest continuously-living organisms on Earth are a few species of plants. If you thought the mighty Sequoia redwoods of northern California were the oldest, think again. Clonal plant species (those that do not reproduce sexually through pollen) such as the quaking aspen, live a prodigiously long time. A colony in Utah has been dated to 80,000 years old. A species of sea grass, *Posidonia oceania* located around the Balearic Islands off the coast of Spain is 100,000 years old. A colony of Siberian actinobacteria is estimated to be 400,000 to 600,000 years old, and remarkably, achieves DNA repair in below-freezing temperatures.

—"The World's Oldest Living Organisms" by Rachel Sussman, a fine arts photographer, FORA.TV, 2011

More than 50% of the world's most damaging invasive plant species escaped from botanical gardens.

—"Data: Science News—Bad News," *Discover Magazine,* June 2011, p. 14

THE INVADERS OF DRY LAND

INTRODUCTION

We finish the story of plants with the two groups that are most successful living in dry environments—the *cone plants* and the *flowering plants*. Both of these groups developed special structural and reproductive mechanisms to master the challenges of living on land.

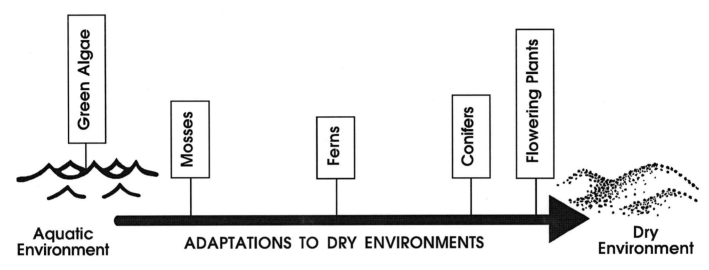

? QUESTION

Can you remember a structural and a reproductive feature of moss and fern plants that would limit their success in very dry environments?

_____

_____

ACTIVITIES

ACTIVITY #1

"REVIEW OF MOSSES AND FERNS"

MOSSES

1. The moss plant that we see growing on a log is haploid. How many *sets* of chromosomes does a haploid plant have? _____

2. A haploid plant is limited to a comparatively simple structure. How does the mutation of genes particularly hurt a haploid plant?

3. What is one example of a simple *structure* in moss plants?

4. What is *simple* about moss reproduction?

FERNS

1. The fern plants that we see growing in the forest are diploid. How many *sets* of chromosomes does a diploid plant have? _____

2. A diploid plant can possess more complex structures. How does having a diploid set of genes contribute to a plant possessing more complex structures?

3. What is one example of a complex structure in fern plants that helps them to be better adapted to dry environments?

4. Remember that the ferns use a simple approach to reproduction just like the mosses. How does this limit fern plant success in dry environments?

CONE PLANTS AND FLOWERING PLANTS

INFORMATION

1. Both the cone plants and the flowering plants owe their reproductive success to an emphasis on the diploid stage of the life cycle.

   As you remember, an emphasis on the diploid stage allows the organism to have many more genes without taking a serious risk to the destruction of traits by mutation. (Refer to the Moss and Fern Lab for a more thorough review of mutation risks.)

2. Both mosses and ferns drop their spores to the ground, and these spores grow into the gametophyte stage. *The gametophyte is the stage that is vulnerable in a dry land environment.* It is this stage that requires water for fertilization in the mosses and ferns.

   Conifers and flowering plants solve some of the reproductive challenges of dry land by not dropping spores to the ground, but by keeping the spores inside of cones or flower parts, which allows the spores to grow into gametophytes in a safe environment. Actually, the gametophyte is being protected by the sporophyte of the cone plants and flowering plants.

3. Conifers and flowering plants also evolved a new reproductive method called *pollination*. They don't have swimming sperm. The male sex cell (called *pollen*) is carried to the female sex cell (called the *egg*) by wind or insects or birds or mammals. Refer to the diagram on the next page.

   How is this new method a giant step forward for land plants?

4. The conifers and flowering plants have *seeds*.

   A seed is an embryo sporophyte plant with a protective and nourishing covering. They are able to live a very long time in the environment until it rains. Then the embryo plant will grow into the adult plant. (Mosses and ferns do not have seeds. They only have a single-cell spore to weather the dry season.)

5. Study the diagram on the following page to be sure you understand the differences in the general life cycles of mosses and ferns as compared to cone plants and flowering plants.

6. There are some structural and reproductive differences between the conifers and the flowering plants. You will discover some of those differences during the Activities in this lab.

COMPARISON OF GENERAL LIFE CYCLES

THIS PART OF THE MOSS AND FERN LIFE CYCLE
IS VULNERABLE TO DRY LAND CONDITIONS.

Sporophyte ⟶ Spores ⟶ Gametophyte ⟶ Swimming Sperm ⟶ Next Sporophyte

THIS PART OF THE CONIFER AND FLOWER LIFE CYCLE
IS PROTECTED FROM DRY LAND CONDITIONS.

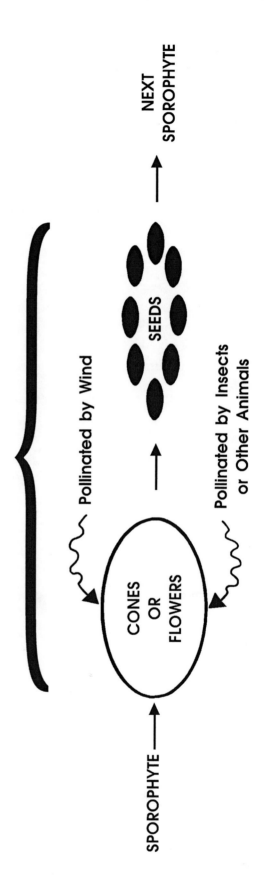

Pollinated by Wind

Pollinated by Insects
or Other Animals

SPOROPHYTE ⟶ CONES OR FLOWERS ⟶ SEEDS ⟶ NEXT SPOROPHYTE

ACTIVITY #2

"CONES"

The word **conifer**, which means "cone-bearing," refers to any plant that uses **cones** as its characteristic reproductive structures. The cone is where the *gametophyte* generation develops. **Remember:** In mosses and ferns the gametophyte has to live independently on the forest floor where it is in danger of drying out and dying.

There are both *male* and *female* cones (the female cone is what people call a "pine cone"). The male cone produces *pollen*, and the female cone produces eggs. Pollen grains contain the male sex cell, and are carried by the wind to the female cones. This is called pollination. After pollination, the pollen grains produce tubes that grow towards the eggs. Fertilization happens when a pollen nucleus (haploid) is transported through the pollen tube and fuses with an egg nucleus (haploid). A diploid seed (pine nut) grows from that union.

MALE CONES

Male cones are small (about 1 to 2 cm in length), and can be found in clusters at the ends of pine branches. They are designed for wind pollination.

GO GET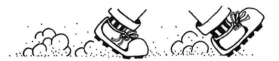

1. A compound microscope.
2. A small sample of pollen from the male cones on display. Look at the design of the male cones when you are at the demonstration table.

Male Cones	Pollen

NOW

1. Draw a simple sketch of a cluster of male cones.
2. Make a wet mount of the pollen and put it under high magnification.
3. Draw a simple sketch of the pollen.

? QUESTION

1. Why is so much pollen produced by each male cone? _____
2. How does the pollen get to the female cones? _____
3. What is the value of the two "ears" on the conifer pollen? _____
4. Which generation is the pollen? (sporophyte or gametophyte) _____

GROWING PINE POLLEN

NOW

1. Ask your instructor if the class will be growing pine pollen, or wait to grow flower pollen in the next Activity.

2. Several hours ago, some pollen from a campus pine tree was put into a weak sugar solution (food).

3. A slide of the growing pollen cells is under the microscope on the Instructor's Table. Look at this slide and draw what you see.

Growing Pollen Cells

? QUESTION

What structure do you see that aids in the delivery of the pollen nucleus to the egg inside the female cone?

FEMALE CONES

Female cones are usually found near the tips and along the higher branches of the pine tree. They start out very small, but there may be more than 100 eggs in each of these cones.

The pollen from the male cone blows onto these female cones when they are very small and the eggs are fairly close to the outside of the cone. Fertilization happens with the union of pollen and egg.

The fertilized egg becomes part of the seed and continues to be protected by the female cone as it grows larger. Eventually the female cone is quite large (what you usually see on a pine tree), and the seeds are now ready to be released into the environment.

GO GET

A prepared microscope slide marked "Pine Megasporangia" (very young female cones).

NOW

1. Put your compound microscope on low power and position the slide.

2. Look for oval structures at the base of the projections from the female cone.

   These are called ovules and each will produce an egg.

   You may be lucky enough to find one with a large egg cell inside.

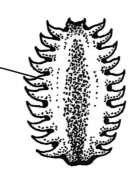

3. Draw a simple sketch of where the egg is found.

4. *Return the slide to where you got it.*

? QUESTION

Which generation (sporophyte or gametophyte) of the conifer life cycle actually produces the egg, and is being protected inside the female cone? _____

(This is the same generation of the moss and fern life cycle that has to live unprotected and on its own.)

SEEDS

Seeds are a "land habitat" feature of both conifers and flowering plants. (There are no seeds in mosses and ferns.)

The seeds of conifers can be found inside the female cone about one year after pollination. The mature seeds are released into the environment and must survive on their own. Because conifers do not have nutritive fruit surrounding the seeds, they are called **gymnosperms** (meaning "naked seeds").

The seeds of flowering plants are found inside the fruit, which gives these plants their name—**angiosperms** (meaning "covered seeds"). The fruit is discussed in more detail in the next Activity.

GO GET

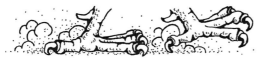

1. A dissecting microscope.

2. A pine seed (soaking in water).

3. A dissecting probe.

1. If your pine seeds haven't been shelled, then carefully crack the seed coat with pliers. Under the microscope, use your probe and carefully remove the seed tissue from the outer part of the pine seed until the *plant embryo* can be seen.

2. Show your instructor.

? QUESTION

1. What function does the seed coat provide?

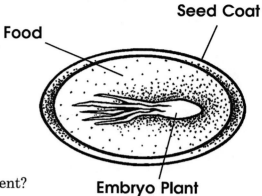

2. Why is this a better adaptation to a dry land environment?

3. The embryo inside the seed is which generation of the conifer life cycle (gametophyte or sporophyte)?

ACTIVITY #3

"FLOWERS AND FRUIT"

Flowers are like "neon signs" to attract pollinators (usually insects, birds, and mammals). Color, fragrance, nectar, and shape are some of the more important features that determine which pollinators will be attracted to a particular flower species.

Examine each flower in this lab to see if you can determine what kind of pollinator might be involved with the reproduction of the plant. If a plant can involve another species to help it with reproduction, then that plant will be more successful than a plant that must rely on the wind for pollination.

GO GET

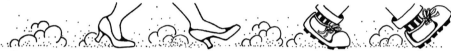

1. A tree-tobacco flower.

2. Dissecting materials—a probe, a pair of tweezers, and a razor blade.

NOW

1. The basic theme of most flowers is: The male organs surround the female organ. The male organs are called the **stamens**, and they contain the pollen. The female organ is called the **pistil**, and it contains the eggs.

2. Use the dissecting microscope to look at the open end of the tree-tobacco flower.

   Does any reproductive organ stick up higher than the others?

   What color is the tip of that organ?

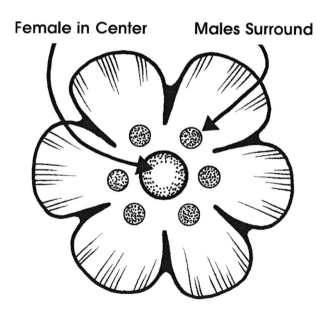

Female in Center   **Males Surround**

Hypothetical Simple Flower

3. Carefully tear open the top half of the flower so that you can better see the reproductive organs. If you see several identical filaments, then you have found the males (*stamens*). *Remember:* There will only be one female (*pistil*).

Can you now determine which organ sticks up highest in the flower?

What would be the value of the female organ being higher than the stamens?

4. Continue to tear the yellow petal until it is removed from the green base of the flower.

Draw a simple sketch of the arrangement of pistil and stamens in the box provided.

Tree-Tobacco Flower

THEN

1. Using the compound microscope, make a wet mount slide of some pollen from the stamen.

2. Draw a simple sketch of what you see.

Does the flower pollen have "ears" like the conifer pollen?

What does this tell you about the mechanism of pollination in this species?

3. Cut open the green base of the flower with a razor blade, and find the eggs using the dissecting microscope.

This part of the pistil is called the *ovary*.

You may see young seeds if your flower is older.

4. Draw a simple sketch of the pistil with its eggs or seeds.

Flower Pollen

Pistil

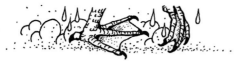

GO GET

1. A citrus flower without the fruit. (You can use the Tree-Tobacco fruits if citrus flowers and fruits are unavailable.)

2. Another citrus flower with the fruit.

NOW

1. *Don't dissect the flowers!* We need to save them for use in other classes.

   Look at the two flowers and determine what part of the flower grows into the fruit.

2. Different species produce fruit from different parts of the flower, and the fruit usually attracts some kind of animal to eat it.

3. *Return the flowers for other students to use.*

? QUESTION

1. What specific part of the flower becomes the fruit?

2. What kind of pollinators might this flower attract?

3. Explain how an animal can disperse seeds by eating a fruit.

4. Flowers typically grow in small clumps scattered in their habitat, whereas conifers typically grow in large groves of trees. How does this difference in distribution relate to your answer in question #3?

ACTIVITY #4

"VASCULAR TISSUE IN STEMS AND ROOTS"

Vascular tissue is an evolutionary invention occurring near the time of the first fern plants. In these early ferns, the conducting tissue was only moderately developed, which is one reason that fern plants can't get water from deep in the ground.

The cone plants and flowering plants developed a much better system of vascular tissue, and their resulting success in dry land environments is obvious.

The vascular system in plants is analogous to the circulatory system in animals. It is a network of vertical tubes that extend from the leaves to the roots. As a general rule, the cell walls forming the tubes are very thick when compared to other cells in the leaves, stems, and roots.

You will be looking at prepared *cross-sections* of the plant parts.

Remember that you are seeing a section cut through the stem. You will have to imagine the three-dimensional vertical tube structure that makes up the vascular tissue.

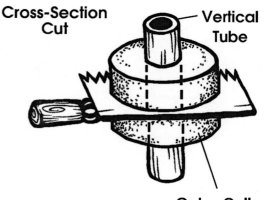

Cross-Section Cut — **Vertical Tube** — **Outer Cells of Stem**

 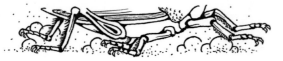

1. A prepared microscope slide of a "Root Cross-Section."

2. A prepared microscope slide of a "Herbaceous Stem Cross-Section."

Look at the root cross-section under low magnification, and determine where most of the vascular tissue is located. (The vascular tubes are *thick-walled* cells.)

Draw a simple sketch of the root showing the location of the vascular tissue.

The nutrients and water in the soil must diffuse into the vascular tubes.

Now that you know where the vascular tubes actually are, what does this tell you about the size of the roots that do the absorption for a plant? (Is it the big roots or the small roots?)

Root

Look at the herbaceous stem cross-section under low magnification, and determine where the vascular tissue is located. (circle your choice)

Stem

Center of the or Towards the outside stem of the stem

Hint: The arrangement in the stem is called "vascular bundles."

This arrangement of vascular bundles is common in plants.

Draw a simple sketch of the distribution of vascular tissue in the stem.

? QUESTION

An unthinking person made a cut with a pocket knife all the way around the trunk of a tree. The tree died soon after.

Explain why the tree died.

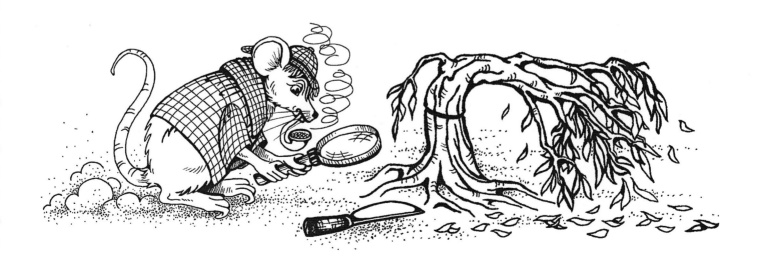

ACTIVITY #5

"WOOD"

The wood that we use to build our houses comes from the stiff cell walls that are a part of the plant's vascular system. This part is called the *xylem*, and it conducts water from the roots in the ground up to the leaves at the tips of every branch. *Remember:* Water is one of the necessary ingredients for photosynthesis, which takes place in the leaves.

The xylem continues to be produced on the inside of an ever-expanding growth ring called the *cambium*. Cambium is just inside the bark of a living trunk or branch. It is shown as a "dashed" circle in the diagram.

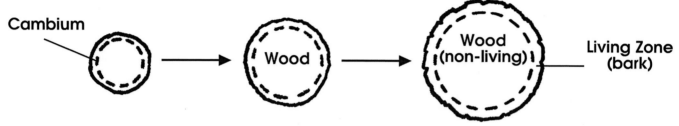

The xylem continues to conduct water even after it dies. This tissue is somewhat like thousands of tiny straws that transport water and provide support for the tree at the same time. The water moves up the xylem by a process called *capillary action*. Your textbook explains the details of capillarity and the osmotic "pushing" forces in the roots. In larger trees, the middle section fills with resin and no longer transports water, but functions only as a supporting structure.

A thin zone of living vascular tubes called the *phloem* is produced on the outside of the cambium. These tubes carry sugars from the leaves to the roots for storage. The outermost part of the bark is the remains of dead phloem that has been pushed out by the ever expanding cambium.

? QUESTION

1. In a forest fire, sometimes the inside of a tree can be badly burned, forming a hollow in the tree trunk, yet the tree doesn't die. How do you explain that?

2. What specific part of the vascular tissue is the wood of the tree?

3. What specific cellular feature of vascular tissue makes it ideal as a building material for our houses?

4. What specific part of the vascular tissue is produced on the outside of the cambium?

5. What specific part of the vascular tissue is produced on the inside of the cambium?

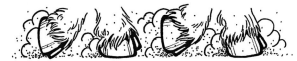

A prepared microscope slide marked "Woody Stem."

NOW

1. Look at the slide under the lowest power of the dissecting microscope and find the annual rings of tissue. These are called *tree rings*.

2. Find these same rings with your compound microscope and look carefully at the individual cells of the rings.

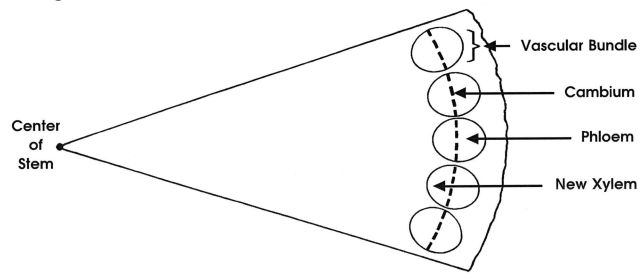

3. Draw the tree rings in the above diagram, and show how the cell *size* changes in these rings. By the way, you should be able to see the vascular bundles that are towards the outside of the stem.

? QUESTION

1. What is the direction of time as you move outward from the center of the tree stem?

2. Where are the youngest tree rings?

3. What would cause these annual rings to show the cell size change that you see?

   a. When would you see big cells? _____

   b. When would you see small cells? _____

ACTIVITY #6

"LEAVES"

The most basic purpose of a leaf is to expose chlorophyll to light so that the plant can perform photosynthesis.

There are a number of problems that a leaf has to overcome to be successful. Some of those challenges include:

1. A leaf has to get water from the roots as a raw material for photosynthesis, and it has to send sugars made during photosynthesis to the rest of the plant.

2. A leaf has to get CO_2 as a raw material for photosynthesis, and this carbon dioxide has to be delivered to all of the cells in the leaf.

3. A leaf has to catch light energy for photosynthesis, but not overheat from absorbing too much sunlight.

4. A leaf must not lose too much water from evaporation, or the plant will dry up.

LEAF VEINS

Leaf veins are vascular bundles leading to various parts of the leaf. The pattern of veins depends on the type of plant and the shape of the leaf. However, in all cases, these veins are used for carrying water to the leaf cells and for carrying photosynthetic sugars away from the leaf cells.

GO GET

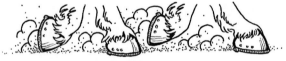

A broad leaf from the *mallow tree*. (We will have it in the lab, or your instructor will tell you where you can find it.)

NOW

1. Look at the leaf under the dissecting microscope, and determine the pattern of leaf veins. You already have some information about these structures from Activity #3.

2. Draw a simple sketch of the pattern of veins in this mallow leaf.

Leaf Veins

What is carried in these mallow leaf veins? (Be specific about the content and direction and purpose.)

LEAF STOMATA

Leaf stomata are openings on the underside of the leaves. We looked at stomata in the *Zebrina* plant during the Cell Lab earlier in the semester.

If you didn't get a chance to see these structures, then make a leaf peel now and search for them.

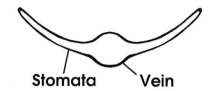

Stomata   Vein

GO GET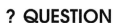

A prepared microscope slide of a cross-section of a leaf.

Cross-Section

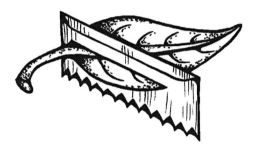

NOW

1. First, locate the vein so that you know where you are.

2. Look for the stomata on the underside of the leaf.

   The guard cells are round in cross-section instead of being like "lips" in the leaf peel. Some of the guard cells are sectioned through the middle so that you can see the stomata opening.

3. Draw a simple sketch of the structural relationship between the stomata and the clear spaces inside the leaf. Also, show the vein. Label each part.

Leaf Cross-Section

? QUESTION

Describe how the CO_2 gets into the leaf and to the interior cells of the leaf.

COMPARISONS OF LEAF TYPES

NOW

We have selected four leaf types to demonstrate different leaf adaptations. Carefully look at each leaf on display, and make a simple sketch of each. Your instructor may use local plants to represent the four leaf types.

Mallow (Broad-flat)

Pine (Needle-like)

Jojoba (Upward pointing)

Buckwheat (Very small)

Study your drawings of these four leaf types and then answer the questions on the next page.

1. Which leaf design is best for catching the most light? _____

2. Which leaf design would absorb the most heat? _____

3. Which leaf design loses water the fastest, and must live in a wetter environment than the rest? _____

4. The jojoba leaf does better than the pine leaf in very dry environments. What features of the jojoba help the leaf lose less water than the pine leaf?

5. Notice the orientation of the jojoba and buckwheat leaves. What time of the day do these two leaf types absorb more light? _____

   What part of the day do they absorb less light and heat? _____

   What advantage is there to this kind of leaf orientation to the sun?

Chapter 13

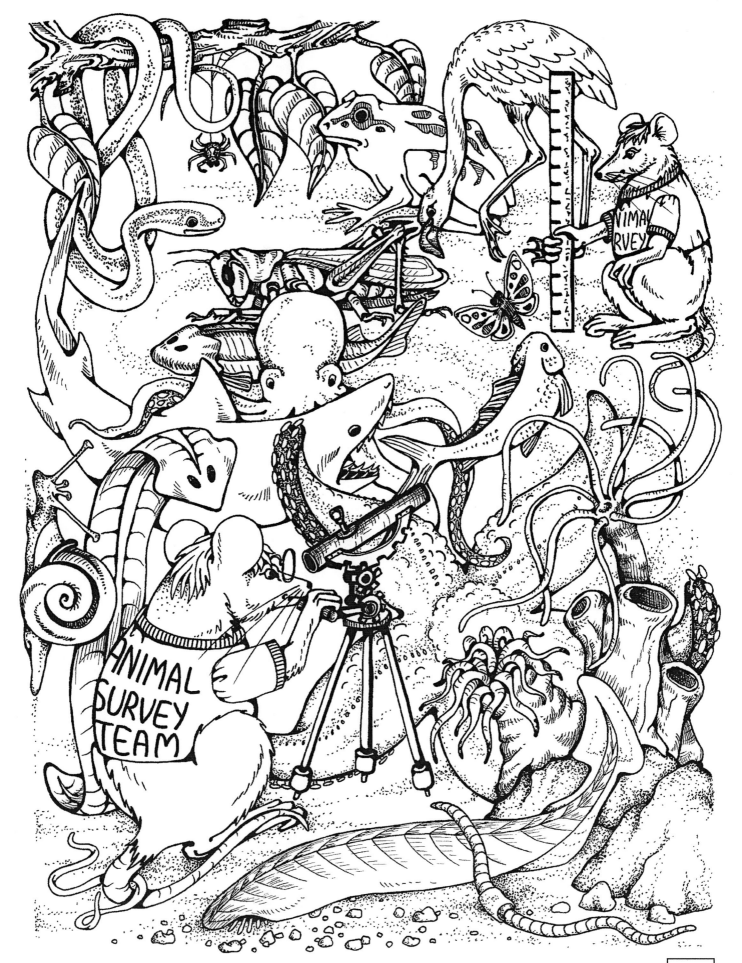

Bergman's Rule: a non-exclusive generalization postulating that smaller species tend to evolve in hot climates and large species evolve in colder climates.

—"MAMMALS AND CLIMATE CHANGE" BY ELIZABETH HADLEY, *FORA.TV ONLINE,* 2010

The oldest known animal organism is a brain coral in the waters around Tabago; it is 2,000 years old.

—"THE WORLD'S OLDEST LIVING ORGANISMS" BY RACHEL SUSSMAN, A FINE ARTS PHOTOGRAPHER, FORA.TV, 2011

Bioluminescence is the largest source of light in the deep oceans. Ninety percent (90%) of all creatures who live below 1,500 feet emit their own light.

—"20 THINGS YOU DIDN'T KNOW ABOUT LIGHT" BY LEEAUNDRA KEANY, *DISCOVER MAGAZINE,* MARCH 2010, P. 80

The Global Ocean Conveyor Belt is crucial to life in the oceans. It wraps around all the continents delivering heat to the polar regions, cooling and sinking, bringing oxygen from the surface to the depths then being drawn up to be warmed again. This cycle continues around and around like a huge circle.

—*UNDERWATER UNIVERSE,* BY LONE WOLF DOCUMENTARY GROUP FOR THE HISTORY CHANNEL, 2011

Volcanos erupting in Siberia 250 million years ago caused a 90% extinction event for the entire planet. The eruptions lasted for 700,000 years, emitting lava gases and CO_2 that heated the earth's atmosphere and oceans. The water temperature increase prevented cooler water at the poles from sinking, slowing the Global Ocean Converyor Belt. This released CO_2 and O_2 gasses carried in the water, warming the atmosphere even more and depleting the oceans of oxygen. Everything began to die. It is estimated that it took 5 million years for the water system—and life—to recover.

—*UNDERWATER UNIVERSE,* BY LONE WOLF DOCUMENTARY GROUP FOR THE HISTORY CHANNEL, 2011

According to the group Global Wildlife Conservation, 32 percent of the world's known amphibian species are threatened with extinction, largely because of habitat loss or pollution.

—HTTP://NEWS.YAHOO.COM/SCIENTISTS-DISCOVER-12-FROG-SPECIES-INDIA-095127170.HTML

Sharks are remarkably resistant to viruses. A molecule called *squalamine,* found in sharks, appears to destroy human liver viruses that cause hepatitis, and may be a future treatment for other viral and microbial infections in humans.

—HTTP://NEWS.YAHOO.COM/SHARK-MOLECULE-KILLS-HUMAN-VIRUSES-TOO-191207486.HTML

SURVEY OF ANIMALS

INTRODUCTION

This lab is a brief survey of the Animals—organisms that are eukaryotic, multicellular, and heterotrophic. You will investigate some of the defining characteristics and evolutionary relationships that divide these animals into subgroups called phylum and class.

The taxonomic story presented in textbooks gives the impression that more complex forms of life were created sequentially during evolution. This portrayal is convenient for viewing life from a human perspective, but evolution doesn't "climb the ladder" toward perfection. In fact, there is evidence to the contrary. For example, the reptiles as a group have enjoyed a much longer and more diverse history than the mammals, your group. Mammals evolved from an early reptile form and so did birds. That poses an interesting question. Evolutionary speaking, which is the more successful lifeform—a lizard or a human?

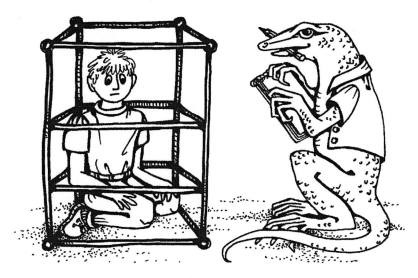

But, before arguing about it or before you place yourself at the top or bottom of the evolutionary heap, consider the one animal group that far out-numbers all of the other animal groups combined. That group is the **arthropods**. By number and diversity, they are the dominant animal in both the aquatic and land environments on this planet!

Although humans are out-numbered and out-diversified, and haven't been on Earth for very long, we are the ones who have begun to figure out the whole story. This lab will explore both the *invertebrates* (animals without a backbone), and the *vertebrates* (animals with a backbone).

ACTIVITIES

ACTIVITY #1

"ORIGIN OF THE ANIMALS"

Modern biology tells the history of life as best as we can with the scientific evidence we have. There are a few accepted generalizations.

▶ The fossils of simple one-celled organisms, called prokaryotes (before the nucleus), date back to almost 4 billion years ago.

▶ The oldest fossils of more advanced cell-types, called eukaryotes (have a nucleus), date between 1–1½ billion years ago.

▶ Fossils of multicellular organisms appear between ¾ and 1 billion years ago.

▶ The DNA comparisons of today's organisms suggest that there could have been four or more different paths of multicellular life.

The diagram below illustrates the interconnectedness of all life.

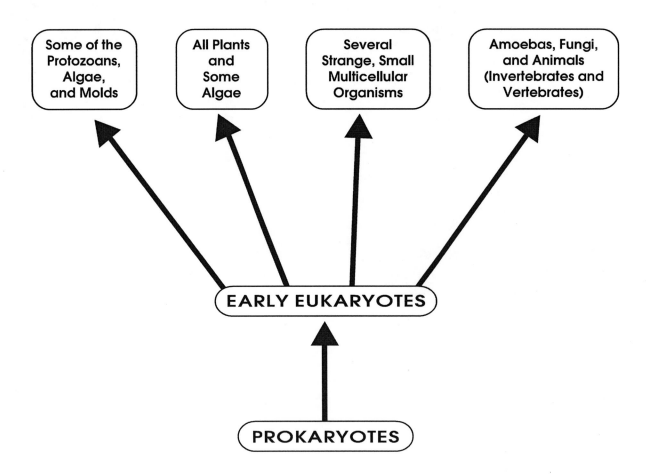

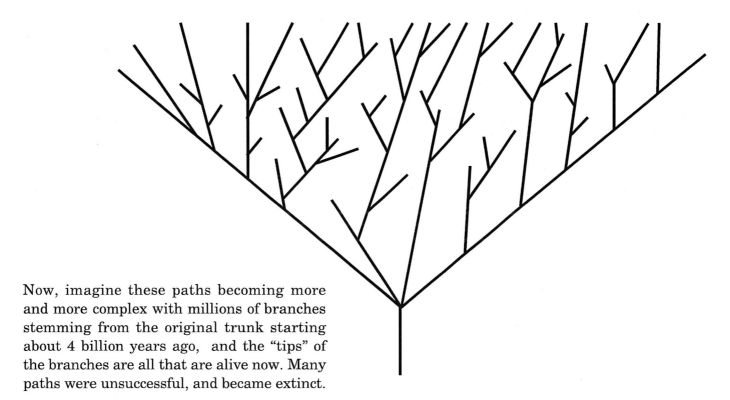

Now, imagine these paths becoming more and more complex with millions of branches stemming from the original trunk starting about 4 billion years ago, and the "tips" of the branches are all that are alive now. Many paths were unsuccessful, and became extinct.

All of this complex branching, with extinct branches, and new branching, etc. happened over and over so many times that we will never know the whole story of life. But we do have three kinds of evidence that will help us to solve parts of this impossible puzzle.

▶ Fossils
▶ Features of living animals
▶ DNA of living animals

We have a long way to go to tell the history of life. We will be working, reworking, and retelling this story for a long, long time to come.

? QUESTION

1. An animal without a backbone is called an _____.

2. An animal with a backbone is called a _____.

3. Which is the most successful animal group? (both by number and diversity) _____

4. The oldest fossils of prokaryotic cells are about how old?

5. The oldest fossils of eukaryotic cells are about how old?

6. The oldest fossils of multicellular organisms are about how old?

7. List the three kinds of scientific evidence that help us to discover the history of animal life.

ACTIVITY #2

"TAXONOMY AND CLASSIFICATION"

Taxonomy is the process of identifying genetic traits (called characters) with the goal being to name animals or plants (if they are unknown) or to find their scientific name (if they are known). This general way of naming an organism is called the binomial system and uses genus and species.

Genus is a collection of different species that share many common features, but these different species cannot interbreed to produce fertile offspring. Humans, for example, are in genus *Homo* and species *sapiens*. Our taxonomic name is *Homo sapiens*. No other species but humans are *sapiens*. In fact, no other hominid still exists but *Homo sapiens*.

In taxonomy there are a number of categories starting with the most general groups (Domains) and ending with the most specific groups (species). An older style of expressing taxonomic classification of humans would list similar groups in a table like that on page 234.

The modern method of grouping organisms is by Phylogenetic Classification. *Phylogeny* is the description of the evolutionary history of a taxonomic group. In other words, it is the story of the steps in evolution that led to a particular group of organisms. We have recently discovered that mammals are evolved from an early reptile group, so the modern phylogenetic classification would have Mammals listed under Reptiles instead of alongside of them as in earlier taxonomic classification.

CATEGORY	EXAMPLE
Domain	Eukaryotes
Kingdom	Animalia
Phylum	Chordata
Class	Reptilia
Subclass	Mammalia
Order	Primate
Family	Hominid
Genus	Homo
Species	sapiens

The most recent method for showing the phylogenetic classification is called *cladistics*. These diagrams of evolutionary history are called *cladograms* (meaning "branch diagram"). Each cladogram has a record of significant new characters (mutations) that caused separation along the "branches" in the diagram. Cladograms organize taxonomic groups not only by what they have in common, but also by how they differ from each other.

Each "bar" in the cladogram represents a defining evolutionary character or trait. The placement of any "bar" on the horizontal line of the cladogram means that the species on the right side of it (including vertical branches) have that character trait or some modification of it. Any "bar" on a vertical branch defines only the species above the bar.

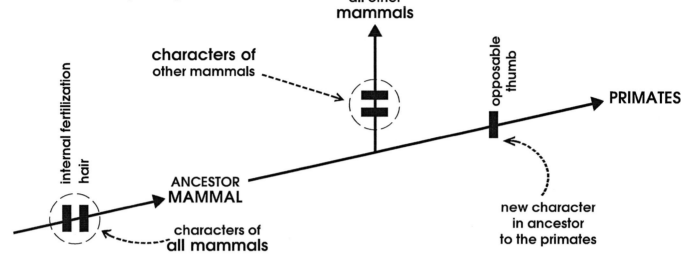

Cladograms present a more detailed history of life. Every new evolutionary character has to be correctly placed. There are rules for this diagram phylogenetic classification. Evolutionary biologists must present direct evidence or a convincing theory when they decide to place a character on a specific branch of a cladogram.

RULE 1	A unique character happens only once. No organism had that particular feature before that point in evolution. All of the taxonomic groups on the branch beyond the new character trait either have that feature or some direct modification of it.
RULE 2	Some features (like wings, or a complete digestive tract, or segmentation) were so valuable for survival that they evolved independently more than once during the history of life. For example, insects, bats, and birds all have wings. However, those wings were created by modifications of different genes. They are not derived from the same ancestral gene, and they develop differently in the embryo. Therefore, each new wing feature occupies a different "bar" in the complete cladogram of animals.
RULE 3	Some evolutionary events are called reversals. A group can lose a character it had before. For example, land vertebrates had four legs. One of the groups lost its limbs and became the ancestor of snakes. (Someone could make a mistake in thinking that snakes are ancestors of legged animals, when actually they are the descendants.)
RULE 4	The more similar the DNA of two groups, the closer they are to a common ancestor. Group placement in a cladogram must reflect these DNA comparisons or the cladogram is incorrect.

1. The process of describing or identifying animal characters with the goals of naming them is called _____.

2. The binomial naming system includes _____ and _____.

3. Arranging organisms into groups and showing their evolutionary history and common ancestors is called _____ classification.

4. Another way of telling the history of life is by using a diagram that illustrates the above arrangement. It is called a _____.

FINALLY

The classification systems we have been discussing are ways to understand and describe *Kingdom Animalia*. The following list is a preview of some of the animals you will cover next.

KINGDOM ANIMALIA

Phylum Porifera: .... sponges

Phylum Cnidaria: .... jellyfish and hydra

Phylum Platyhelminthes: .... flatworms

Phylum Nematoda: .... roundworms

Phylum Mollusca: .... mollusks

Phylum Annelida: .... segmented worms

Phylum Arthropoda: .... arthropods

Phylum Echinodermata: .... echinoderms

Phylum Chordata: .... *Amphioxus*

Subphylum Vertebrata:

Class Agnatha: .... jawless fishes

Class Chondrichthyes: .... cartilage fishes

Class Osteichthyes: .... bony fishes

Class Amphibia: .... frogs

Class Reptilia: .... lizards

SubClass Aves: .... birds

SubClass Mammalia: .... mammals

HISTORY OF LIFE CHART

Times When Various Life Groups Occurred on this Planet

Group Name	Earliest Fossil Evidence	Time of Greatest Success for Group
Anaerobic Life	4 billion years ago	3.9 to 3.3 billion years ago
Stromatolites (photosynthetic bacteria and aerobic bacteria)	3.5 billion years ago	3 billion to 700 million years ago
Eukaryotic Cells (Protists)	2 billion years ago	1 billion years ago to today
Invertebrate Animals	1 billion years ago	500 million years ago to today
Early Chordates	600 million years ago	_____
Jawless Fish	500 million years ago	480 to 370 million years ago
Cartilage Fish	400 million years ago	380 to 240 million years ago
Bony Fish	380 million years ago	66 million years ago to today
Lobe-Finned Fish	370 million years ago	_____
Lung Fish	370 million years ago	
Amphibians	350 million years ago	320 to 240 million years ago
Early Reptiles	300 million years ago	230 to 210 million years ago
Dinosaurs	210 million years ago	180 to 66 million years ago (extinct 66 million years ago)
Mammals	200 million years ago	66 million years ago to today
Birds	180 million years ago	66 million years ago to today
Humans	1.5 million years ago	today

THE HISTORY OF LIFE

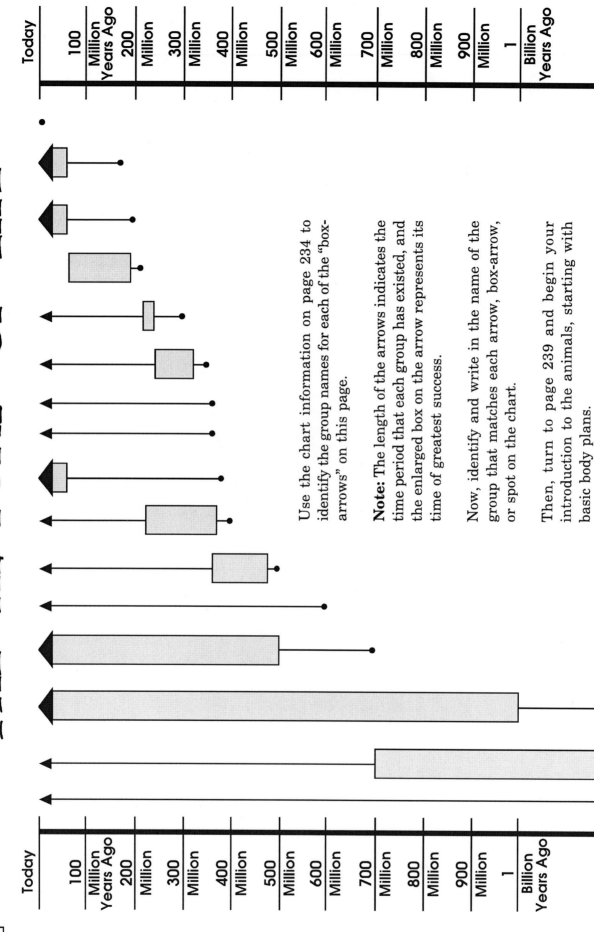

Use the chart information on page 234 to identify the group names for each of the "box-arrows" on this page.

Note: The length of the arrows indicates the time period that each group has existed, and the enlarged box on the arrow represents its time of greatest success.

Now, identify and write in the name of the group that matches each arrow, box-arrow, or spot on the chart.

Then, turn to page 239 and begin your introduction to the animals, starting with basic body plans.

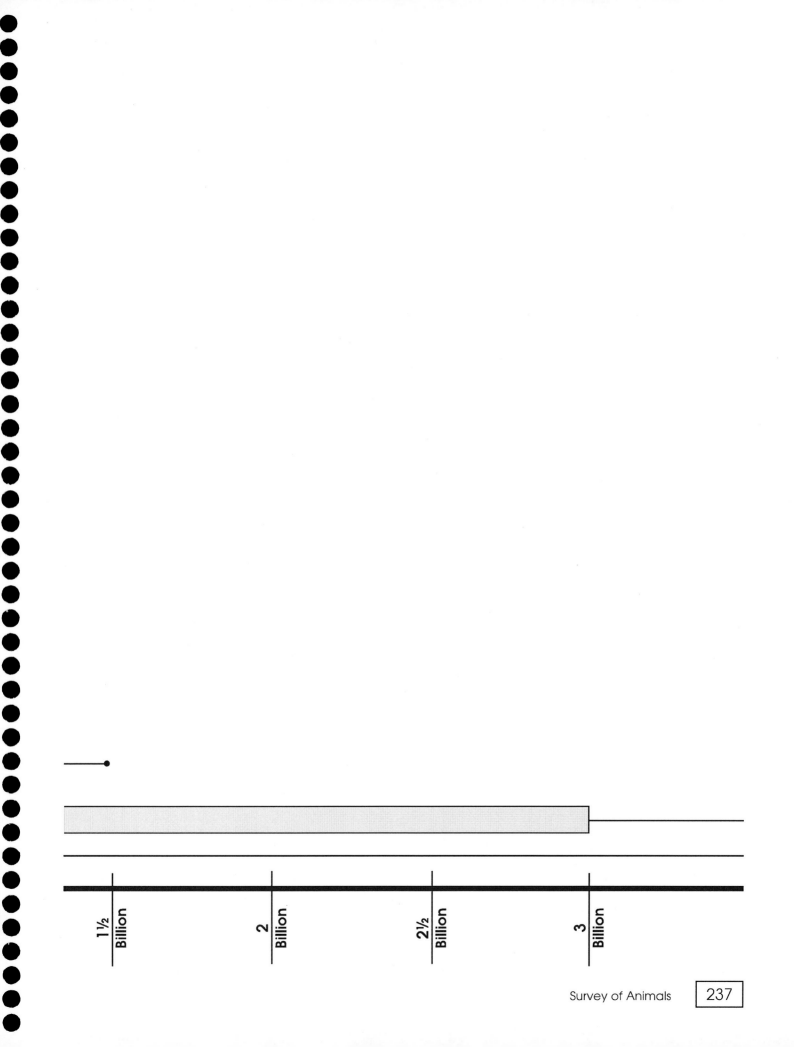

1½
Billion

2
Billion

2½
Billion

3
Billion

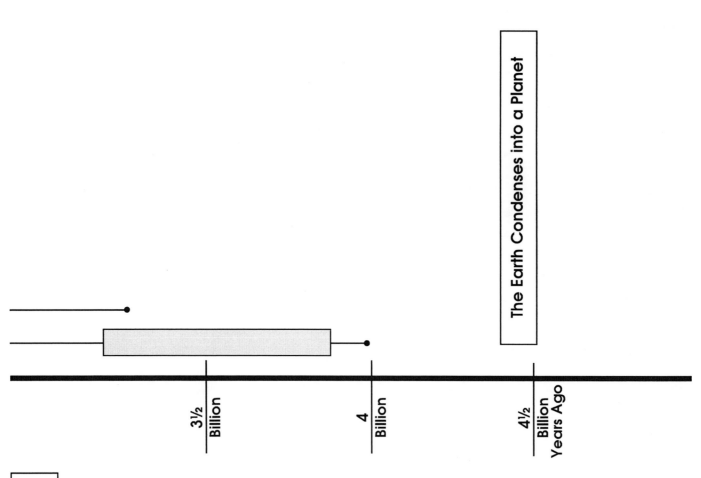

The Earth Condenses into a Planet

3½
Billion

4
Billion

4½
Billion
Years Ago

ACTIVITY #3

"BASIC BODY PLAN"

There are three basic body plans found in the animal groups—*no symmetry*, *radial symmetry*, and *bilateral symmetry*.

NO SYMMETRY

(no directionality)

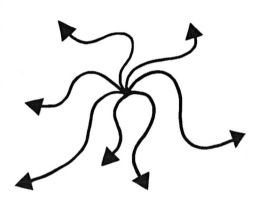

An animal with this design grows in all directions, usually on the surface of something else, and typically has no particular defining form.

These organisms do not respond to stimuli in their environment because they don't have a nervous system.

Each part of the organism can act independently of the other parts.

We will look at only one group with this design—the sponges.

RADIAL SYMMETRY

(radial directionality)

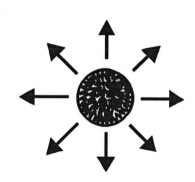

An animal with radial symmetry can be divided into two equal-looking halves by any cut through the longitudinal axis (like cutting a pie or a ball in half).

These animals move or react to the environment equally in all directions.

This design does not have a head end and a tail end, and does not search for and locate its food like the next group does. To get food, this animal is usually stationary or is carried by water currents, capturing the food that passes by. Jellyfish and sea anemones are examples of radial symmetry.

To get food, this animal is usually stationary or is carried by water currents, capturing the food that passes by. There are some predators with radial symmetry, like the seastars, but their sense organs are dispersed over the surface of the animal and are not concentrated at one end of the animal.

BILATERAL SYMMETRY

(head and tail ends)

Bilateral means "two sides," and there is only one way to cut the animal into two equal-looking halves.

An animal with this design responds to its environment by using directional movement. Its head end is the location of the sense organs, and orients to different kinds of environmental stimuli such as light and food. Flatworms are the first example of bilateral symmetry that we will consider.

This organism is designed to search for and locate things in its habitat, including its food.

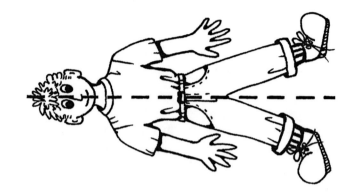

SPONGES

The oldest animal fossils discovered are sponges from the late Precambrian Era (nearly 600 million years ago). A biochemical residue of sponges has been found in geologic sediments more than a billion years old. Of all organisms, the sponges may represent the first multicellular animals on our planet. They have no symmetry.

The phylum name for sponges is Porifera which means "to have holes." Water flows in through some of the openings and flows back out of others. As the water percolates through the sponge various small particles of food and bacteria are removed from the water and engulfed by special amoeba-like cells. The water canal system through a sponge is one of three types from very simple to quite complex. And the skeletal structure is provided by a meshwork of spicules made of either glass, calcium, or spongin (a protein fiber).

1. A dissecting microscope.

2. A small glass dish for the specimen.

3. A small piece of preserved sponge.

NOW

1. Place the piece of the sponge onto the dish, and add enough fluid to cover the specimen.

2. Use the dissecting microscope to observe the general symmetry and structure of the sponge. Notice the many holes.

3. Draw a picture of the sponge and label its parts.

4. Return the sponge sample for other students to use.

JELLYFISH TYPES

Jellyfish and sea anemones belong in a phylum named Cnidaria which means "to sting." There are two unique evolutionary characters found in this group: stinging cells and radial symmetry. Radial symmetry orients an animal to its environment in all directions at the same time. The jellyfish types and all groups following them also have tissues. Tissues are groups of identical cells that work together to perform a particular function. The Cnidarians have two primary tissue layers, with various other cell types scattered through the organism.

These organisms feed by stinging their prey and pulling them into a gastrovascular cavity where they are digested. There are two body forms: polyp (the sea anemone) and medusa (the jellyfish form). Many species alternate between both forms as parts of their life cycle.

GO GET

1. A dissecting microscope.

2. A living hydra or preserved small jellyfish.

NOW

Cnidaria

1. Compare the two body forms at the demonstration table.

2. If you are to examine a living hydra, follow the specific directions of your lab instructor. Otherwise, obtain a preserved specimen of a small jellyfish, and follow the same general procedure you used to examine the sponge.

3. Draw a picture of your Cnidaria.

4. Return your specimen for other students to use.

FLATWORMS

You've seen no symmetry as represented by the sponges, and radial symmetry exemplified by jellyfish types. The next step in evolution comes with bilateral symmetry. The first group illustrating that feature is the flatworm. These worms are flat and we'll use that as their unique trait on the cladogram later. Although the word bilateral means "two sides," the importance of this symmetry is that it results in a head end and a tail end. Bilateral animals are directional. As such, bilateral animals are better designed to focus on where they are going. And because they have a head end they very effectively search through their environment.

Flatworms have three primary tissue layers. And they have organs. The earlier groups did not. An organ is made of a group of tissues working together for a united function. However, because flatworms are not complex organisms, they do not have organ systems like a circulatory system. This limitation means that flatworms depend on diffusion to move nutrients and waste products around their bodies. They are forced to be very flat in order to facilitate diffusion.

GO GET

1. A dissecting microscope.

2. A plasti-mount of a flatworm.

3. A living planarian flatworm.

NOW

1. View the flatworm from the top and the side. You should easily see why they are called flatworms. Using the dissecting microscope, see if you can identify any of the organs or structures that are shown in the anatomical diagram on the demonstration table.

2. If there are living planarian flatworms, carefully remove one with a probe or dropper. Include a small amount of water from the container for the flatworm to move through. Examine with the dissecting microscope.

3. Draw a picture of the flatworm.

4. There are also examples of parasitic flatworms (tapeworms and flukes) at the demonstration table.

5. When you have finished, please return all specimens to their appropriate containers for other students to use.

Flatworm

1. Which type of symmetry is displayed by the sponge?

2. The taxonomic name of the sponges is phylum *Porifera*, which means "hole bearing." Is your sponge full of holes?

3. Which type of symmetry is displayed by the hydra and jellyfish?

4. Jellyfish and hydras are in the phylum *Cnidaria*, which means "stinging cells." How are stinging cells used by these animals?

5. Which type of symmetry is displayed by the flatworm?

6. The flatworms are in the phylum *Platyhelminthes*, which means "broad, flat stem." What does this definition tell you about the shape of these organisms?

7. What are the two most obvious characteristics of flatworms?

    _____ and _____

8. Put the three animal subgroups (hydra, flatworm, and sponge) in order of increasing complexity or symmetry.

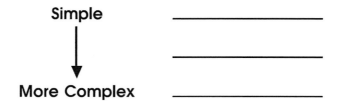

Simple   _____

↓   _____

More Complex _____

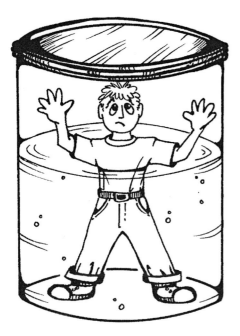

Please return all specimens to the specimen table so that the other labs may also use them.

Do not throw away any preserved animals or *you* will be added to our collection!

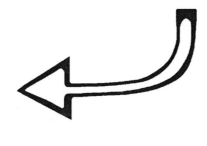

ACTIVITY #4

"TYPE OF DIGESTIVE SYSTEM"

There are two basic designs for the digestive system within the Animal phyla—incomplete and complete gut.

INCOMPLETE GUT

Basically, this digestive system consists of a tube with only one opening to the outside. The food is taken into the tube through the mouth and it is digested. After digestion is completed, the waste products are ejected from the animal through the same opening.

Animals with an incomplete gut do not have excretory and circulatory systems. Therefore, they are dependent on diffusion to obtain nutrients from digestion and to get rid of waste products. Example phyla are sponges, jellyfish, and flatworms.

COMPLETE GUT

This digestive system consists of a tube extending completely through the organism. There are two openings-one for taking in food, and another for eliminating the waste products of digestion. These animals have excretory and circulatory systems to transport nutrients to all body cells and to remove wastes from those cells for transport to the outside of the organism.

The complete gut trait was so efficient at processing food that it evolved independently at least two different times in evolution-once in the evolutionary branch leading to roundworms, mollusks, annelids, and arthropods (the Protostomes); and again in the branch leading to the echinoderms and chordates (the Deuterostomes). The names of these two branches refer to the way the digestive system forms in the developing embryo. Protostome means "first mouth"; Deuterostome means "second mouth."

ROUNDWORMS

Roundworms are Protosomes and can be found in almost all environments. Roundworms are in phylum Nematoda, which means "thread-like." Most are very small-just visible with a magnifying glass. They consume dead plants and animals, and are important in the ecological recycling of organic matter in both soil and water. Some are parasitic. The example used in this lab is Ascaris, the "dog roundworm." It is unusually large and easy to dissect.

Special evolutionary traits include the complete digestive tract and the round body shape. That shape formed because this group evolved body systems. Systems are groups of organs that work together for a united function-like digestive, circulatory, and excretory. Roundworms and all the following groups are not forced to have a body shape devoted to diffusion like their precursors.

1. Dissecting microscope.

2. Preserved Ascaris specimen.

3. Dissecting equipment.

NOW

1. The instructions at the demonstration table will indicate whether you are to do your own dissection, or observe the previously dissected specimen instead. Now, observe the dissected Ascaris roundworm.

2. Notice the general appearance of the roundworm and compare it to the form of the flatworm. What obvious difference do you notice?

3. Try to identify some of the internal organs as indicated on the anatomical diagram at the demonstration table.

4. Draw a simple sketch of the roundworm, and label some of its organs.

Roundworm

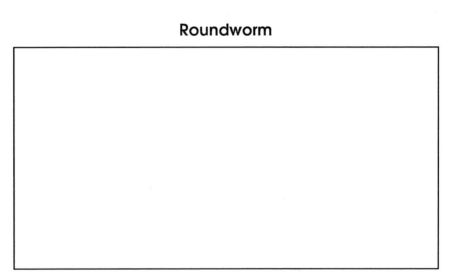

5. If you dissected, please discard all remains appropriately.

1. Sponges are full of holes, jellyfish are big open sacs, and flatworms are flat. How are these features important in facilitating the process of diffusion?

2. Roundworms are round. Is a round shape a better shape for diffusion than a flat shape? Explain.

3. If the basic body design of an animal like the roundworm is not designed for diffusion, then how do they transport nutrients and waste products?

4. The shape of roundworms would favor . . . (circle your choice)

   Swimming   or   Burrowing

5. Which digestive system would you call an "eating machine"-one more efficient at getting nutrients? (circle your choice)

   Incomplete gut   or   Complete gut

6. If an animal group is more efficient at getting nutrients, then it will probably be . . . (circle your choice)

   More successful   or   Less successful

7. Draw a simple sketch of an incomplete digestive tract.

   Which animal groups have an incomplete gut?

   Example   **Phylum**

   _____   _____

   _____   _____

   _____   _____

8. Draw a simple sketch of a complete digestive tract.

   Which animal group has a complete gut?

   Example   **Phylum**

   _____   _____

9. Which digestive system type do you belong to?

ACTIVITY #5

"SEGMENTATION"

Segmentation is a body design resulting from a radical change in the normal development of an animal. This unique evolutionary feature allowed a "new" kind of animal to develop.

In segmentation, blocks of embryonic tissue are duplicated instead of remaining as one single block.

 Original Animal 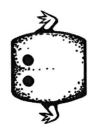 **Segmented Animal**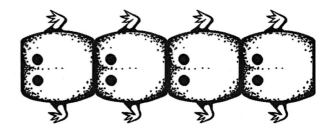

These repetitive blocks result in an organism that is a combination of segments. This "new" animal is like making a chain of the original animal, linked together, one after the other.

Segmentation is another trait so valuable to animals that it may have evolved at least twice—once in the evolutionary branch leading to annelids and arthropods, and again in the branch leading to chordates.

GO GET

Go to the specimen table.

NOW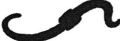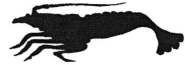

1. Put a roundworm, an earthworm, a millipede, and a crayfish next to each other in that order.

    You have just laid out an important evolutionary arrangement!

2. The earthworm is called the *segmented worm* (phylum **Annelida**, meaning "ringed"). The millipede and crayfish are the phylum **Arthropoda** (meaning "jointed foot"), the most successful animal group today. Arthropoda includes many body designs based on segmentation.

? QUESTION

1. A segmented animal would be _____ (smaller or larger) than the early "pre-segmented" animal form.

2. What would be the benefit to the animal that developed from the above change?

3. Based on your observations of the segmented worm, what evolutionary changes happened to the individual segments?

4. Use your knowledge of *basic body plan*, *digestive systems*, and *segmentation* to put the animal subgroups in order of increasing complexity (hydra, sponge, arthropod, roundworm, flatworm, and segmented worm).

Simple

More Complex

_____

_____

_____

_____

_____

_____

5. How do you think the evolutionary development of segmentation applies to human development?

OTHER PHYLA

Evolution is not a "directional game," even though we humans find it easier to talk about the process that way. Evolution is more like an experiment. Some experiments succeed; others fail. And some go on and on because there are no big obstacles to prevent their continuation.

So, many creatures resulting from evolution's experiments may be interpreted by us to be "exceptions" to the rule, or "special examples." But, in evolutionary reality, all organisms are exceptions depending on your point of view.

The mollusks and echinoderms are two more evolutionary groups that fit somewhere in the animal story.

MOLLUSKS

Phylum *Mollusca*, meaning "the soft ones," includes animals that have a *shell* during some stage of their lives. They evolved at about the same time as segmentation was evolving, perhaps a bit before the segmented worms.

ECHINODERMS

Members of the phylum *Echinodermata,* which means "spiny skin," are very complex animals that have returned to a modified radial symmetry. (Originally, they came from a bilateral marine group.) Echinoderms have an unusual arrangement of tube-feet that are moved by a hydraulic system within the body.

The larval stage of echinoderms is more like the larva of simple chordates. The complete gut seems to have developed from the same evolutionary mutation in both groups. This embryonic similarity means that echinoderms are one of the closest invertebrate relatives to the phylum *Chordata* (the animal group to which you belong).

 GO GET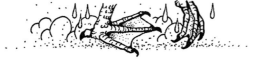

Go to the specimen table.

NOW

1. Look at the examples of mollusks on the specimen table.

2. Look at the examples of echinoderms.

3. Draw a simple sketch of an example of each organism.

Mollusk

Echinoderm

MATCHING INVERTEBRATES

Make the correct match between the two columns.

Group Names

_____ Sponge

_____ Jellyfish Types

_____ Flatworm

_____ Roundworm

_____ Mollusk

_____ Segmented Worm

_____ Arthropod

_____ Echinoderm

Defining Features

(A) This group has blocks of duplicated embryonic tissue that develop into different parts in the adult organism.

(B) This invertebrate group is more closely related to chordates than to other invertebrates. Their larval stage is bilateral, but the adult phase has a modified radial symmetry.

(C) This group is by far the most successful animal group living on this planet today. And they have an exoskeleton.

(D) This group includes clams, squids, octopuses, slugs, and snails. There is a shell during some stage of the animal's development.

(E) This animal has stinging cells, and has radial symmetry in the adult form.

(F) This animal is the first multicellular animal of the groups considered in this course.

(G) This is the first group with a complete digestive tract—food in one end and waste out the other end.

(H) This is the first group with a head-end and a tail-end. They have bilateral symmetry.

INVERTEBRATE CLADOGRAM

Use the evolutionary character information in Exercises #3, #4, and #5 to label "bars" and boxes that are not labeled in this diagram.

To correctly view this cladogram, rotate this page so that the taxonomic boxes are at the top.

Ancestor Prokaryotes

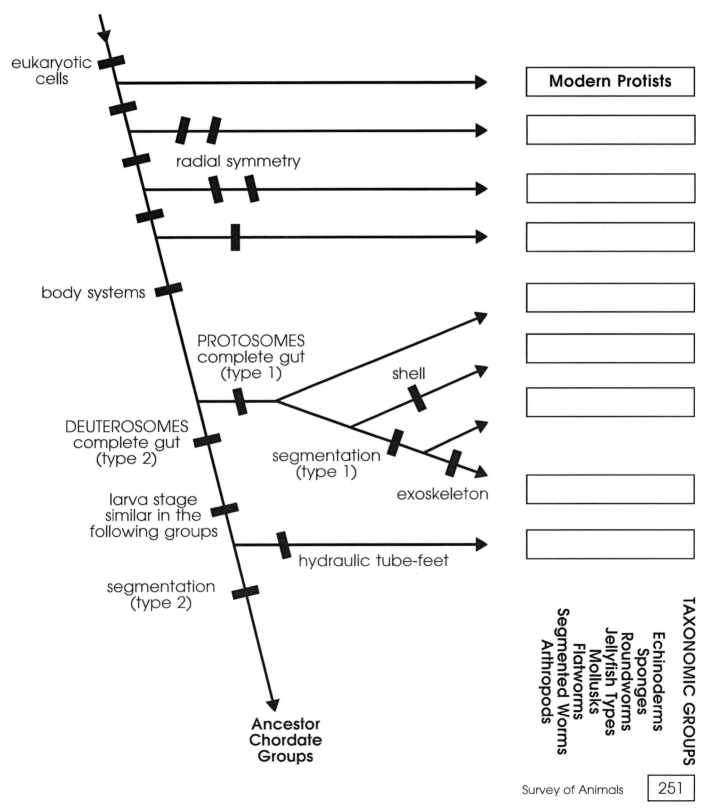

eukaryotic cells

Modern Protists

radial symmetry

body systems

PROTOSOMES
complete gut
(type 1)

shell

DEUTEROSOMES
complete gut
(type 2)

segmentation
(type 1)

exoskeleton

larva stage
similar in the
following groups

hydraulic tube-feet

segmentation
(type 2)

**Ancestor
Chordate
Groups**

TAXONOMIC GROUPS

Echinoderms
Sponges
Roundworms
Jellyfish Types
Mollusks
Flatworms
Segmented Worms
Arthropods

ACTIVITY #6

"SKELETONS"

A skeleton is a supporting structure made of different pieces that can be individually moved by muscles. The evolutionary success of animals with skeletons is an expression of the capacity for refined movement. The better you are at moving on this planet, the better off you are in terms of survival.

There are two basic kinds of skeletons in the animal kingdom—the *exoskeleton* and the *endoskeleton*. Both types are successful. The main difference is in the size of the organism that can be supported by each.

EXOSKELETON

"Exo" means outside. An **exoskeleton** is on the outside surface of the animal. The animal group that has most successfully utilized the exoskeleton is the *arthropod*.

Name an example of an arthropod: _____

ENDOSKELETON

"Endo" means inside. An endoskeleton is inside an animal, and there are three variations of the endoskeleton.

INTERNAL FLEXIBLE ROD (NOTOCHORD)

This doesn't exactly fit our definition of skeleton because it is a one-piece structure, but it is the beginning of a skeleton. The notochord has many muscle fibers attached along its length for control of swimming movements. The first animal with a notochord was something like *Amphioxus* which was followed by another group (Jawless Fish) with a larger notochord and brain.

CARTILAGE SKELETON

This doesn't exactly fit our definition of skeleton because it is a one-piece structure. It is the precursor of an internal skeleton. The notochord has many muscle fibers attached along its length for controling swimming movements. The first animal with a notochord would have been something like the current-day Amphioxus. This small fish-like chordate has gill slits, a dorsal nerve cord, and a notochord. These evolutionary character traits link them to all other chordates. The earliest chordates were followed by the Jawless Fish, which had a larger notochord and brain. Jawless fish dominated the seas 400 million years ago, and some of them were extremely large (10 meters or more).

BONY SKELETON

This type of skeleton is made of many hard bony pieces that can be individually moved by separate muscles. Movement is much more refined than what a cartilage skeleton will allow. Bony Fish are the first evolutionary group with a bony skeleton, and they are the dominant fish found in today's seas. Theirs was the beginning skeleton for all other vertebrates that followed.

 GO GET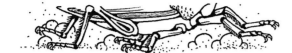

Go to the specimen table.

 NOW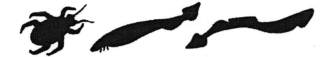

1. Put an insect, an *Amphioxus*, a jawless fish, a cartilage fish, and a bony fish in that order.

2. Put the cartilage skeleton and the bony skeleton plastic mounts next to the appropriate fish.

3. Study these animals carefully, observing their particular skeletal structures.

? QUESTION

1. Compare the insect to the other four animals. What is the most obvious difference?

2. What kind of skeleton does the insect have? _____

3. Which type of skeleton looks like it would present a problem to a growing animal? (circle your choice)

    Exoskeleton   or   Endoskeleton

4. Explain why you think it would be a problem.

5. Which skeleton is designed to grow along with the animal? (circle your choice)

    Exoskeleton   or   Endoskeleton

6. Can a fish have a *jaw* if it doesn't have a multi-piece skeleton? _____

7. What does that tell you about an animal we call a jawless fish?

8. Which two organisms are examples of animals with a one-piece skeleton (internal flexible rod)?

_____ and _____

9. Which type of skeleton is capable of more refined swimming movements? (circle your choice) Explain why you think so.

Cartilage skeleton   or   Bony skeleton

10. Do you think that *Amphioxus* can swim as well as an aquarium fish? _____ Explain why or why not.

ACTIVITY #7

"LAND ADAPTATIONS"

About 350 million years ago the vertebrate fish had already evolved, and there were large areas of the planet with shallow seas and lowlands. These conditions favored the evolution of any group with features suited to land.

Several environmental challenges had to be overcome before any organism could survive in the land environment. Among those challenges were: *movement on land*, *breathing air*, *preventing water loss*, and *reproduction*.

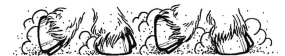 **GO GET**

Go to the specimen table.

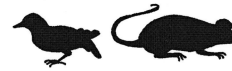 **NOW**

Put a bony fish, a frog, a lizard, a bird, and a mammal in that order. This order represents a series of land adaptations that were made by the vertebrate groups.

? QUESTION

1. Compare the bony fish to the frog. What is the most obvious structural difference?

2. Those structures found on the frogs evolved from what parts of the fish? _____

3. The frog is in the phylum ***Chordata*** (meaning "notochord"), is part of the subphylum ***Vertebrata*** (meaning "having a backbone"), and is a member of the class ***Amphibia***. The word *amphibian* means "living both lives."

    What process in the amphibian life cycle depends on water? (Recall the situation you studied with moss and fern plants.)

4. The fact that a frog can live out of water and a fish cannot tells you that the frog has solved the problem of _____.

5. What structure in the frog solves that problem? _____

6. Compare the frog to the lizard. What is the most obvious difference?

7. The lizard belongs to the vertebrate subgroup class **Reptilia**, which means "creeping." Modern reptiles have legs that are positioned out to the side of the animal, which makes them appear to creep as they move. One of the early reptiles had legs positioned under the body, and that group gave rise to what are now mammals.

   Now you know why it is inappropriate to call some of the mammals you know "creeps." Unless the legs are positioned out to the side of the body, the name does not apply.

   The land success of reptiles resulted from two improvements over the amphibians—waterproof skin and significant changes in reproduction. Reproductive improvements included *internal fertilization* and the *amniotic egg*.

   What two features allowed the reptiles to be so successful in dry environments?

   _____ and _____

8. How did the two special changes in reproduction improve land success for the reptiles? (Ask your instructor.)

9. Compare the lizard to the bird and the mammal. What are the most obvious external differences?

   _____ and _____

   Discuss the advantages of having insulating features that allow for regulation of body temperature.

10. Birds and mammals are descended from early reptile groups, and are classified as subclasses under **Reptilia**. The subclasses are **Aves** (which means "birds") and **Mammalia** (which means "breast"). Mammals are given their name because they are the only animals with mammary glands for feeding their young. And their embryos develop within a special structure called the *placenta*. The external features of birds (feathers) and mammals (hair) are important evolutionary character traits that separate them from the other reptilian groups. Discuss how these external differences allow birds and mammals to live in places where reptiles can't survive.

11. Using your knowledge of skeletons and land adaptations, put the subgroups of chordate animals in order of complexity (reptile, jawless fish, mammal, amphibian, bony fish, bird, and *Amphioxus*).

Simple

↓

More Complex

MATCHING VERTEBRATES

Make the correct match between the two columns.

Group Names

_____ Chordate (*Amphioxus*)

_____ Jawless Fish

_____ Cartilage Fish

_____ Bony Fish

_____ Lung Fish

_____ Lobe-Finned Fish

_____ Amphibian

_____ Reptile

_____ Bird

_____ Mammal

Defining Features

(A) First animal with both legs and lungs.

(B) One of two groups that can regulate body temperature.

(C) Has hair. It is the only group with internal development of the embryo supported by a placenta.

(D) A small (5 to 7 cm) fishy-looking creature (but not a fish) that has a notochord, gill slits, and a dorsal nerve cord.

(E) First animal with internal fertilization. First to lay an energy rich and protective egg to support the next generation.

(F) First fish with a lung.

(G) First fish with limbs.

(H) The most successful fish today.

(I) The first fish with a skeleton and a jaw.

(J) A fish creature that can be a foot long or so today. This group has a vertebral column and a brain, but no skeleton beyond that. It dominated the seas 400 million years ago and some were very large.

VERTEBRATE CLADOGRAM

Taxomomic groups are completed for this cladogram. However, your job is to label the correct evolutionary character at each point indicated in the diagram. (Put the correct letter in each box.)

To correctly view this cladogram, rotate this page so that the arrows point up.

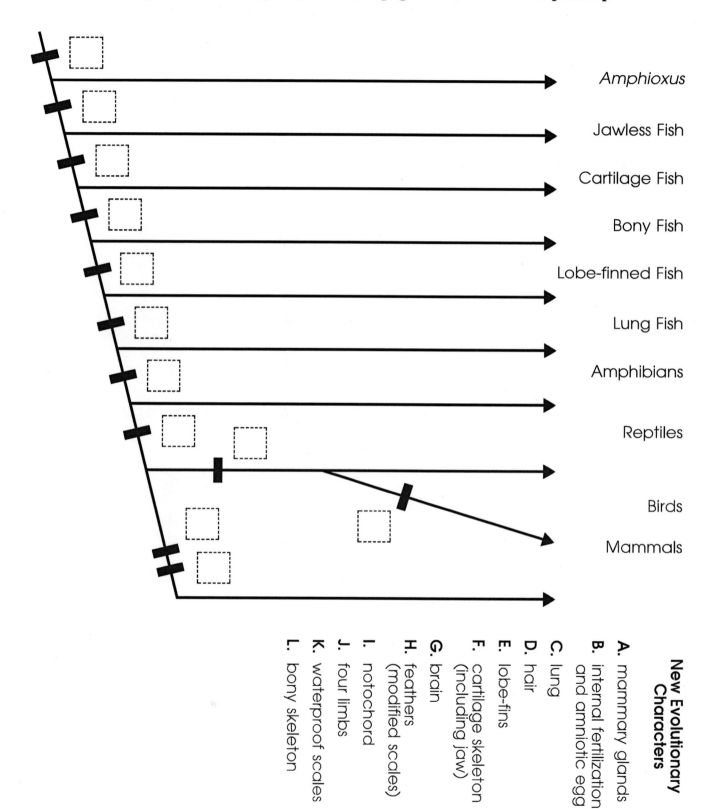

Amphioxus

Jawless Fish

Cartilage Fish

Bony Fish

Lobe-finned Fish

Lung Fish

Amphibians

Reptiles

Birds

Mammals

New Evolutionary Characters

A. mammary glands
B. internal fertilization and amniotic egg
C. lung
D. hair
E. lobe-fins
F. cartilage skeleton (including jaw)
G. brain
H. feathers (modified scales)
I. notochord
J. four limbs
K. waterproof scales
L. bony skeleton

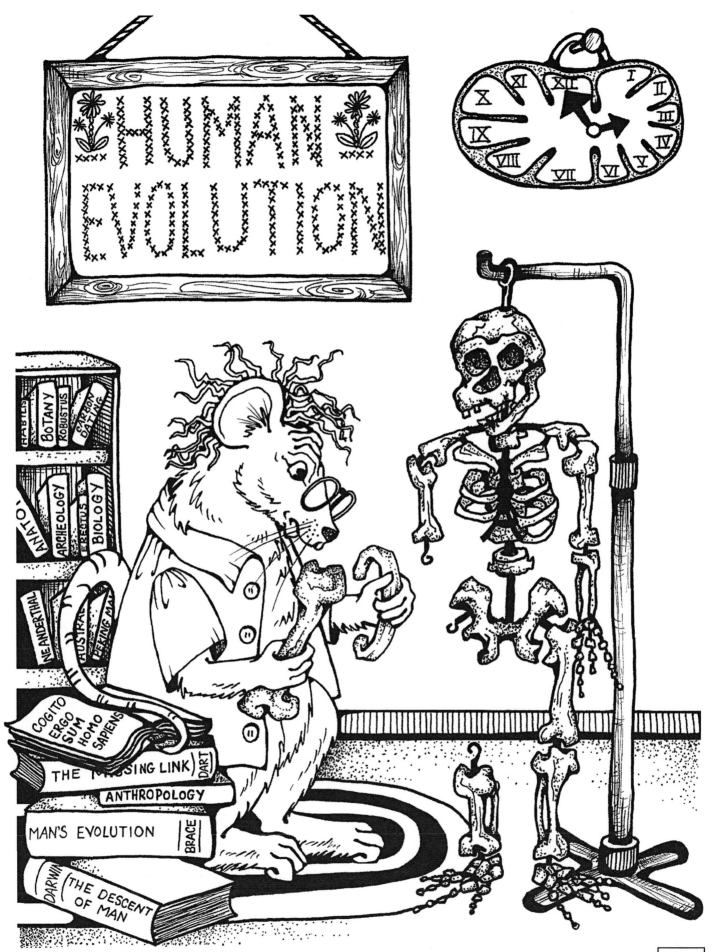

Roughly 10% of all human beings ever born are alive at this very moment.

—HTTP://WWW.SKYGAZE.COM/CONTENT/FACTS/BIOLOGY.SHTML

Genetic studies verify that 1% to 4% of *Homo sapiens'* genome contains Neanderthal DNA. *Homo sapiens* mingled and mated with Neanderthals after early modern humans migrated out of Africa as long as 80,000 years ago, significantly earlier than scientists who support the interbreeding hypothesis would have expected.

—HTTP://ESCIENCENEWS.COM/TOPICS/PALEONTOLOGY.ARCHAEOLOGY

—HTTP://NEWS.NATIONALGEOGRAPHIC.COM/NEWS/2006/10/061030-NEANDERTHALS.HTML

HUMAN EVOLUTION

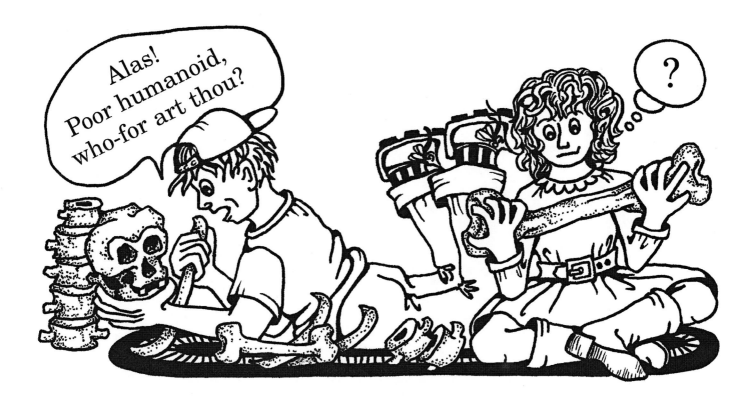

Alas! Poor humanoid, who-for art thou?

?

INTRODUCTION

People are very curious about where they come from. Written and oral stories are all we had to tell us about our past, until discoveries by anthropologists and molecular biologists revealed what happened before written history. This new evidence comes from four main sources: 1) cultural artifacts; 2) fossils; 3) comparisons of human traits with other primates; and 4) DNA similarities among living humans and other primates, and DNA extracted from fossil remains.

We are now able to present a scientific story about human evolution. During this lab you will learn to develop a scientific history of humans, using several techniques of thinking, map-making, and group discussion.

ACTIVITIES

ACTIVITY #1

"TRAILS OF THE CROSS-COUNTRY HIKERS"

This first problem will develop your thinking method for understanding a scientific history of modern humans.

The information provided may seem to be brief. But, as you think through the problem, you will be able to draw a map of the different paths taken by the five students, indicating when they separated from each other, and the trails they took.

Your time map will look something like this, using branches to represent when the different hikers separated from each other.

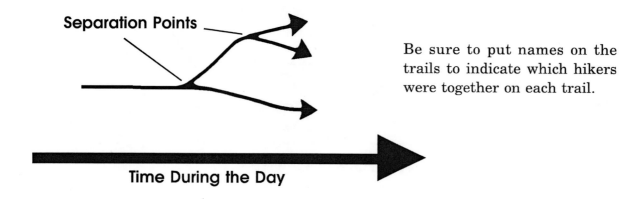

Be sure to put names on the trails to indicate which hikers were together on each trail.

NOW

1. Divide into groups of 3 or 4 people.

2. Your group may need some quiet space to do this Activity, so don't hesitate to work outside or in another room if necessary.

GO GET	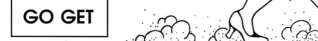

1. Refer to the worksheet at the end of this lab titled, "Trails of the Cross-Country Hikers."

2. A five-card set of names. You can use these name cards as an aid to physically keep track of the hikers during your analysis of the problem.

Five members of the Cross-Country Running Team decided to have a rugged day of fun last Saturday. They drove out a long dirt road, and parked the car at a grove of trees that was 12 hours of hard hiking away from the freeway. All they had to do was to walk west and they were guaranteed to reach the Highway 8 Freeway, where they could hitch a ride back to their parked car.

Your task is to figure out the general paths that were taken by the individual people using the limited information provided below, and to draw those paths on a map.

INFORMATION

1. The five hikers started out together, but divided into smaller groups, taking different paths as they went along.

2. Below you will find clues about the different people. The clues tell you when particular hikers separated from each other and took different paths. You will have to use those clues to figure out and draw their approximate paths to the highway.

3. The hikers names are: Bill, Hector, Julie, Tom, and Maria.

4. The hikers all began to walk at about 6:00 a.m. All of the hikers reached Highway 8 at around 6:00 p.m., but they did not necessarily arrive together.

CLUES

A. Tom and Maria arrived at Highway 8 together.

B. The last time Hector was with Julie was 5 hours before he reached the highway. (This clue does not tell you whether or not Hector or Julie were with anyone else when they separated from each other. You will have to figure that out—read on!)

C. The last time Julie was with Tom was 8 hours before she arrived at the highway. (Again, this clue does not tell you whether or not Julie or Tom were with anyone else when they separated from each other.)

D. The last time Bill was with Hector, they were 10 hours away from the highway. (Was Hector or Bill with anyone else at the time they last saw each other? Again, this clue does not tell you. Work it out!)

NOW

1. Draw a map of the trails taken by these five hikers. Show when they split up during the day, and how they were grouped when they arrived at the highway at 6:00 p.m.

2. Make a practice map to work out the problem, then draw your final map on the "TRAILS" worksheet at the end of this lab.

3. You may find it helpful to use the name cards to keep track of the hikers. Lay them on your paper, on the ground, or on the table, and move them along the trails as you work through the clues.

FINISHED

1. Check with your instructor to make sure you got the correct answer to this problem before going on.

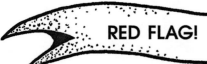

RED FLAG!   WARNING!   WARNING!

2. The next problem is going to take more calculation and time, and will use the same kind of thinking you used for the Cross-Country Hiker problem.

3. *Good advice:* Have the best reader in your group read aloud as the rest of your group reads Activity #2, "The Mitochondrial DNA Clock."

   Work together.

   Work slowly.

   When you have questions, check with your instructor.

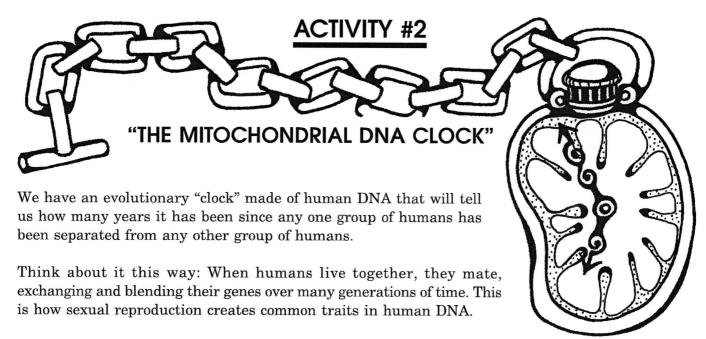

ACTIVITY #2

"THE MITOCHONDRIAL DNA CLOCK"

We have an evolutionary "clock" made of human DNA that will tell us how many years it has been since any one group of humans has been separated from any other group of humans.

Think about it this way: When humans live together, they mate, exchanging and blending their genes over many generations of time. This is how sexual reproduction creates common traits in human DNA.

Now, what happens if one group splits into two separate groups that migrate far away from each other, and they never get a chance to interbreed with each other again?

As you would expect, the two groups are no longer mixing genes (and DNA), and over time they will begin to look somewhat different from each other.

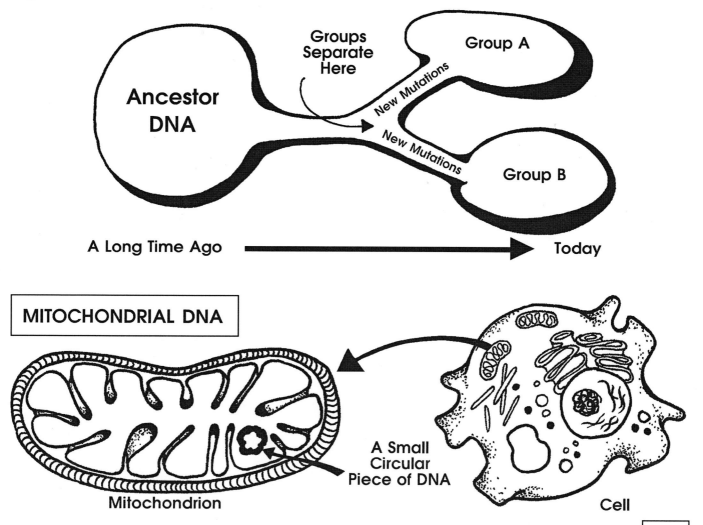

MITOCHONDRIAL DNA

Humans have DNA in the mitochondria. This mitochondrial DNA does not mix with the DNA in the cell nucleus during sexual reproduction. So, the only way it gets passed onto the next generation is through the mitochondria in the *mother's egg*. The father's sperm does not give mitochondria to the egg during fertilization. This strange situation means that mitochondrial DNA (passed on by the mother) stays the same, and cannot change except by "new" mutations. These mutations occur randomly as a natural process of living on this planet.

By comparing DNA patterns, chemists can detect any new mutations that have been added to the small piece of original mitochondrial DNA that was passed on from mother to child through thousands of human generations.

If a group of humans splits off from a common ancestral group, then both groups will begin to accumulate different mutations from each other. Each group is genetically separated from the other group. This starts at the point where they no longer interbreed.

The easiest way to show that two groups have separated in the past is to count the number of *new* mutations found in the DNA of one group and *not* found in the DNA of the other group.

The *greater* the number of *different* mutations, the longer is the amount of time that the two groups have been separated from each other. (**Remember:** Mutations take a lot of time to happen.) If however, the DNA of the two groups is quite similar, then they have not been separated very long.

COMPARATIVE DNA ANALYSIS

Diagrammed below is a comparison of the mitochondrial DNA of three geographically separate human racial groups. Each **bar** represents a mutation.

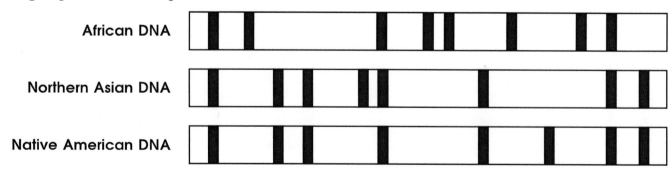

? QUESTION

1. Which two groups are the most similar?

2. Which one of the three groups is the most different from the other two groups?

3. So, which group has been separated from the others for the longest time?

4. And, which two groups haven't been separated from each other for very long?

THE "CLOCK"

Biologists have studied many different species, including humans, and have estimated that it takes 500,000 years for 1% of the mitochondrial DNA to be changed by mutation. (This estimated mutation rate is currently being debated, but we will base our calculations on it. Perhaps more research will clarify our understanding of evolutionary timelines.)

This mutation rate is a kind of "clock."

Researchers have gone around the world collecting mitochondrial DNA samples. They have counted the total number of small mutations that have occurred in the humans of today. Each one of those mutations represents an amount of "time" on the mitochondrial clock.

? QUESTION

A representative sample of different human geographical/racial DNA has been collected and analyzed. When all of the different mutations were counted, scientists found that only 0.4% of the DNA of modern humans has been mutated. How many years have *modern* humans been on this planet?

Remember: It takes 500,000 years for 1% of the DNA to be mutated.

? QUESTION

Can you estimate how long geographical/racial groups have been separated from each other?

HOW TO DO IT

If you want to estimate how long it has been since two racial or geographical groups have been separated, you must:

1. Use the figure for the % of genetic difference between the two groups (as determined by genetic researchers).

2. Multiply the % of genetic difference by 500,000 years. (It takes 500,000 years for 1% of the mitichondrial DNA to be mutated.)

3. *Practice Example:* If Group A and Group B have 0.1% genetic difference, then it has been about _____ years since they separated, and have not had the opportunity to interbreed.

500,000 years x 0.1% genetic difference = 50,000 years

Answer: 50,000 years

Calculate the answer to the following problem:

Group A, the "Altitudinals," have lived in the high mountain ranges of Nepal for longer than anyone can remember. Group B, the "Basinals," have lived on the flat river delta plains of Southern India for hundreds of centuries according to their written history.

A genetic researcher has measured a 0.05% genetic difference in the mitochondrial DNA of Group A and Group B.

How long would you say it has been since these two groups lived together and had the opportunity to interbreed? In other words, how long ago was it that the Altitudinals and the Basinals split company, one moving to the highlands and the other moving to the lowlands?

_____ years

Show your work here:

FINISHED

1. It's time to move on to Activity #3, the "Time Trails of *Homo Sapiens*" and test your understanding of the "Mitochondrial Clock."

2. If you are having trouble understanding the mitochondrial clock, then *now* is the time to get help from your instructor!

ACTIVITY #3

"TIME TRAILS OF *HOMO SAPIENS*"

Archaeologists have found skeletal evidence of a modern-type human (looks like people today) who lived on this planet about 100,000 years ago. There is a question as to exactly how long modern humans have been here, and where they might have originated.

You will investigate a partial answer to these questions. Modern human types are known as *Homo sapiens*. They are somewhat lighter in build, with a bit larger brain size than the previous human fossils. Evidence also suggests that they lived much like the hunter-gatherer peoples of today. If you were to bring some of these skeletal remains back to life, put some modern clothes on them, and put them on a bus, you could not tell them apart from anyone else on that bus.

Where did modern humans originate on this planet?

What is the "trail" that modern humans took when spreading out to the different continents on this planet?

Figuring out the answers to these questions is somewhat like doing the "Trails of the Cross-Country Hikers" problem. Here, you will follow five geographical/racial groups instead of five hikers.

You must calculate when these groups separated from each other, and relate those times of separation to a world map. From that information, you will be able to tell a story of modern human migration and origin.

HOW TO DO IT

Answer the following questions using what you learned about the Mitochondrial DNA Clock.

1. When genetic researchers compare the DNA of *Northern Asian* populations versus *Native American* populations, they find a 0.07% difference. The "Mitochondrial Clock" formula tells us that there has been about _____ years since the separation of these two groups.

2. When comparing the DNA of *Northern Asian* and *European* populations, they discover a 0.10% difference. The "Mitochondrial Clock" formula tells us that there has been about _____ years since the separation of these groups.

3. When comparing the DNA of *Indonesian* peoples to either the *European* group or the *Northern Asians*, they find a 0.12% difference. The "Mitochondrial Clock" formula tells us that there has been about _____ years since separation.

4. When researchers compare the DNA of *African* populations to any other group, they find a 0.20% difference. The "Mitochondrial Clock" formula tells us that there has been about _____ years since the separation of Africans from other groups.

GO GET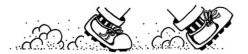

1. Refer to the "Time Trails of *Homo sapiens*" worksheet at the end of this lab.

2. Refer to the "World Map" worksheet at the end of this lab.

NOW

Use the "years since separation" information you just calculated on the previous page for the different geographical/racial groups, and . . .

Fill out the map of the "Time Trails of *Homo sapiens*" on your worksheet. Show when each group split off from the original group (just like you did for the Cross-Country Hikers).

THEN

Using the "World Map" worksheet and the "Time Trails" map you just completed, draw your best interpretation of the trail taken by humans as they separated and spread out on this planet. Show where the original population started and show the sequences of where they separated and where they went after that. There may be more than one possible trail based on the genetic information presented in this Activity.

FINALLY

Below is a table of information about the general anthropological evidence of the earliest settlements of modern humans that have been excavated so far.

Region	Time of the Earliest Settlements
Americas	less than 35,000 years ago
Indonesia	50,000 years ago
Europe	35,000 years ago
Asia	60,000 years ago
North Africa	100,000 years ago

How does your story, illustrated by the Migration Map, compare to this evidence?

If you think that all of this is hard to figure out, remember that many researchers have spent their careers just to give you the small amount of information you are working with in this lab. There is a great deal more to know that will make the picture more accurate. Anthropology is one of the sciences of biology. Archeology is another. If you are enjoying what you are learning in this lab, consider studying in these other fields of biology as well.

ACTIVITY #4

"THE STORY OF THE EARLY HOMINIDS"

Dating back to before Homo sapiens (modern humans) appeared on Earth, hominid fossils give clues to our origin and evolution. Comparison of human and gorilla DNA evidence suggests that the gorilla line branched off the human ancestral line about 7 million years ago. Then approximately 6 million years ago the chimpanzee and human lines separated.

1. Earliest hominid

Two fossils were vying for earliest hominid, but one of them has been declared an ape, leaving *Orrorin tegenensis* as the oldest discovery in our lineage. The bones of this hominid suggest that it is about four feet tall and bipedal. The fossils were found in Kenya (east Africa) and date to more than 6 million years ago.

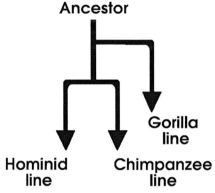

2. Other early hominids

Originally all early hominid fossils were called Australopithecines. New research has subdivided them into ten or more species within three separate genuses. The oldest is called *Ardipithecus* (about 6 million years ago). It is followed by several species of *Australopithecus* (2–4 million years ago) that are lighter-boned. A branch off *Australopithecus* apparently led to a heavy-boned species named *Paranthropus*.

All of these hominids were smaller than modern humans, standing about four feet high, walking slightly bent over, and had smaller brains. Their skeletal comparisons suggest there were different lineages and niches. These fossils occur between 6 and 1.5 million years ago, and one or more of these early hominids are in the ancestral line leading to *Homo habilis* and *Homo erectus*.

3. *Homo habilis*

The *Homo habilis* group was a tool maker. They had somewhat larger brains than Australopithecines, stood more erect, and were slightly bigger in size. Compared to *Homo erectus*, who also made tools, the *Homo habilis* group had a smaller brain. These fossils occur between 1.5 and 2.5 million years ago.

4. *Homo erectus*

The original fossil groups were designated as Peking, Java, and Heidelberg Man. They stood fully erect (for which they are named), and had the same general height and brain size as modern man. The earliest fossils of *H. erectus* (1.8 million years ago in Africa) are sometimes referred to by the name *Homo ergaster*. They have been found with more artifacts than earlier hominids, telling us something about how they lived. Apparently, they were very much like *Homo sapiens*, but may have had less ability to speak because of some throat structure differences. This is currently being debated. There is evidence suggesting that *Homo erectus* may have included more subgroups, and their lineage and migration out of Africa might be a much more complex story. Some of them, including Neanderthals, survived until 30,000 years ago, and may have interbred to a small extent with some *Homo sapiens*. (Researchers estimate that 60% of modern humans carry some Neanderthal genes.) The *Homo erectus* group started to die out about 200,000 years ago as *Homo sapiens* evolved and migrated around the world.

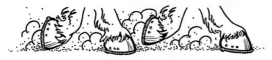

GO GET

Refer to the second World Map worksheet at the end of this lab.

NOW

Using the information provided below and the World Map worksheet titled "Trails of the Early Hominids," put a dot on the map for each of the groups. See if the dots suggest a story of how these human-like species might be related to each other, and where they developed and migrated.

INFORMATION

Fossils	Age of Fossils	Where Found
Orrorin tegenensis	*6.2 million years ago*	*Africa*
Ardipithecus ramidus	5.5 million years	Africa
Australopithecus anamensis	4.2 million years	Africa
Australopithecus afarensis	3.5 million years	Africa
Australopithecus africanus	3.0 million years	Africa
Homo habilis	2.5 million years	Africa
Homo erectus	1.8 million years	Africa
Homo erectus (Peking)	500,000 years	China
Homo erectus (Java)	1.5 million years	Southeast Asia
Homo erectus (Heidelberg)	800,000 years	Germany

1. How long ago did the human and chimpanzee lines separate?

2. How old is the oldest known hominid?

3. Based on fossil evidence, where did the early hominids originate?

4. A branch off the Australopithecines led to a heavy-boned type that is not considerd a direct ancestral group to us. The name of that group is _____.

5. How long ago did *Homo habilis* live?

   Where did they live?

6. Which group first migrated out of the continent of their origin?

   How long ago?

   How far did that group spread?

7. Was there another group that came out of the continent of origin after the group in Question #6? (See Activity #3.)

   Which species was that group?

   When did the migration of the new species happen?

   Indicate that event on your map.

FINISHED

Show your completed map to your instructor.

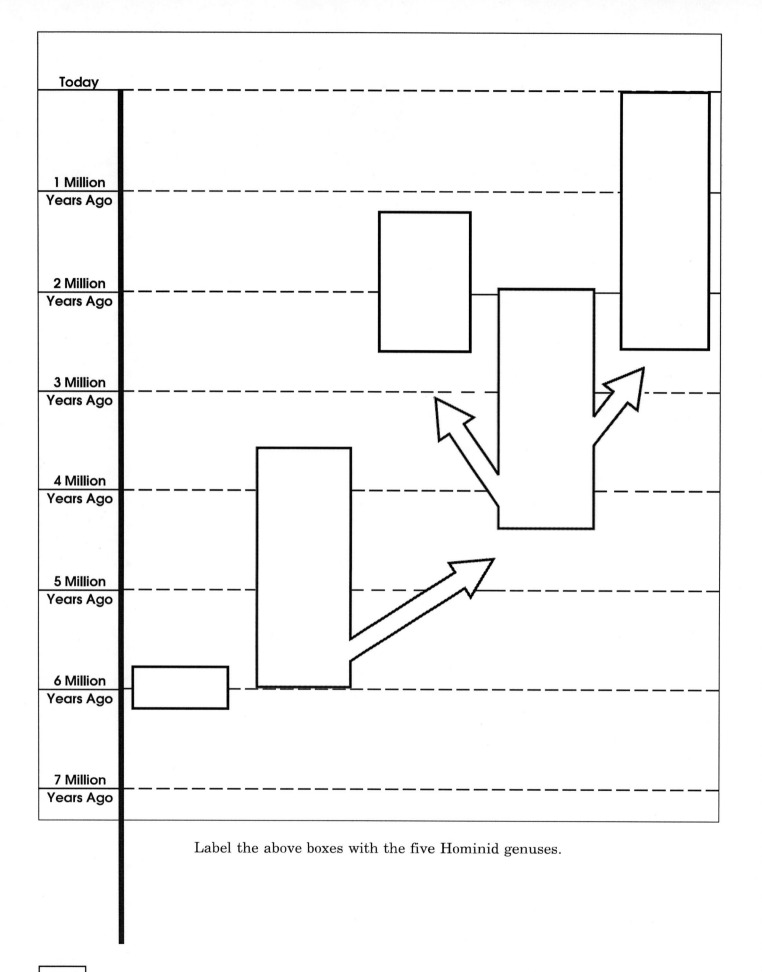

Today

1 Million
Years Ago

2 Million
Years Ago

3 Million
Years Ago

4 Million
Years Ago

5 Million
Years Ago

6 Million
Years Ago

7 Million
Years Ago

Label the above boxes with the five Hominid genuses.

" TRAILS of the CROSS-COUNTRY HIKERS "

(Use for Activity #1)

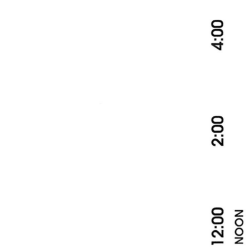

— HIGHWAY 8 —

Bill
Hector
Julie
Tom
Maria

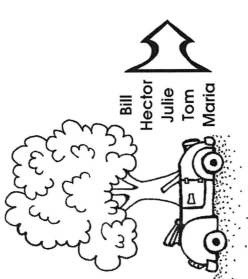

| 6:00 | 8:00 | 10:00 | 12:00 | 2:00 | 4:00 | 6:00 |
| A.M. | | | NOON | | | P.M. |

" TIME TRAILS of *HOMO SAPIENS* "
(Use for Activity #3)

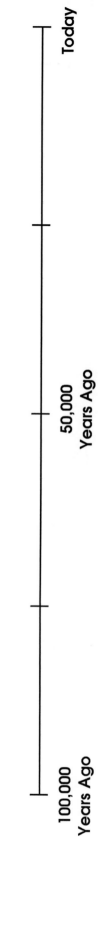

Today

50,000
Years Ago

100,000
Years Ago

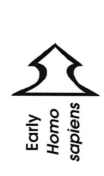

Early
*Homo
sapiens*

WORLD MAP

" *Migrations of Homo sapiens* "
(Use for Activity #3)

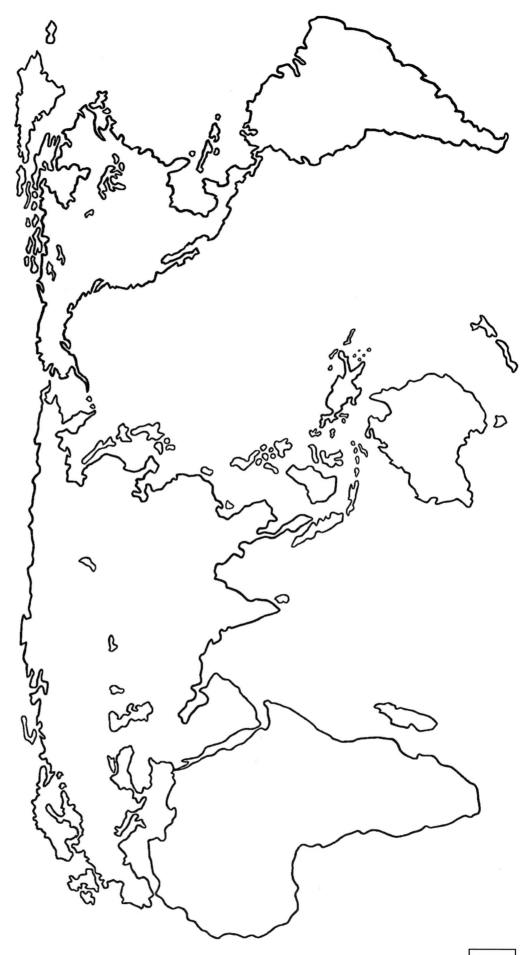

WORLD MAP

" Trails of the Early Hominids "
(Use for Activity #4)

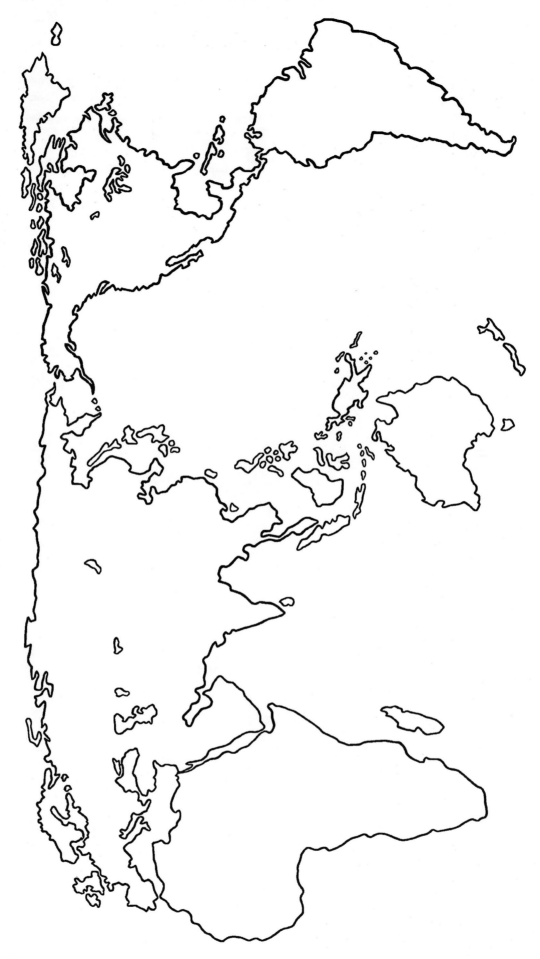

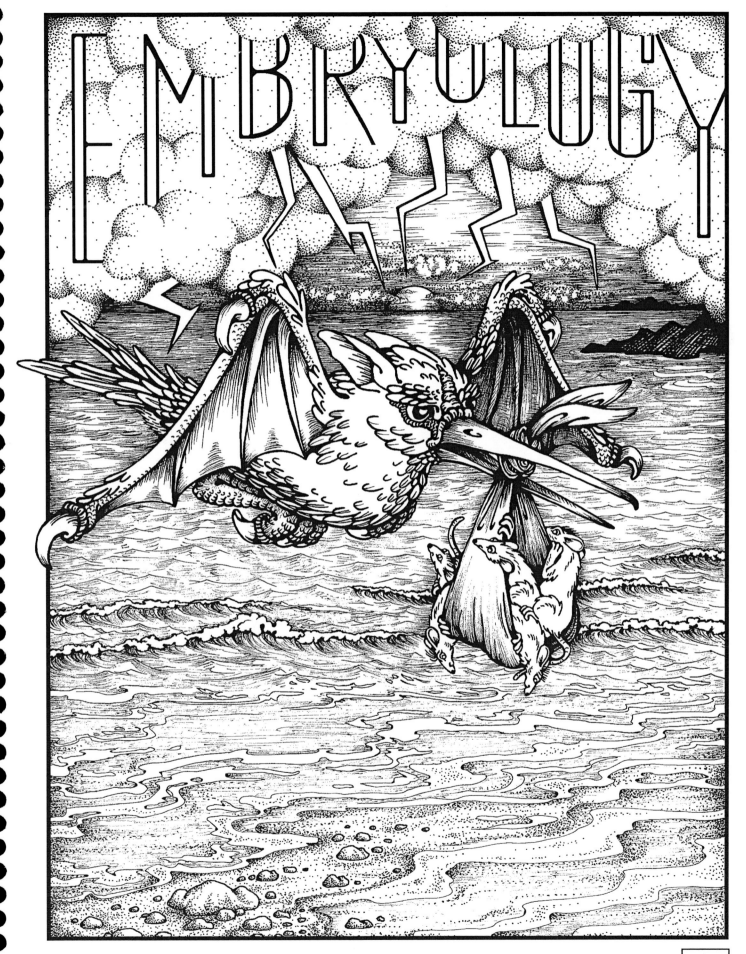

EMBRYOLOGY

DYNAMIC DEVELOPMENTS
AND
FASCINATING FACTS
IN BIOLOGY

The embryonic development of gills slits is a fascinating process. In fish, the gill slits become what you'd expect—gills that filter water for oxygen. In other animals and especially humans, the same structures in the embryo modify into the tiny middle bones of the ear, the hyoid bone in the throat that allows for swallowing, and facial nerves. Comparative anatomy is an enlightening study in how all life is related.

—SHUBIN, NEIL, *YOUR INNER FISH: A JOURNEY INTO THE 3.5-BILLION-YEAR HISTORY OF THE HUMAN BODY*,
PANTHEON BOOKS, 2008

EMBRYOLOGY

INTRODUCTION

Embryology is the study of early developmental phases in plants and animals. An *Embryo* is any stage after the egg becomes fertilized, but before the developing organism looks like the adult form (about 8 weeks for humans). In advanced vertebrates, any stage after the embryo and before birth is called a *fetus*.

A century ago, there were two contrasting theories about development. One view (*preformation*) held that a miniature version of the adult existed in the egg and grew into the adult form. This theory is incorrect. The second theory (*epigenesis*) stated that new structures and body systems are continually being created during embryonic development. This description is correct. All vertebrates begin as a single cell, but develop amazing degrees of complexity by the time they are born.

Scientific research has revealed two very important embryological concepts. First, the study of embryos shows how simple life-forms could have evolved into complex life-forms. The developing traits provide biologists with the opportunity to observe how genetic mechanisms operate to create an organism. The second concept is that there are developmental processes common to all vertebrates. This means that studying the embryos of simpler organisms can help us to understand development in human embryos.

In today's lab, you will learn the general terminology and descriptions of embryonic stages, and you will compare the embryos of various organisms at similar stages found in human development.

ACTIVITIES

ACTIVITY #1

"ONTOGENY RECAPITULATES PHYLOGENY"

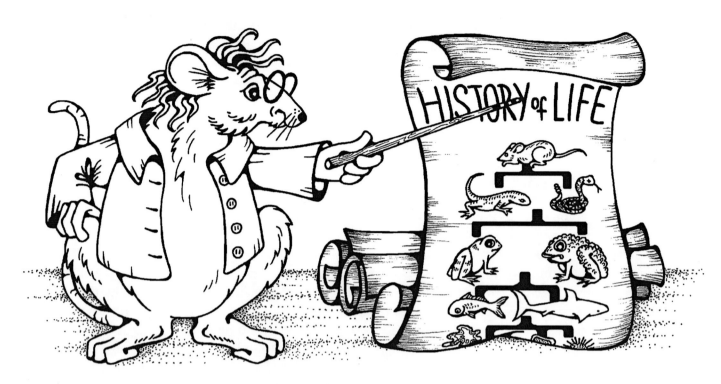

The title of this Activity has been a recurring TV quiz-show question. The quote is from Ernst Haeckel, a German scientist at the turn of the 20TH century. He thought that embryonic development replayed the entire evolutionary history of a species. In other words, watching the development of a frog would be like seeing a movie of the evolution of vertebrates leading to the frog. Since Haeckel's time, science has discovered that both evolution and development are far more complicated than his original idea suggested.

The human embryo does proceed through various levels of complexity similar to those of earlier vertebrates. There is certainly as much change in the human embryo from conception to birth as there is change in the fossil record from one-celled organisms to complex land vertebrates. The situation faced by the human embryo is similar to the challenges presented to vertebrate groups that evolved from a water environment to dry land conditions. But, we do not first become a fish, then a frog, followed by a reptile, and finally a mammal. The developmental "movie" is much more blurred than that.

NOW

1. Read the brief descriptions of human embryonic stages on the next page, and then refer to the "Ontogeny Recapitulates Phylogeny" chart on the following page.

2. Then, complete the chart by writing the name of the appropriate human embryonic stage that compares in complexity to organisms in evolutionary history.

HUMAN EMBRYONIC STAGES

Name	Description
Zygote	A diploid cell formed by the union of egg and sperm.
Morula (3–4 days)	A small solid ball of identical cells.
Blastocyst (1 week)	Cells begin differentiating into tissues.
25-Day Embryo	The heart begins to beat, but there are no organ systems yet (i.e., circulatory systems, etc.).
4-Week Embryo	The *notochord* has formed. This is the very beginning of a skeletal system that will develop in later weeks.
4–5-Week Embryo	Organ systems have developed including a primitive type of kidney called the *mesonephros*. This kidney will soon degenerate and be replaced by a new one.
5–6-Week Embryo	Organ systems are developing very rapidly. A new type of kidney appears called the *metanephros*. This will eventually grow into the adult human kidney.
6–8-Week Embryo	There is a rapid development of a brain lobe called the telencephalon which grows into the *cerebrum* in later weeks.
8-Week Fetus	This stage is now called the *fetus* because it looks like the adult form.

ONTOGENY	RECAPITULATES	PHYLOGENY
(Developmental Stages)	(Repeat)	(Evolutionary History)

Pig and Primate Embryo
(developed cerebrum of brain)

_____

Chick Embryo
(has dry land kidney called *metanephros*)

_____

Frog Embryo
(has aquatic kidney called *mesonephros*)

_____

Early Vertebrates
(beginning of internal skeleton)

_____

Flatworms and Roundworms
(definite organs present)

_____

Jellyfish
(cells organize into tissues)

_____

Colonial Protozoa
(cluster of identical cells)

_____

Eukaryotic Cells
(unicellular with organelles)

_____

(no comparable stage
in human development)

Prokaryotic Cells
(no cell organelles)

1. Define *embryo*.

2. Define *fetus*.

3. What week of development marks the beginning of the fetus stage in humans?

4. What is meant by "ontogeny recapitulates phylogeny"?

5. Is it true that the human embryo first looks like a fish, a frog, and then a reptile before reaching the fetal stage? Explain your answer.

ACTIVITY #2

"EGGS, SPERM, AND FERTILIZATION"

EGGS

By the fifth week, a human female embryo already has pre-egg cells multiplying in her ovaries. These pre-egg cells begin meiosis and develop into a cell stage called the *oocyte*. Each oocyte is surrounded by a small cluster of cells called the **follicle**. There are about a million oocytes in the ovary of a female baby at birth. These immature eggs are stopped at Prophase I of meiosis until she reaches puberty. This is a significant vulnerability because the chromosomes of oocytes are exposed to many environmental chemicals during childhood. Chromosomes can be damaged by these chemicals.

The oocytes mature into eggs beginning at puberty. Usually one egg is released (called **ovulation**) each lunar month. This monthly process, called the **menstrual cycle**, is initiated by follicle stimulating hormone (**FSH**), which is produced by the pituitary gland (one of the glands of the endocrine system).

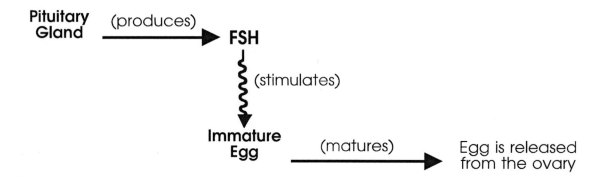

As the egg matures, the other cells surrounding it divide and grow. Most of this growing cellular mass remains in the ovary after the egg is released. It is called the **corpus luteum**. There is a fatty substance stored in the corpus luteum that contains the hormones **estrogen** and **progesterone**. These hormones are released into the bloodstream and stimulate the growth of the inner uterine wall (**endometrium**) for possible implantation of an embryo.

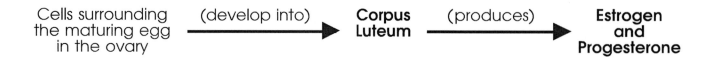

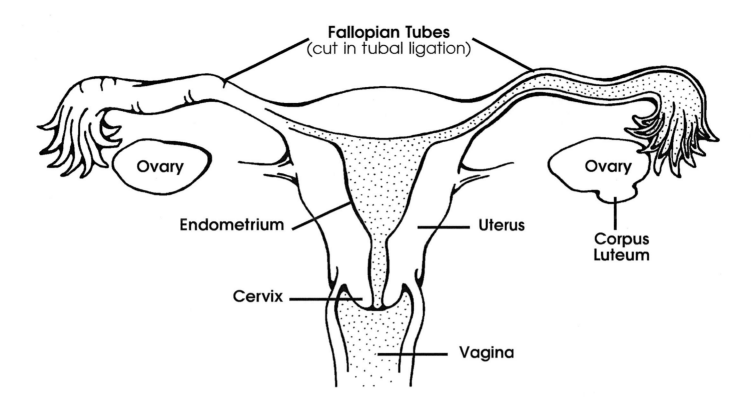

Fallopian Tubes
(cut in tubal ligation)

Ovary

Ovary

Endometrium

Uterus

Corpus
Luteum

Cervix

Vagina

The monthly menstrual cycle is fairly complex but can be summarized as:

Day 1   Menstrual flow begins from previous month's cycle. One egg begins
                  to mature in the ovary for release in the next cycle.

Day 14–15   Ovulation. (Ovary releases an egg.) The corpus luteum produces
                  hormones that stimulate the endometrium of the uterus to grow.

Day 28   If the egg isn't fertilized, then the uterus lining is shed with the
                  menstrual flow.

? QUESTION

1. Health officials warn: "The eggs of your daughters can be damaged by certain chemicals you are
   exposed to during pregnancy." How can the eggs of your daughter be damaged when she won't
   start menstruating until 12 or 13 years after her birth?

2. Which endocrine gland produces the hormone that stimulates an egg to mature?

3. Where does the corpus luteum form, and what hormones does it produce?

4. What day of the menstrual cycle does ovulation usually happen?

5. The menstrual flow is a shedding of the _____ lining.

| GO GET |

1. A compound microscope.

2. Three microscope slides: Immature Egg
Mature Egg
Corpus Luteum

| NOW |

1. Work with two other lab groups. Put a different slide on each microscope, and use low magnification to get an overview of the sectioned ovaries.

2. The immature eggs are bigger than most other cells in the ovary. A maturing egg cell is larger and has a ring of cells surrounding it. The spherical mass of cells is called the follicle. The corpus luteum is even larger than the follicle, and is a solid mass of cells without an egg inside. (The egg has been released.)

3. Look back and forth among the three slides until you can see the difference in the structures.

4. Draw each structural stage in enough detail so that you can find it again (perhaps on a test) with the help of your picture.

| Immature Egg | Mature Egg | Corpus Luteum |

5. *Return the slides.*

SPERM

The reproductive system of the human male embryo is noticeably differentiated by the eighth week. However, the male fetus does not begin meiotic division of sex cells as does the female fetus. The female has immature eggs that are stopped at Prophase I of meiosis. The male doesn't begin sperm production until puberty.

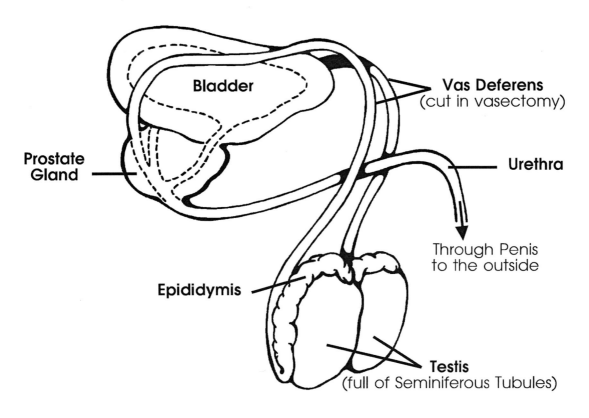

It takes about three weeks for sperm to be produced. If a male is exposed to damaging chemicals, only the current "batch" of sperm is affected. After a month, sperm production could be back to normal. Of course, chromosome damage does sometimes happen in the male gametes as in the female. But, consider how little time sperm chromosomes are exposed to potential damage by environmental factors compared to egg chromosomes.

Sperm are produced (200–500 million daily) along the inside of an extensive system of tubes (*seminiferous tubules*) in the testes. They are stored in enlarged tubes called the *epididymis*.

SPERM

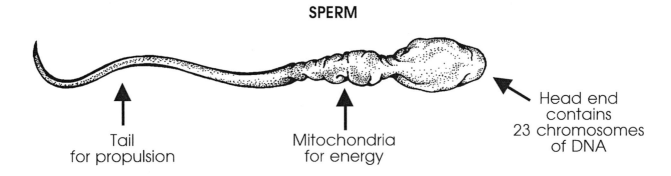

Tail for propulsion

Mitochondria for energy

Head end contains 23 chromosomes of DNA

1. Explain how sperm are less vulnerable to chromosome damage than eggs.

2. Where specifically are sperm produced?

3. Where are they stored?

GO GET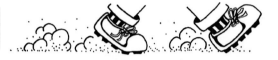

Two microscope slides: Testis
                           Human Sperm

NOW

Testis

1. Examine the cross-section of a testis, and find the seminferous tubules filled with various stages of sperm production.

2. Draw a picture of the testis. Label the seminiferous tubules and sperm.

3. Examine the slide of human sperm. Identify the head, mitochondrial region, and tail. Make a sketch and label it.

4. *Return the slides.*

Sperm

FERTILIZATION

The human egg is released from the ovary with a layer of follicle cells stuck to its outside. Sperm cannot fertilize the egg until this layer of cells has been removed. Each sperm cell produces a small amount of enzyme that dissolves the jelly-like glue holding the small cells to the egg. Much of this enzyme is necessary to separate the follicle layer from the outside of the egg.

Eventually, enough of the protective layer surrounding the egg is dissolved, and one of the sperm penetrates the egg. Once that happens, the egg membrane reacts by forming a new layer of jelly around the egg, thereby preventing any more sperm from entering it. If more than one sperm fertilizes an egg, the resulting embryo dies.

Fertilization usually occurs as the egg moves through the fallopian tube towards the uterus. The embryo continues to develop for about one week before it implants in the wall of the uterus. After implantation, a hormone from the growing embryo signals the corpus luteum (in the ovary) to produce large amounts of estrogen, which then stimulates the mother's reproductive system to prepare for pregnancy. Estrogen also prevents new eggs from developing during pregnancy. (This is why estrogen can be used for birth control.)

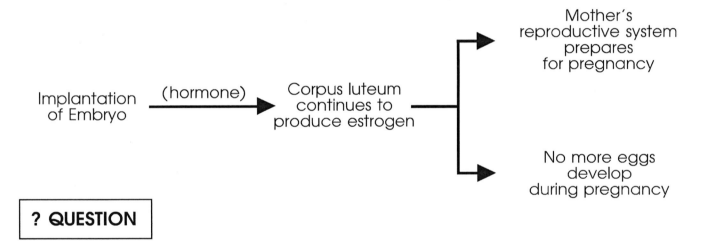

? QUESTION

1. It is necessary for a male to have a high sperm count to be fertile. If only one sperm is necessary to fertilize the egg, then what function is served by the other sperm?

2. What event signals the mother's reproductive system to prepare for pregnancy?

3. What prevents more than one sperm from fertilizing the egg?

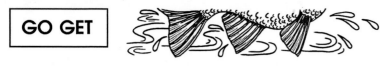

GO GET

A depression slide and coverslip.

NOW

If your instructor has been able to get mature sea urchins, then this is the time to watch fertilization actually happen.

1. Your instructor will inject the urchins with a salt solution that stimulates the release of their gametes. The urchins are then placed upside-down in a beaker of sea water. The gametes will flow out of the animal.

2. Sperm looks milky. The eggs are granular and usually have a slight pink or yellow color.

3. Put a drop of the eggs into a depression slide (no coverslip). Carefully place the slide on your microscope and examine the unfertilized eggs using the 10x objective lens.

4. The sperm must be diluted with sea water because too many sperm causes abnormal fertilization. If the sperm collection beaker looks slightly milky, then dilute the sperm further. Add a drop of the sperm to your egg slide. Cover the slide with a coverslip, and immediately observe the events under the microscope. A *fertilization membrane* usually forms within 2 minutes.

5. When you've seen the membrane form, put this slide aside, and recheck it every 30 minutes. Don't leave the slide on the microscope with the light on because fertilized eggs will soon overheat. If everything goes well, the first *cleavage* (division) should happen in about an hour. Watch for it!

6. Draw pictures of the following:

Unfertilized Egg	**Fertilization Membrane**	**Cleavage**

ACTIVITY #3

"METHODS OF FEEDING THE EMBRYO"

QUICK-DEVELOPMENT
SELF-FEEDING

Invertebrates usually give no special care to their embryos. The only source of food during the first stages of development is provided by the cytoplasm in their eggs. After fertilization, there is rapid cell division and development to allow the embryo to feed on its own. As one example, the sea urchin embryo develops to a self-feeding stage in 24 hours or less. There are many small pieces of organic matter and micro-organisms in water for young embryos to eat. (You will see sea urchin embryos during Activity #4.)

YOLK

Nutrition in the form of *yolk* is another way of giving food to the embryo. Fish are examples of organisms that have small amounts of yolk in the egg. Birds and reptiles have much more yolk in their eggs. Larger amounts of yolk provide longer possible times for development. This is especially necessary for the more advanced land vertebrates.

**Sea Urchin
& Human
Egg Cell**
(very little yolk)

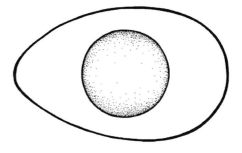

**Reptile & Bird
Egg Cell**
(very large yolk)

O

**Frog
Egg Cell**
(a little more yolk)

PLACENTA

Mammals provide nutrition to their embryos through a specialized integrated feeding structure called the *placenta*. It is formed partly by the embryo and partly by the mother. Nutrients, wastes, and blood gases are exchanged between the embryo's blood system and the mother's blood system. The placenta begins as a few specialized cells on the outside of the implanting embryo. These special cells digest their way into the wall of the uterus. Soon after implantation, finger-like projections begin the formation of a more efficient structure. By the second month, the placenta is well developed, and continues to grow with the fetus.

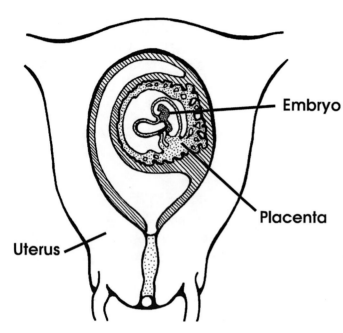

Embryo

Placenta

Uterus

The human embryo, from the zygote to blastocyst stage, must survive on the cytoplasm of the original egg cell. The egg divides but cells don't grow in size. In about one week the developing human embryo begins to implant into the uterine wall for the next stage of feeding (the placenta).

? QUESTION

1. List three methods for feeding early embryos by different organisms.

    a.

    b.

    c.

2. Why do complex animals require more specialized embryonic feeding mechanisms?

3. Why do most land animals require a more developed embryonic feeding mechanism than aquatic animals?

ACTIVITY #4

"STAGES OF DEVELOPMENT"

During this Activity, you will examine 10 stages of vertebrate development using various organisms from sea urchin to pig embryos to illustrate each stage. We will skip many of the details, and focus only on a few structures as examples of the events.

CLEAVAGE, MORULA, AND BLASTOCYST

The first divisions in development are called *cleavage* because the zygote divides (or cleaves) into two cells, then four, then eight, etc. Eventually, a small solid ball of cells forms called the *morula*. Cells of the morula continue to divide, producing a hollow ball of cells called the *blastocyst*. The human blastocyst develops in about one week after fertilization. You can get an idea of what these early stages look like by observing early embryos of sea urchin and frog.

GO GET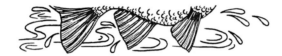

Two microscope slides: Early Sea Urchin Development
                           Frog Blastula (stage 8)

NOW

1. Examine the early developmental stages of the sea urchin.

2. Compare the sizes of the earliest embryos undergoing cleavage. Are the stages from zygote to morula about the same size? _____ Are these early cells growing or just dividing?

   _____

3. Draw pictures of these stages:

Zygote	Early Cleavage	Morula

NEXT

1. Examine the early frog embryo.

2. The frog blastocyst (also called *blastula*) is a partial hollow ball of cells. You should be able to see several different cell types. These cells are changing into new kinds of cells for the next stage of development.

3. Draw a picture of the frog blastocyst, and show the different cell types.

4. *Return the slides.*

Frog Blastocyst

EARLY CHICK EMBRYOS

GO GET

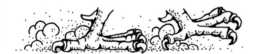

Two microscope slides: 21-Hour Chick Embryo

28-Hour Chick Embryo

NOW

1. Work with another lab group. Put the two slides on different microscopes so that you can look back and forth between them.

2. The 21-hour embryo shows early development of the nervous system. The long **neural fold** becomes the spinal cord in a later stage. Perhaps you can see that the head end is slightly larger.

3. The 28-hour embryo has a more developed neural fold, and you can see that the brain end has enlarged. Also, there are several paired blocks of tissue along the **neural tube**. These blocks are called **somites**. The somites develop into the internal organs, skeleton, and muscles of the adult body.

4. Draw pictures of the two embryonic stages, and label the neural fold, neural tube, head end, and somites.

21-Hour Chick Embryo

28-Hour Chick Embryo

5. *Return the slides.*

LATER CHICK EMBRYOS

GO GET

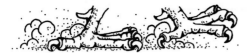

Two microscope slides: 56-Hour Chick Embryo

72-Hour Chick Embryo

NOW

These chick embryo stages are comparable to three and four-week-old human embryos.

1. Put the two slides on different microscopes for comparison. These are side views of the embryos, which are shaped like a question mark (either forward or reversed depending on how the slide was made).

2. You should be able to see changes in the brain development between the two embryonic stages. The brain consists of several lobes. In the 72-hour stage there is a lobe in front of the lobe with the eye in it. That front lobe is the **cerebrum**.

3. The somites are easy to see. How many are there? _____

4. There is a structure bulging from the middle of the embryo, and positioned below the brain. This is the developing heart. In the older embryo, the bottom chamber of the heart is larger. That larger chamber is the *ventricle*.

5. Draw a picture of the 72-hour embryo showing brain and spinal cord, eye, heart, and somites. Label your drawing.

6. *Return the slides.*

72-Hour Chick Embryo

PIG EMBRYO

GO GET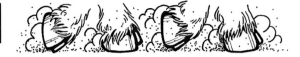

The slide of the 10-mm pig embryo.

NOW

The 10-mm pig embryo is comparable to a human embryo stage at six to eight weeks.

1. You should recognize a well developed nervous system, including backbone, large brain, but smaller eyes than in the chick embryo.

2. Can you find the *limb buds*? In the human embryo these buds will develop into arms and legs.

3. Just below the heart is a large dark structure, the *liver*.

4. Draw a picture of the pig embryo showing brain, eye, vertebral column, heart, liver, and limb buds. Label your drawing.

5. *Return the slides.*

10-mm Pig Embryo

ACTIVITY #5

"DISRUPTION OF NORMAL DEVELOPMENT"

Considering all the events that must go exactly right during embryonic development, it is easy to see that events can go wrong. The general principle for understanding developmental disorders is:

The earlier the disruption, the more serious are the consequences.

Some researchers estimate that one-third of conceptions do not make it to birth. Women are usually unaware of the earliest embryonic failures, which are also the most common. However, there are several disruptions of later development that are very serious and reveal themselves at birth (4–5% of births), or as late-term miscarriages.

GENE MUTATIONS

Gene mutations can destroy the normal production of essential enzymes controlling basic metabolic processes in the fetus.

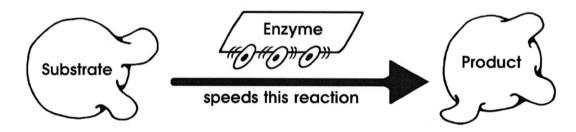

Most states require the immediate testing of all babies for PKU (phenylketonuria), which is a deficiency of an enzyme responsible for the metabolism of the amino acid *phenylalanine*. This disorder is similar to other gene mutations—no product is formed, and there is a buildup of the substrate. High concentrations of these substrates are usually toxic or disruptive, and often the product is essential for other processes. Tay Sachs, galactosemia, and tyrosinosis are other metabolic disorders resulting from gene mutations.

CHROMOSOMAL ABERRATIONS

When mistakes occur during meiosis of sperm or egg production, abnormal numbers of chromosomes in the embryo are possible. These events are almost always lethal. However, some chromosomal aberrations (X, XXY, and three #21 chromosomes) occur in about 1% of births. These babies have serious health problems. The *trisomy* of #21 chromosomes produces Down's syndrome, the most common form of mental retardation. The other chromosomal aberrations also result in similar problems.

ECTOPIC PREGNANCY

Occasionally, the embryo implants in the wall of a fallopian tube, or on the outside of the uterus or intestine. There are two serious consequences of this abnormal event. First, the child will have to be delivered by Cesarean section. The second serious problem is that the placenta can attach to the wall of the wrong organ. That organ may be damaged or destroyed by placental development. This condition can be so dangerous to the mother's life, that termination of pregnancy may be her only chance of survival.

POSSIBLE SITES OF IMPLANTATION

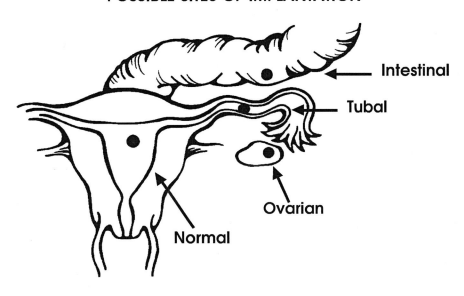

Intestinal

Tubal

Ovarian

Normal

INCOMPLETE DEVELOPMENT OF ORGAN

Sometimes an organ does not develop completely during early development. The cause can be a foreign chemical like thalidomide, or a disease like measles. Common examples are spina bifida (neural tube doesn't close), or holes between the heart chambers.

The general principle of developmental disorders applies especially in these cases. The earlier the problem happens, the more serious are the consequences.

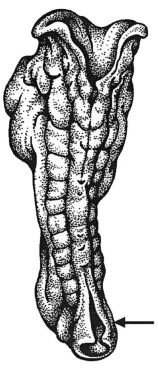

Spina bifida occurs if this part of the neural tube does not close during early development.

BAD HABITS DURING PREGNANCY

We have very little control over the previously described disruptions of normal development. In fact, many early miscarriages are the result of the mother's hormonal system "warming up" for future reproductive success.

However, there are disruptions in development that we *can* control—bad habits during pregnancy. Science makes a certain direct statement about bad habits during pregnancy:

"Drink alcohol, smoke cigarettes or marijuana, use drugs, or have poor nutrition, and your child will be below normal in mental abilities, and may be physically deformed."

FETAL ALCOHOL/DRUG SYNDROME

This fetal damage is predictable and results from the mother's drinking or drug habit. Fetal Alcohol/Drug Syndrome includes characteristic facial deformations, a degree of mental retardation, and defects in internal organs (especially the heart and liver).

CIGARETTE SMOKING

The majority of babies born by mothers who smoke, have a smaller placenta, lower birth weight, and lower overall health. The effects on the fetus are not usually as extreme as with alcohol or drug use by the mother, but the birth results are 100% predictable.

POOR NUTRITION

The usual problem with poor nutrition in this country is not a lack of Calories, but an unbalanced diet (not enough protein, vitamins, and minerals). The effects of poor nutrition are lower birth weight, lower overall health, and below-average mental ability.

If the nutritional problems during pregnancy are severe, as seen in overpopulated parts of the world, all of the detrimental effects during embryonic and fetal development are greatly magnified.

1. What is the general principle for understanding developmental disorders?

2. Perhaps as many as _____ of all embryos don't survive to birth.

3. What is the percent of births with developmental defects?

4. What is the most serious potential risk in an ectopic pregnancy?

5. List the two immediate biochemical effects of most gene mutations.

   a.

   b.

6. What is the usual result of chromosomal aberrations?

7. What are the common effects on embryonic development caused by alcohol, drugs, cigarettes, and poor nutrition?

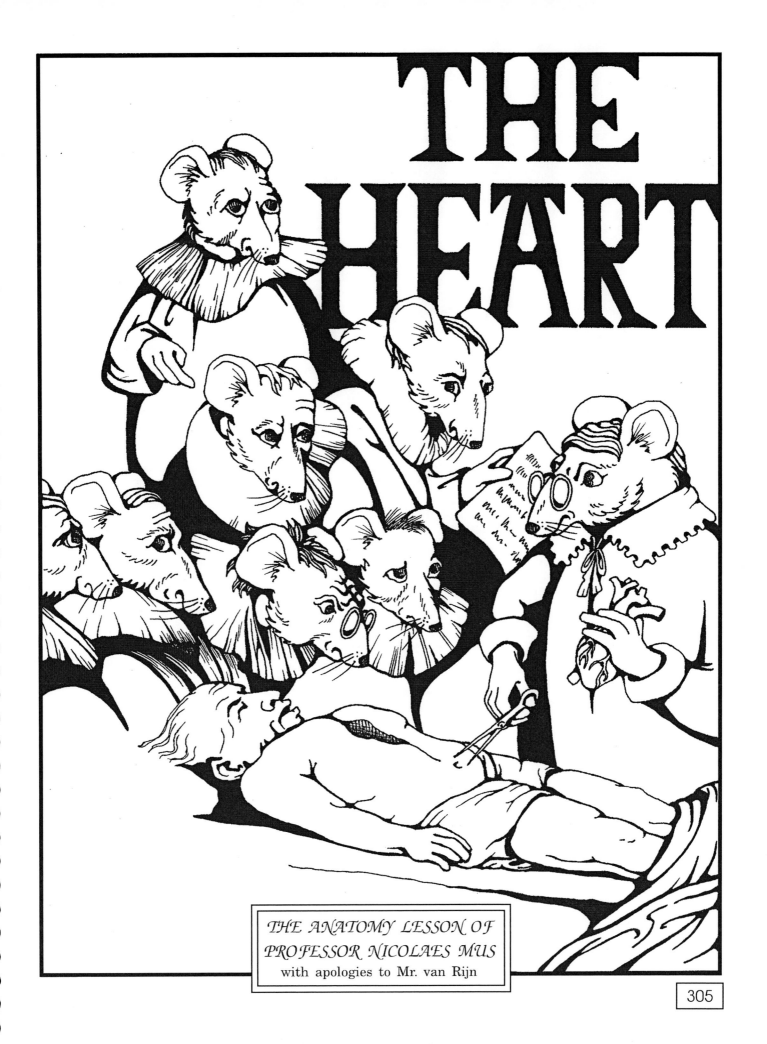

THE HEART

THE ANATOMY LESSON OF
PROFESSOR NICOLAES MUS
with apologies to Mr. van Rijn

305

Cardiomyocytes (heart muscle cells) will beat all by themselves in a petri dish. Most astonishingly, they will beat synchronously (in unison). Heart cells grafted to a synthetic scaffold of biodegradable mesh will beat like a heart, which may in the future lead to repair patches that can be applied to human hearts damaged by myocardial infarction.

—HTTP://WWW.YOUTUBE.COM/WATCH?V=RO4PAC21M24

In one year the average human heart circulates from 770,000 to 1.6 million gallons of blood through the body—4000 gallons of blood each day. The heart creates enough pressure to squirt blood 30 feet (9 m). Blood travels 60,000 miles (96,540 km) per day on its journey through the body.

—HTTP://WWW.SKYGAZE.COM/CONTENT/FACTS/BODY.SHTML

THE HEART

INTRODUCTION

The heart is an incredible pump. It can beat 2.5 billion times in a lifetime, pumping 35 million gallons of blood. Furthermore, the heart is capable of varying its output between 50 ml and 250 ml per stroke. It can contract at rates from 60 to 160 beats per minute. You can't buy a better pump!

This week's lab will include some aspects of heart structure and function. Also, you will learn to measure blood pressure, and discover the medical implications related to heart function.

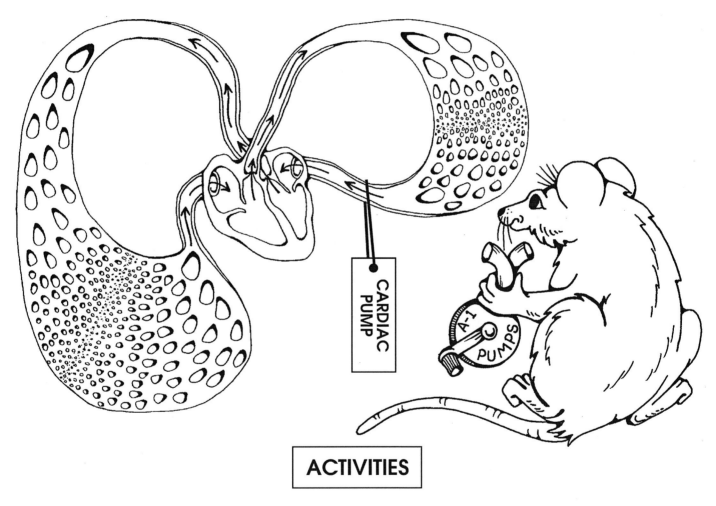

CARDIAC PUMP

A-1 PUMPS

ACTIVITIES

ACTIVITY #1

"THE HEART AS A PUMP"

When you are resting, your heart pumps about 5 liters of blood per minute. This is about the same rate as a slow flow of water from the bathroom faucet when you brush your teeth. During strenuous exercise your heart can pump 30 liters of blood per minute. This is about equal to the water flow when you fast-fill the bathtub. The heart is capable of this wide range of performance because of its structure.

TWO PUMPS IN ONE

The heart is actually two pumps—a *right pump* and a *left pump*. The right pump delivers blood to the lungs; this route is called the *pulmonary circuit*. The left pump pushes blood to the rest of the body; this route is called the *systemic circuit*.

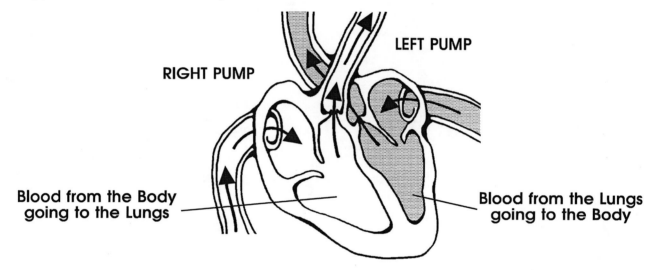

Notice that this diagram is drawn as if the heart is facing you. This means that the right side of the heart is on the *left* side of the drawing. All anatomy diagrams are drawn in this view. Remember this whenever you look at a medical picture.

TWO CHAMBERS PER PUMP

There are *two* chambers in each of the two heart pumps. The top one is a temporary storage chamber called the *atrium*, and the bottom one is a pumping chamber called the *ventricle*. Blood from the body tissues flows into the atrium of the right heart pump. This blood is then pushed through a valve and enters the right ventricle. The ventricle does the hard work of pumping blood out of the heart. The right ventricle pumps blood to the lungs where it is *oxygenated*. While the ventricle is pumping blood out of the heart, the atrium fills with blood entering the heart. This efficient design allows the atrium to quickly refill the emptied ventricle, resulting in a fast-pumping heart.

Oxygenated blood from the lungs enters the atrium of the left heart pump. This blood is then moved into the left ventricle, which pumps the blood to all of the body tissues.

1. Which chamber has to do the most work? (circle your choice)

   Atrium   or   Ventricle

2. Which chamber would have a thicker muscle wall? (circle your choice)

   Atrium   or   Ventricle

3. Which pump has to do the most work? (circle your choice)

   Right Ventricle   or   Left Ventricle

4. Which pump has a thicker muscle wall? (circle your choice)

   Right Ventricle   or   Left Ventricle

5. The right heart pump moves blood to the _____.

6. The left heart pump moves blood to the _____.

HEART VALVES

Four heart valves are strategically located to prevent backflow as blood moves through the heart. These valves are like one-way doors—they only open in one direction. There is a *chamber valve* between each atrium and ventricle. These two chamber valves ensure that blood will not flow back into the atria when the ventricles contract.

Blood is pushed out of the ventricles and into the two big arteries leaving the heart. There is a valve in each of these arteries. The *artery valves* prevent backflow into the ventricles once blood has been pumped into the arteries. The four heart valves ensure that blood moves in only one direction through the heart circuit. Each of the heart valves has its own special name, but we'll leave those details to an anatomy class.

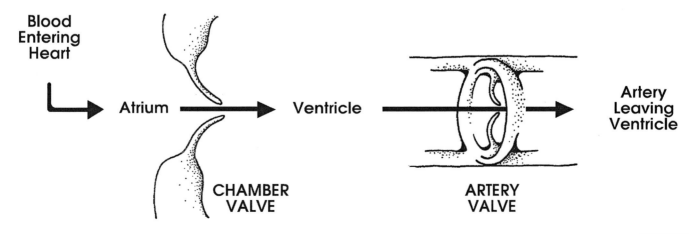

A heart valve is designed to plug an opening when blood moves in the wrong direction. Think of a valve as being something like a parachute that is attached to the heart or artery wall. If blood moves in the wrong direction, the "parachute" (valve) fills with blood and expands to plug the opening. When the blood moves in the correct direction, the valve collapses like an upside-down parachute. This allows the blood to easily pass through the valve.

EXAMPLE

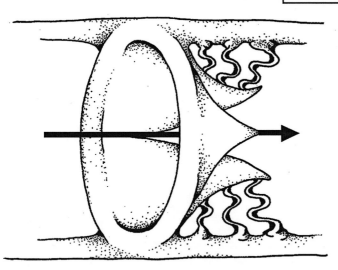

Blood moving in the correct direction pushes the valve aside, and blood enters the ventricle.

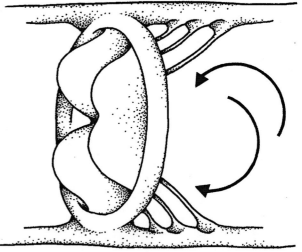

Blood moving in the wrong direction fills the valve which plugs the opening so that blood cannot re-enter the atrium.

The heart valves are *flexible* so that they can fill with blood as shown above. There are *special cords* attaching the valve to the heart wall. These cords operate similar to the ropes of a parachute.

? QUESTION

1. What would happen to blood flow if one of the valve "cords" broke? Be specific.

2. What would happen to blood flow if one of the valves was scarred by disease, narrowing the opening?

3. If you had a moderate heart valve problem, what would the heart have to do to compensate?

4. On which side of the heart would a moderate heart valve problem have more consequence to your health? Explain your answer.

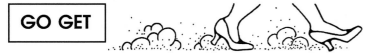
A sectioned sheep heart from the display table.

NOW

1. See if you can identify the four chambers of the heart. *Remember:* One of the ventricles should have a thicker muscle wall.

2. Find a heart valve and feel the valve to determine its flexibility. Can you find the valve "cords"?

3. Show your instructor when you can identify all of these structures.

4. Draw a simple sketch of the dissected heart. This will remind you of what you saw in case you are tested on it later.

Dissected Heart

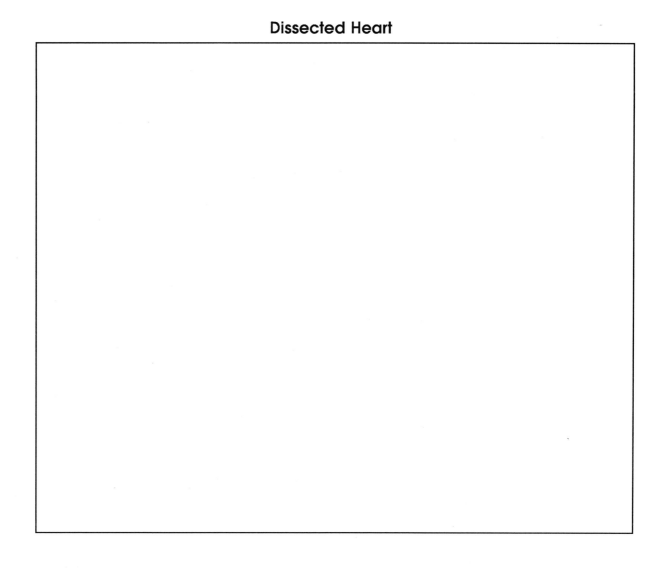

ACTIVITY #2

"HEART SOUNDS"

The heart sound is often described as "lub-dub." You might think that the two parts of this sound come from the separate contractions of the upper and lower chambers of the heart. That is not correct. Actually, these sounds are more closely associated with the closing of the heart valves.

The first sound, *lub*, happens when the blood vibrates after the **chamber valves close** between the atria and ventricles. The second sound, *dub*, occurs when the blood vibrates just after the heart **artery valves close**. The sounds are created by vibration waves. With the aid of a stethoscope, a physician can hear these heart sounds and determine if there has been any damage to the valves.

GO GET	

A stethoscope.

NOW

1. Clean the earpieces of the stethoscope with a cotton ball soaked in alcohol. *Always repeat this procedure whenever another person uses the stethoscope.*

2. Fit the stethoscope earpieces in your ears so that they are comfortable and point slightly forward in the ear passage. (Your ear passage points forward before it turns inwards to the ear drum.)

3. Move the bell of the stethoscope around the *left* side of your chest starting at the lower center notch of your rib cage.

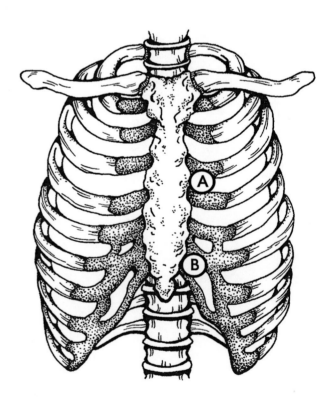

As the stethoscope is moved around the heart area, you will hear the "lub" sound better at some places and the "dub" sound better at other places. An experienced physician or nurse can position the stethoscope to hear each heart valve and determine whether there is an abnormal sound. Abnormal sounds indicate possible valve damage or other circulation problems.

THEN

This part gets a little tricky, so read carefully.

Most people expect that the two big heart arteries would exit from the bottom of the ventricles, but they don't. These arteries come out of the top of the ventricles, and arch upwards above the heart. Refer to the diagram under "Two Pumps in One" in Activity #1, and notice the location of the two heart arteries. The artery valve allowing blood flow out of the ventricle is next to the chamber valve controlling flow from the atrium into the ventricle.

The **"dub"** sound of the heartbeat resonates *upward*, which is the direction that the heart arteries leave the heart. In which position of the stethoscope (A or B) do you hear mainly a "dub" sound? _____ This would indicate that you are located near the top of the heart where the heart artery valves make their sounds.

Continue to move the stethoscope to *both sides* of this position until the heart sounds quiet. You are mapping the general location of the top of the heart. Mark the extent of this "dub" zone on the rib cage diagram. The sound zone is bigger than the heart because the sound spreads outward.

The **"lub"** sound of the heartbeat resonates *downward* from the chamber valves, so you hear it best at the bottom of the heart. In which position of the stethoscope (A or B) do you hear mainly a "lub" sound? _____ This would indicate that you are located nearer the bottom of the heart where the sound of chamber valves is loudest.

Continue to move the stethoscope to the *left* of this position until the loud "lub" sound quiets. You are mapping the general location of the bottom of the heart. Mark the extent of this "lub" zone on the rib cage diagram.

FINALLY

Draw an arrow from the center of the "dub" zone to the center of the "lub" zone on the rib cage diagram. That arrow is the general orientation of the heart. The orientation is (circle your choice)

vertical (straight up and down).

to the left of vertical (bottom of the heart points to the left).

to the right of vertical (bottom of the heart points to the right).

This sound technique of inferring the orientation of the heart is less accurate than the EKG method used in hospitals. The EKG can reveal whether the heart has enlarged on its left or right side. Enlargement is an indication of a heart or circulation abnormality.

ACTIVITY #3

"HEART RATE AND THE PULSE"

The heart of a resting person contracts somewhere between 60 and 80 times per minute. These contractions can be counted with the aid of a stethoscope, which you will do in a few minutes. Heart rate can also be determined by counting the number of pulse waves that pass by a spot on an artery. Counting these waves by touch is how you measure the *pulse*.

THE PULSE WAVE

The *aorta* is the large artery that supplies the blood to all other arteries that feed the body tissues.

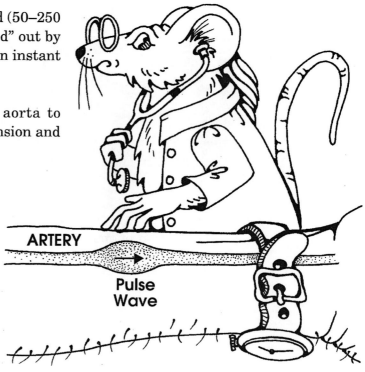

Each heart contraction forces a volume of blood (50–250 ml) into the aorta. First, the aorta is "ballooned" out by blood, then the elastic artery wall snaps back an instant later.

The recoil causes the adjacent area of the aorta to balloon out and snap back. The alternate expansion and recoil of the aorta wall "pulses" outward from the heart to the other arteries of the body.

You can feel these waves passing by whenever you press a finger on an artery.

The *carotid pulse* is felt when you press your fingers against the side of your throat. The *radial pulse* is felt when you press your fingers on the thumb side of your upward-turned wrist.

ARTERY

Pulse Wave

NOW

1. Use the stethoscope to count your heartbeats for 30 seconds.

    Stethoscope Heart Rate = _____ beats per minute

2. Count both your radial pulse waves and carotid pulse waves for 30 seconds.

    Radial Pulse = _____ waves per minute

    Carotid Pulse = _____ waves per minute

? QUESTION

1. Which had the stronger pulse waves? (circle your choice)

    Carotid   or   Radial

2. Which is closer to the heart? (circle your choice)

    Carotid   or   Radial

3. Which would produce a stronger pulse wave? (circle your choice)

    A smaller heart   or   A bigger heart

4. Arteriosclerosis hardens the artery wall with scar tissue. If arteries have been partially injured by arteriosclerosis and the arterial wall is less flexible than normal, then would the pulse be stronger or weaker than normal?

5. If a person has arteriosclerosis, what happens to the blood pressure near the end of the arteries? (circle your choice) *Hint:* Is some of the energy of the heart contraction "used up" by the pulse wave?

    a. it is the same as normal

    b. it is higher than normal

    c. it is lower than normal

    What would be the consequences?

6. Half of the people have a smaller-than-average sized heart and half have a larger-than-average sized heart. In which group would you expect the *heart rate* to be higher? Explain your answer.

7. In general, females have a higher heart rate than males. What explanation can you give for this difference?

HEART RATE AND LONGEVITY

Research in comparative physiology suggests that the average mammal heart beats about 1.5 billion times before it wears out. Although there are exceptions to this heart longevity rule, it seems to be generally true whether you're a mouse or an elephant. A mouse's heart beats about 10 times faster than an elephant's heart, and a mouse lives about $\frac{1}{10}$ as long.

Based on the mammalian average for total heart beats, the modern human species is predicted to live about 35 years. Humans score above most other species for longevity. This is probably because we are smarter and can avoid more hardships than the average mammal. However, we also have a limit—somewhere around 2.5 billion beats—if we are lucky enough to survive disaster and illness. How you spend these heartbeats is partly determined by the activities in your lifestyle.

Let's assume that the longevity rule is generally true for humans. A woman who is already doing enough daily activity to keep her heart healthy, asks the question, *"If I train in a very strenuous sport for 4 hours a day beyond my normal activity, then how much might I shorten my life by doing this extra sport?"* Assume that her normal heart rate of 70 is elevated to 120 during the heavy training.

? QUESTION

1. How many *extra* heartbeats does she use per day of sport training? _____

2. Her normal heart rate of 70 per minute means that she would use 100,800 heart beats on a normal day without sport. If an extra 100,800 beats shortens her life by one day, then how many days of sport training does it take to shorten her life by one day? _____

3. How many years of sport would shorten her life by one year? _____

4. Let's assume that this person is considering 8 hours of strenuous sport per day. How many years of this sport activity would it take to shorten her life by one year? _____

    Before we ascribe too much importance to a higher heart rate, remember that females generally live 10% longer than males even though females have a 10% higher resting heart rate. Obviously, other important factors affect longevity.

5. Smoking elevates the heart rate about 10% above normal; so does drinking 2 to 4 cups of coffee per day. If you were a smoker or a coffee drinker for 40 years, how many years of longevity might be lost due to the increased heart rate alone (not taking into account the obvious health risks of tobacco and caffeine)? _____

6. Negative stress can elevate the heart rate 10–20% above normal. How many lost years of longevity might result from a 20-year stress-filled job that elevated heart rate 20% above normal?

ACTIVITY #4

"HOW TO MEASURE BLOOD PRESSURE"

Knowing how to measure your blood pressure is one of the best health-maintenance tools you can learn to use. We offer this Activity to promote your good health.

BLOOD PRESSURE

Blood pressure in body arteries is created by the contraction of the left ventricle. As you would expect, the pressure is highest when the chamber contracts. Pressure during heart contraction is called the *systolic pressure*. When the ventricle relaxes the blood pressure drops. However, instead of dropping to zero, the blood pressure is partially maintained by the recoil of artery walls that are stretched by blood pumped out of the heart. The lower artery pressure during the relaxation of the ventricle is called the *diastolic pressure*.

Medical books state that the typical resting blood pressure is 120 over 80. The 120 refers to the systolic pressure and the 80 refers to the diastolic pressure.

MEASURING BLOOD PRESSURE

The method we will use to measure blood pressure is fairly simple. It is easier to show you how to measure blood pressure than to explain all of the details in writing. Therefore, most of the instructions will come from your lab teacher.

Read through the general steps of the procedure and the hints that follow before you begin practicing.

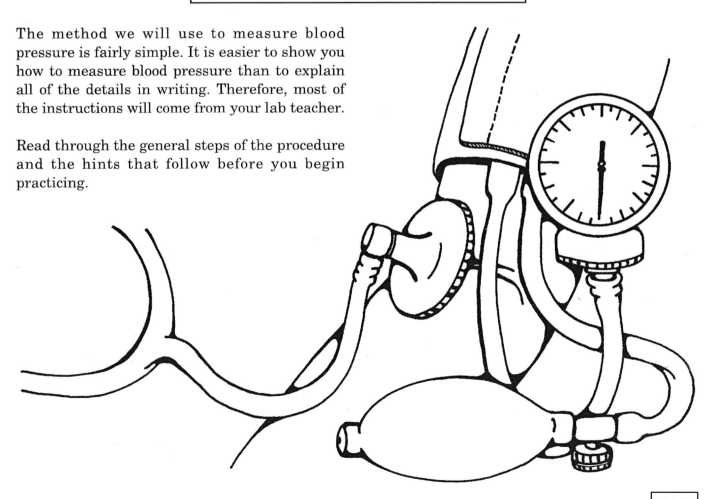

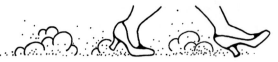

GO GET

A blood pressure cuff.

STEP 1
Fasten a pressure cuff around your upper arm. Place the stethoscope diaphragm over the brachial artery (*inside bend of elbow*). Pump the cuff full of air until all blood is stopped in the brachial artery. The thumping heart sound that you hear through the stethoscope will fade and disappear as the cuff pressure is pumped above the systolic pressure.

STEP 2
Release the pressure on the cuff by slowly opening the valve. Listen to the brachial artery with the stethoscope.

STEP 3
When you first hear a "thumping" sound, read the gauge on the pressure cuff. This is the *systolic pressure*. The blood is just starting to squirt past the cuff during the contraction of the heart.

STEP 4
Continue to release the pressure on the cuff until the thumping sound disappears. Read the pressure gauge. This is the *diastolic pressure*. The blood flows past the cuff during both the contraction and relaxation of the ventricle. The sound disappears when the flow changes from a pulsating squirt to a constant flow.

HINTS

1. Don't pump the pressure cuff over 150 until you've practiced the technique several times.

2. Don't keep pressure on your arm for more than 30 seconds.

3. Let your arm rest for at least 2 minutes after each reading before taking another measurement. This is especially important while you are learning the technique.

4. Take your time. Learn this procedure well. It is important that you know how to measure your own blood pressure. Checking your blood pressure every few months provides you with a thorough understanding of your normal physiology. When an abnormal change occurs, you can seek medical advice.

NOW

Record your blood pressure while sitting: _____ B.P.

With the blood pressure cuff still on your arm but not pumped up, run in place for 30 seconds. Measure your blood pressure after exercise: _____ B.P.

COLD WATER TEST

This test is used to determine the effect of a sensory stimulus (cold) on blood pressure. The normal reflex response to a cold stimulus is a slight increase in blood pressure (both systolic and diastolic). In a normal individual, the systolic pressure will rise no more than 10 mm Hg, but the increase in a *hyper-reactive* individual may be 30 to 40 mm Hg. We will discuss the implications of these responses later.

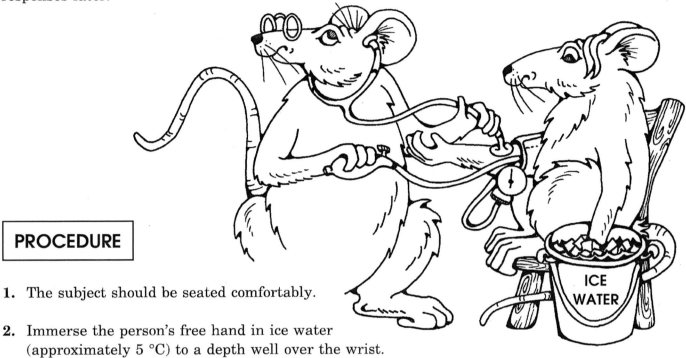

PROCEDURE

1. The subject should be seated comfortably.

2. Immerse the person's free hand in ice water (approximately 5 °C) to a depth well over the wrist.

3. After waiting 30 seconds, measure the blood pressure.

    Your normal resting blood pressure is _____.

    Your blood pressure after cold water is _____.

    Are you a normal or a hyper-reactive
    individual based on the cold-water test? _____

IMPLICATIONS

There is some evidence that people showing a hyper-reaction to a cold stimulus may have a greater chance of developing high blood pressure later in life. Perhaps there is some minor defect in the physiology of these people. Or they may have inherited a more reactive nervous system—favored in hunter-gatherer times—but more easily overstimulated by our modern chaotic life. We just don't know.

Before giving too much importance to the results of the cold water test, remember that lack of exercise, high salt intake, unhealthy diet, and stressful situations are known causes of high blood pressure, and are mostly under your control.

ACTIVITY #5

"MEDICAL IMPLICATIONS"

There are many medical implications related to what you have learned about the heart, and several of these health issues are discussed in this Activity. *Remember:* Always ask your physician to explain health-related problems in a way that you can easily understand. And go to the library. Inform yourself.

ABNORMAL HOLES IN THE HEART

The heart in a normal fetus has a hole between the right and left atria. This opening allows fetal blood to partially bypass the lung circuit since the lungs aren't needed to get oxygen during life in the womb. Usually, the atrial hole closes shortly after birth. A birth defect results if this hole does not grow closed. Another birth defect occurs when there is an abnormal opening between the right and left ventricles. Both of these heart abnormalities can have serious health implications if left uncorrected.

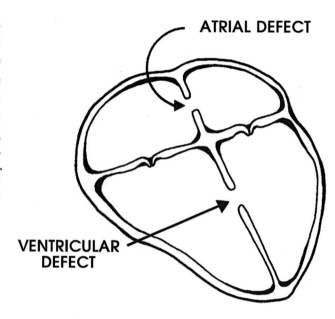

ATRIAL DEFECT

VENTRICULAR DEFECT

? QUESTION

1. What important molecule is carried by blood entering the left heart pump and is not in the blood entering the right heart pump?

2. If the fetal hole between the right and left atria does not close, what happens to the blood in these two chambers?

3. Which ventricle operates under the most pressure (does the most work)?

4. What would happen to the pressure in the two ventricles if there was a hole between them?

5. What would the heart do to compensate for the pressure problem created by a ventricle hole? *Hint:* People with this abnormal hole must have it repaired while they are young or they won't live long.

CORONARY ARTERIES

The heart muscle works very hard and it must be supplied with oxygen and nutrients just like any other part of the body. The vessels that supply blood to the heart muscle are called the *coronary arteries*.

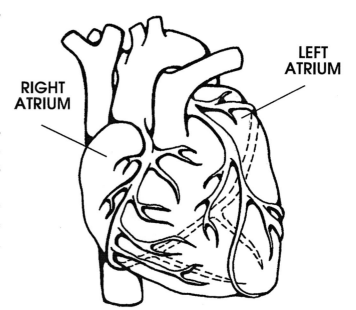

RIGHT ATRIUM

LEFT ATRIUM

There are two important circulation patterns that you can see in this diagram. The right atrium is fed only by the right coronary artery, and the left atrium is supplied only by the left coronary artery. However, each coronary artery supplies blood to parts of *both* ventricles. The ventricles do more work than the atria, and must be supplied with more blood.

Another important aspect of vessel structure in the coronary arteries is the connection between the arteries. Connections between arteries are called *collateral circulation*. These connections are alternate routes of blood flow to tissue if one path is blocked. Some parts of the heart have no collateral circulation. Other parts have only very small-diameter collateral vessels because they are unused. Also, there are different amounts of collateral vessels among people. Can you find a collateral vessel in the heart diagram above? Color that vessel. **Hint:** It is called the posterior circumflex.

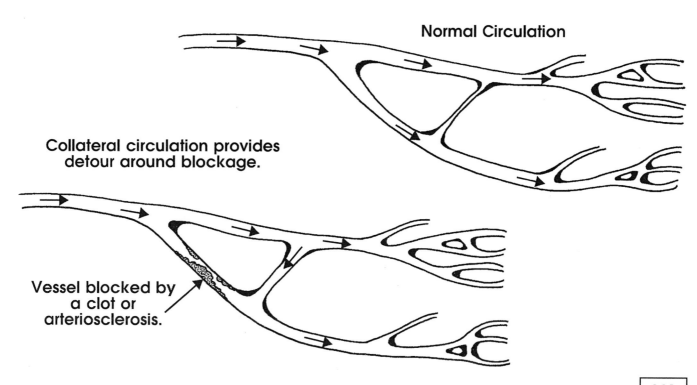

Normal Circulation

Collateral circulation provides detour around blockage.

Vessel blocked by a clot or arteriosclerosis.

1. A patient is told that she has a narrowing of the right coronary artery. Which chambers of her heart are going to be affected the most by this disorder? _____

   Which chamber on the right side has to do the most work and could be the most serious health concern? _____

2. A group of patients were told that they had plugged arteries in their hearts. In addition, they had all suffered a similar size of heart attack. All of these patients survived. Some of them had parts of their injured hearts return almost to normal after several months, while other patients had no such luck. Explain these differences in terms of coronary circulation.

3. A heart attack on which side of the heart would probably cause the most serious immediate risk to the person?

EKG

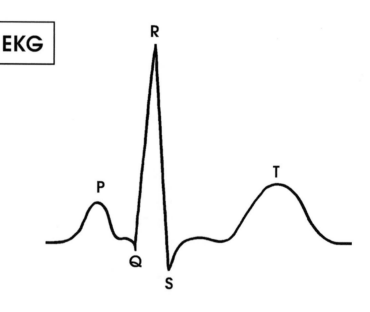

The *electrocardiogram* (called *EKG* or ECG) is a recording of the small electrical currents produced by the contracting and relaxing heart muscle. These electrical patterns indicate whether there is a normal or abnormal functioning of the heart. A normal EKG is shown here.

The *P wave* is a recording of the electrical activity in the atria, and it is especially important in diagnosing problems in the heart's natural *pacemaker*.

The *QRS wave* is a recording of the activating current in the ventricles. This current travels along a special conducting pathway 10 times faster than it would be transmitted through normal heart muscle. The result is that all the muscle cells in both ventricles are stimulated at the same time, causing these chambers to contract quickly and strongly.

The *T wave* occurs just after the ventricles contract, and is a recording of the normal recovery phase of the ventricles. This is a period when the muscle cells perform various biochemical reactions that prepare the ventricles for the next contraction.

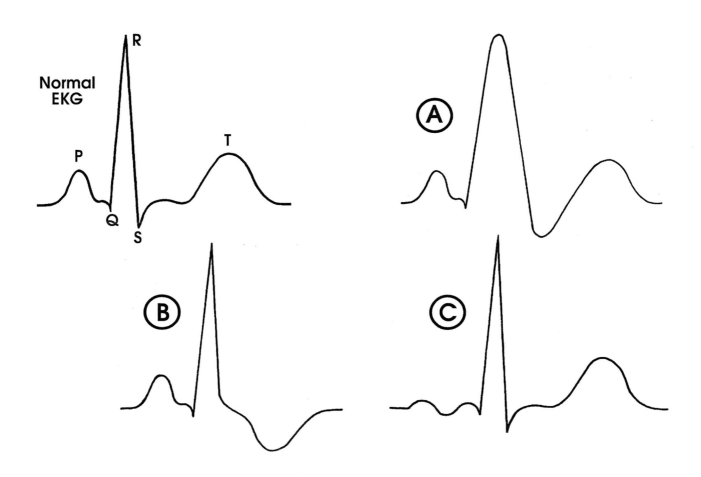

Normal EKG

R
P
Q
S
T

Ⓐ

Ⓑ

Ⓒ

? QUESTION

1. A person who drinks a lot of coffee complains that his heart beats irregularly. Which one of the above EKG waves reflects this problem? _____ Explain your answer.

2. A person has a greatly enlarged heart from the overwork created by long term high blood pressure. Which abnormal EKG wave reflects this problem? _____ Explain your answer.

3. A person with poor coronary circulation to the heart muscle has some heart injury, but may not have suffered death of the heart muscle. Which abnormal EKG wave above reflects this problem? _____ Explain your answer.

4. Why is a heart attack sometimes called a "coronary"?

Chapter 17

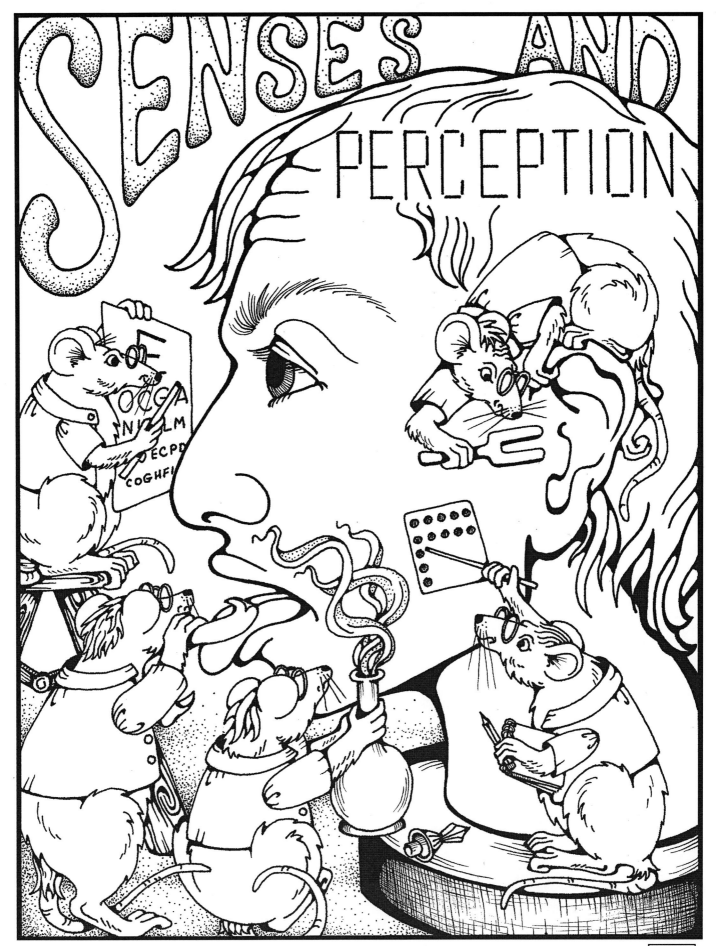

DYNAMIC DEVELOPMENTS AND FASCINATING FACTS IN BIOLOGY

We all know about sweet, salty, sour, and bitter taste sensations. Less widely known is the fifth taste: *umami,* the savory flavor of soy sauce, tomatoes, meats, and many other foods high in glutamate. Umami receptors have also been found throughout the digestive track; their function in digestion and nutrition is unknown.

About 15 to 25 percent of all Americans are *supertasters,* having more papillae and taste buds than the rest of us. Supertasters tend to dislike broccoli and kale, and are more prone to colon polyps because they avoid bitter-tasting vegetables, many of which contain cancer-fighting phytonutrients.

—"20 Things You Didn't Know About Taste" by Kirsten Weir, *Discover Magazine,* December 2010, p.80

—http://discovermagazine.com/2010/dec/20-things-you-didn.t-know-about-taste

Your **enteric nervous system** (ENS) is the intrinsic nervous system of the gastrointestinal tract, in which there are 100–500 million neurons. This enteric nervous system is often referred to as a "second brain." Enteric neurons are mediated mostly by the neurotransmitter serotonin, and secondly by acetylcholine.

—"Enteric nervous system" by John B. Furness (2007), Scholarpedia, 2(10):4064

—http://www.scholarpedia.org/article/Enteric_nervous_system

Our brains and our guts communicate with each other. In fact, most of our intense emotions are signaled through our intestines, leading to visceral manifestations of anxiety, anger, sadness, love, and elation ("butterflies," nausea of apprehension, gut-wrenching dread, etc.) that elicit "the feeling of what happens." This pathway is the foundation of intuition, an important "preconscious" mechanism often regarded as an unnecessary—even bothersome—brain process.

—*The Feeling of What Happens: Body and Emotion in the Making of Consciousness,* Antonio Damasio, 2000

Pain sensation in one part of your body can partially block pain signals from another part. This is the reasoning behind "counter-irritants" and other folk pain remedies that instruct sufferers to endure pain somewhere else to reduce pain in another area. For example, if you plunge your bare foot into freezing water, touching a hot surface with your hand will hurt less.

—"The Brain: Pain" by Carl Zimmer, *Discover Magazine,* June 2011, p. 20

Taste receptors are actually modified skin cells. Taste receptors have excitable membranes just like neurons and release neurotransmitters to excite neighboring neurons.

—Biological Psychology by James W. Kalat, p. 216

SENSES AND PERCEPTION

INTRODUCTION

Humans must be aware of and adjust to environmental demands. Our *senses* provide information about the physical environment. Our **perception**, developed the experiences of trial and error, evaluates sensory information, allowing us to make the appropriate adjustment to the environment. Working together, these two processes have contributed to the success of the human species.

Our senses result from specialized receptors located in various parts of the body. These *receptors* are activated by only one kind of *stimulus* (sound, touch, light, chemicals, etc.). The information from one receptor is kept separate from that sent by another sense organ. In the brain, particular areas are specialized for processing and interpreting the information pertaining to each sense.

Today's lab is designed to demonstrate some of the sensory and perceptual mechanisms of your nervous system.

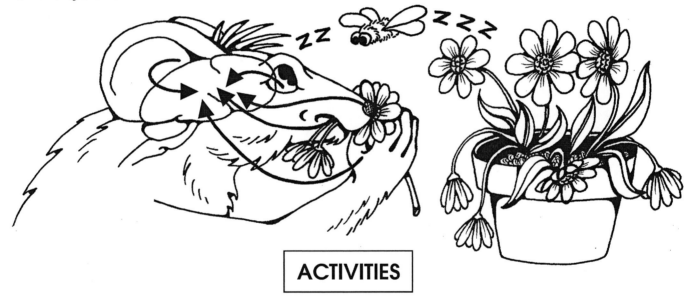

ACTIVITIES

ACTIVITY #1

"TOUCH"

A string-line that loops over on the top of your head from ear to ear approximately separates the *motor area* of the brain (which controls movement) from the *touch area* of the brain (which interprets touch signals). The touch area is behind this line and the motor area is in front of it.

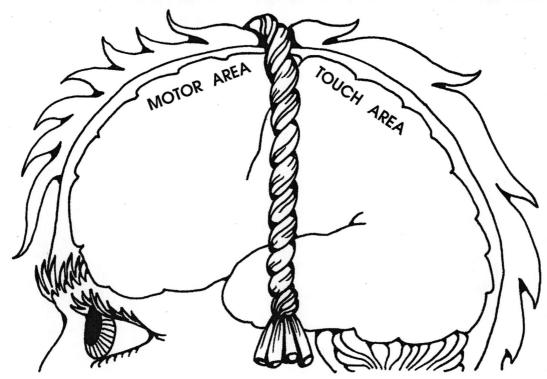

You will determine the density of touch receptors in several areas of your body. Using that information, you can test the idea that *areas of greater sensitivity contain more touch receptors.*

 GO GET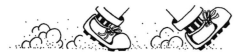

1. A horse hair.

2. A metric ruler.

3. A compass.

NOW

1. Be sure to perform all the tests on each person in your lab group.

2. Mark off a 1 cm x 1 cm square on your fingertip, back, and another area of your body that you would like to test. You might choose an area that itches often or feels strange when touched.

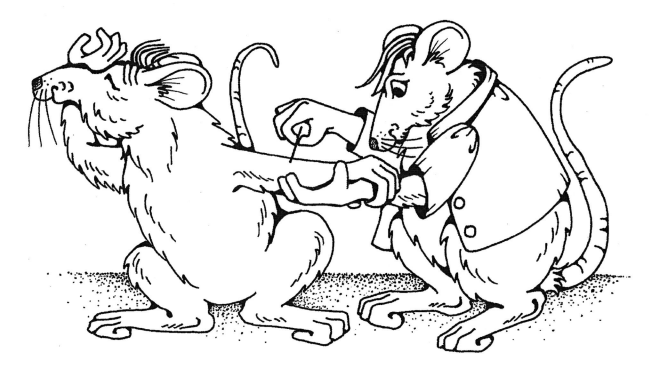

3. Close your eyes while your lab partner lightly touches you 25 times with the horse hair. The touching should be done in a grid-like pattern that covers all of the square you have marked.

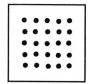

4. Each time you feel the touch of the horse hair, say so. Record the number of positive responses in the Touch Experiment Table on the next page.

5. Next, use the points of a compass to *lightly stimulate* the subject's skin in the area of the marked boxes. The compass points must be blunt and not poke through the skin. (File the points if necessary.) Start with the points close together, then increase their distance apart until the subject definitely feels *two distinct points*. Be sure that the two points are applied simultaneously each time, and retest to see if there is error due to imagination.

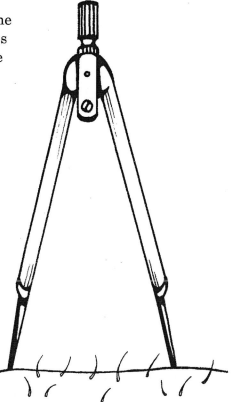

6. Measure the distance between the two compass points when the subject clearly perceives two points. This is called **two-point discrimination**. Record the results for each area of the body that you mapped for touch receptor density. Include the results from everyone in your lab group.

TOUCH EXPERIMENT TABLE

Part of the Body	# of Positive Responses During 25 Touches in 1 cm²	Two-Point Discrimination (in cm)
Fingertip		
Back		
(Other) _____		

? QUESTION

1. Which test area had the greatest density of touch receptors?

2. Which test area had the best two-point discrimination? Explain.

3. How is *two-point discrimination* related to *density* of touch receptors?

4. When you have an itch somewhere on your back, why does it take so much scratching before you finally find it?

ACTIVITY #2

"TEMPERATURE SENSATION"

During this Activity you will determine whether your body detects the *actual* temperature of the environment or only the *change* in environmental temperature.

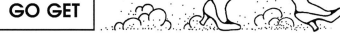

GO GET

1. A large beaker of cold water (10 °C).

2. A large beaker of hot water (50 °C).

3. A large beaker of 30 °C water.

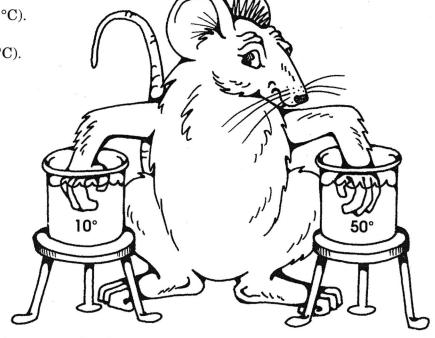

NOW

1. If the water beakers are already set up at the demonstration table, then check and adjust the temperatures using water from the hot plate or ice cubes in order to maintain the three temperature conditions listed above.

2. Place the index finger of one hand into the cold water, and the index finger of the other hand into the hot water for 15 seconds.

3. After 15 seconds, quickly place both fingers into the 30 °C water. Record the sensations.

    Cold-water Finger = _____.

    Hot-water Finger = _____.

? QUESTION

What seems to be the most important factor related to your perception of skin temperature? (circle your choice)

    actual temperature   or   *change* in temperature

ACTIVITY #3

"HEARING"

The ear is divided into three parts: *outer*, *middle*, and *inner* ear. When sound waves enter the ear, the **eardrum** (between the outer and middle ear) is shaken and special small bones vibrate. These **middle ear bones** transmit the sound vibrations into the inner ear where the **auditory nerves** leading to the brain are activated. The area of the brain that is specialized for interpreting sounds is next to the ears.

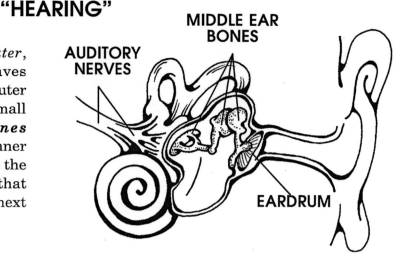

AUDITORY NERVES

MIDDLE EAR BONES

EARDRUM

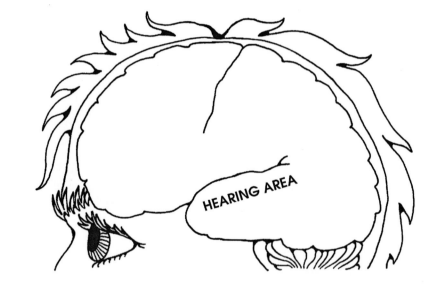

HEARING AREA

GO GET

1. Some cotton for ear plugs.

2. A set of tuning forks.

3. A meter stick.

NOW

1. Do this test in a quiet room. Have the subject close one ear with cotton and close his eyes. Strike the tuning fork against the table and hold it in line with the open ear. Move the tuning fork away from the ear until the subject just loses the ability to hear it. Measure the distance. Repeat the test again to validate your first measurement. Record the hearing distance for the other ear. *Be sure to strike the tuning fork with equal force each time you do the test.*

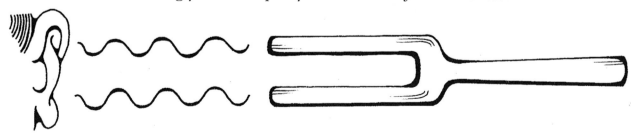

2. Repeat the test with each of the six tuning forks of different tones to determine if you have hearing loss in any of the six ranges. If one of your ears has a hearing loss at a particular tone range, then do the next test.

3. This next test should not be performed in a quiet room. Place the handle of a vibrating tuning fork on the midline of the subject's forehead.

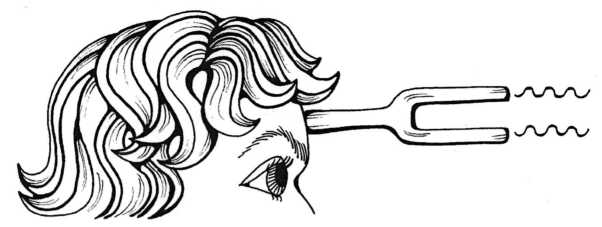

A person with normal hearing will localize the sound as if it were coming from the midline. If one ear has defective middle-ear function (ear bones), then the sound will be heard much better in the defective ear than when the tuning fork is not in contact with the forehead. If there is an affliction of the auditory nerve in the ear, then touching the tuning fork to the forehead won't improve hearing in the defective ear.

RESULTS OF HEARING TESTS

Sound Frequency (cycles per second)	Farthest Distance sound heard from Left Ear	Farthest Distance sound heard from Right Ear
128 cps fork		
256 cps fork		
512 cps fork		
1024 cps fork		
2048 cps fork		
4096 cps fork		

ACTIVITY #4

"SMELL"

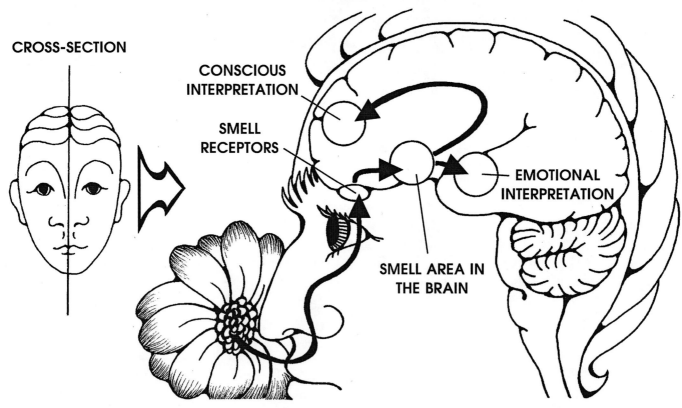

Recent studies show that smell is much more important in human behavior than was previously thought. Some researchers suggest that the evolutionary specialization of the mammal forebrain began with the sense of smell. The exact role of smell in our lives is not understood. This sense seems to be more closely linked to emotional memories than to the conscious activities of our brains. As you experiment with the various odors in the exercise below, describe the type of *emotional reaction* you have to each.

 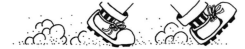

A smell kit.

NOW

1. Close your eyes. Have your lab partner pass an open odor vial about 3" under your nose for a couple of seconds. Repeat the test if necessary.

2. *First*, determine if you can smell the odor. *Second*, determine if you can correctly identify the smell. *Third*, describe any special memories associated with the smell.

3. Record the results of your test in the Odor Recognition Table.

ODOR RECOGNITION TABLE

Vial Number	Detects Smell	Identifies Smell	Memories Associated with the Smell
1	_____	_____	_____
2	_____	_____	_____
3	_____	_____	_____
4	_____	_____	_____
5	_____	_____	_____
6	_____	_____	_____
7	_____	_____	_____
8	_____	_____	_____
9	_____	_____	_____
10	_____	_____	_____
Totals	_____	_____	

? QUESTION

1. How many of the smells were associated with emotional memories?

2. List three examples of how specific smells might be used to sell you a product.

   a.

   b.

   c.

ACTIVITY #5

"TASTE"

The tongue has at least four different taste receptors (*salty*, *sweet*, *bitter*, and *sour*). However, the taste of many chemicals is also influenced by your interpretation of their *smell*. In this Activity, you will examine different aspects of your ability to taste.

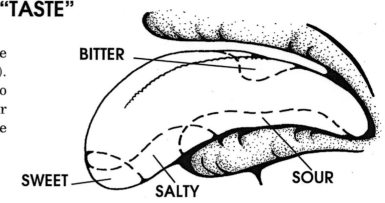

BITTER

SWEET   SALTY   SOUR

GENETICALLY DETERMINED TASTE

Your ability to taste certain chemicals is not influenced by previous eating habits, but is determined by whether or not you have inherited the *gene* controlling the taste response to that particular substance. This is an important lesson to remember when certain foods don't taste bitter to you, but other people complain about them (especially your children). They may have the gene to taste it, and you don't!

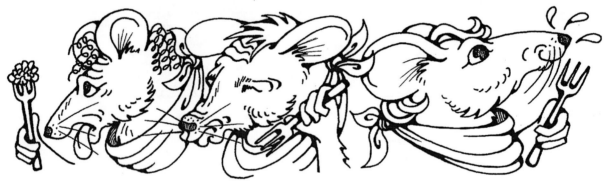

GO GET

The special taste papers for PTC and thiourea.

NOW

1. Take one taste paper, and touch it to your tongue. You will immediately know if you are a taster!

2. Do the same test with the other taste paper.

3. *Put the used taste papers in the trash.*

4. Your lab may have a setup for making a "food coloring" tongue print to count the number of taste buds in different people.

1. Are you a taster for thiourea?

2. Are you a taster for PTC?

3. If you are a non-taster and you want to be a high-class chef, what might you do to compensate for this genetic limitation?

SUGAR TASTE THRESHOLD

This experiment should give you insight about why some people prefer more sugar in their foods.

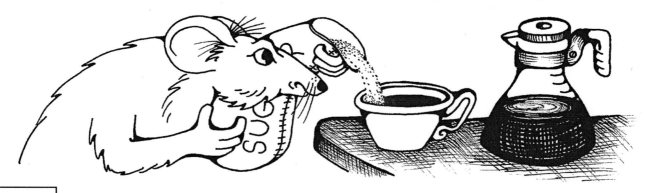

NOW

1. Go to the demonstration table and determine your sugar taste threshold (minimum percent of sugar you can taste).

2. Dip a strip of tasting paper into each solution, and record whether or not you can detect a sweet taste. *Discard the used taste papers.*

3. After testing all of the solutions, go to the front desk for the key to the sugar concentration of each solution.

4. Record your results in the summary chart on the front chalkboard.

? QUESTION

1. What was the lowest percent of sugar tasted by your classmates?

2. What was the highest threshold in the class for tasting sugar?

3. Do the people with a high taste threshold also like more sugar in their food? (Perhaps you could determine this by asking your classmates how much sugar they add to their coffee.) Your lab may have a setup for making a "food coloring" tongue print to count the number of taste buds in different people.

ACTIVITY #6

"VISION"

Human beings are primarily visual animals. This is the dominant sense you use to relate to the environment. Furthermore, most human behavior is strongly influenced by visual perception. There is a lot of scientific literature on visual perception and we encourage you to investigate this information when you have time to do so. What you don't know can be used against you!

PREFERRED EYE

This Activity is designed to reveal which one of your eyes is used for certain visual functions. Your *preferred eye* is the one your brain chooses to use when both eyes can see the same object.

NOW

1. Pick an object that's about 30 feet away. Make a circle with your thumb and first finger of both hands.

2. Straighten and raise your arms from your waist to a position where the circle surrounds the object. Keep your head and feet positioned straight ahead.

3. Without further movement, close one eye. Then open the closed eye, and close your other eye.

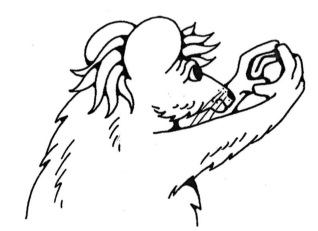

4. Which eye has the *same view* as the view with *both eyes* open? This is your preferred eye. ***Hint:*** When you close your preferred eye, the distant object will move out of the circle formed by your hands.

? QUESTION

1. Which eye is your preferred eye?

2. If you are left-eyed, what problem will you have in shooting a rifle?

3. Why should you use your preferred eye when looking through a monocular microscope?

EYE WITH BEST VISION

Use the classroom eye chart to determine which of your eyes has the best vision (without glasses).

? QUESTION

1. Which of your eyes has the best vision?

2. Talk with other lab students, and discover whether the eye with the best vision is always the same one as the preferred eye. Results: _____

EYE WITH BEST DEPTH PERCEPTION

There are fairly simple ways of determining which of your eyes has the best depth perception. If this equipment is available, then determine the depth perception for each of your eyes. If this equipment is unavailable, then refer to the information chart to answer the questions below.

INFORMATION

Vision Tests	13 Left-Handed People	11 Right-Handed People
Eye with Best Depth Perception	9 left eye 3 right eye 1 same in both eyes	2 left eye 8 right eye 1 same in both eyes
Preferred Eye	7 left eye 6 right eye	5 left eye 6 right eye
Eye with Best Vision	1 left eye 1 right eye 11 same in both eyes	2 left eye 1 right eye 8 same in both eyes

? QUESTION

The preferred hand (whether left-handed or right-handed) is most closely associated with . . . (circle your choice)

Eye with Best Depth Perception   or   Preferred Eye   or   Eye with Best Vision

ACTIVITY #7

"REFLEXES"

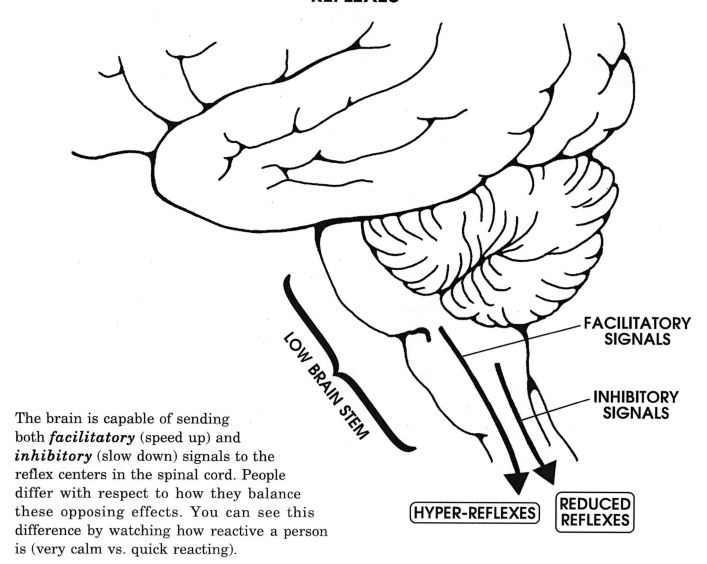

LOW BRAIN STEM

FACILITATORY SIGNALS

INHIBITORY SIGNALS

HYPER-REFLEXES

REDUCED REFLEXES

The brain is capable of sending both *facilitatory* (speed up) and *inhibitory* (slow down) signals to the reflex centers in the spinal cord. People differ with respect to how they balance these opposing effects. You can see this difference by watching how reactive a person is (very calm vs. quick reacting).

A reading reflex test can be used to determine which reflex type you are. *Concentrating on reading should reduce the effect your brain normally has on your reflex centers.* If reading reduces your reflex response, then normally your brain must be stimulating reflexes (you are a quick-reacting person). If reading increases your reflex response, then your brain normally inhibits reflexes (calm reacting). Your brain's reflex emphasis can change. No person is 100% one type or the other all of the time.

GO GET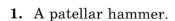

1. A patellar hammer.

2. A meter stick.

1. Before beginning the test, ask your lab partner to evaluate whether you are the calm or quick-reacting type.

        Lab Partner's Opinion: _____

        Your Opinion: _____

2. Sit on a table so that your legs hang freely over the edge. Have your lab partner hit the patellar ligament (just below the knee) with the reflex hammer. *Don't hit too hard.* This may take some practice. Measure the amount of leg movement several times to get an average estimate of the reflex intensity.

        Normal Reflex: _____

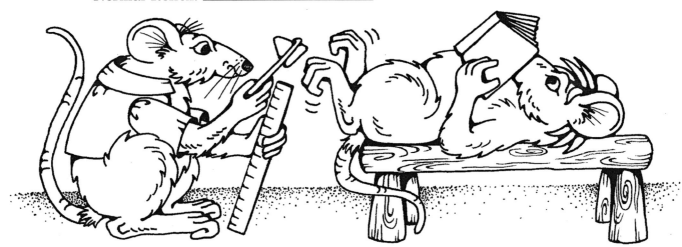

3. Next, read from a textbook while your lab partner measures the amount of reflex leg movement. Is the reflex more intense or less intense during the reading conditions?

1. Under normal circumstances, does your brain activate or inhibit spinal reflexes?

2. So, which reflex type are you?

3. Does this agree with how you evaluated yourself before the test?

4. Compare your conclusions with those of other students in the class. What did you discover?

Chapter 18

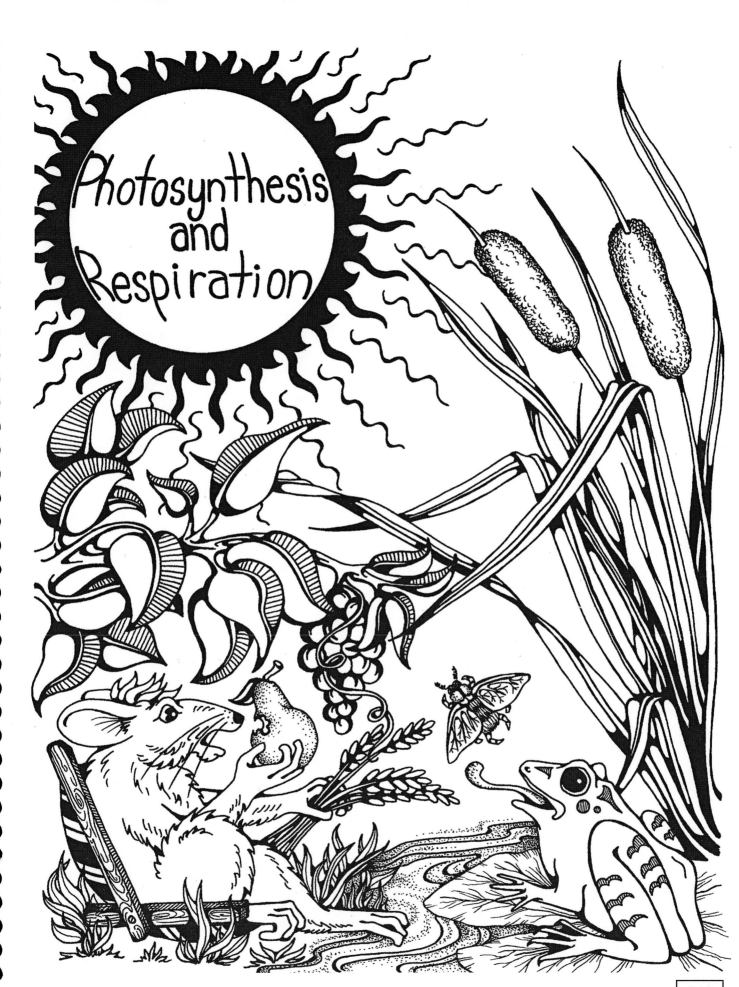

Photosynthesis
and
Respiration

PHOTOSYNTHESIS AND RESPIRATION

Physicists have developed two ways of describing the universe: One of these is energy, and the other is matter. Matter is anything that has mass and occupies space. Energy is non-material, travels in waves, and has the capacity to change matter.

Life can be described from both of these points of view. Life is an assemblage of atoms and molecules. It is also an energy process. The following Activities present highlights of energy conversions and substance changes in living systems.

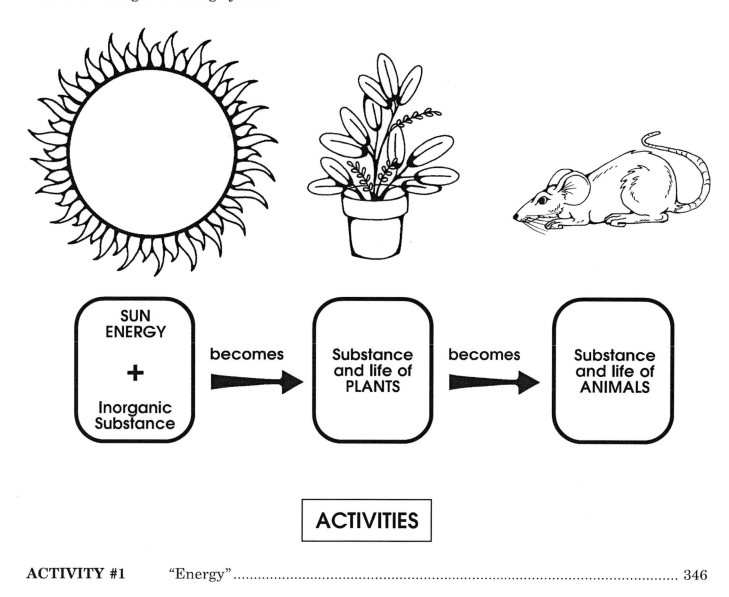

SUN ENERGY + Inorganic Substance →becomes→ Substance and life of PLANTS →becomes→ Substance and life of ANIMALS

ACTIVITIES

ACTIVITY #1

"ENERGY"

Energy can move and change matter, and can exist in different forms. Some of these forms include heat, light, electrical, chemical, and mechanical energy. In addition to describing the form of energy, we can measure the *amount* of it. The amount of energy can be measured using various experimental methods. For example, we can estimate the amount of heat energy in a flame by observing how fast that flame can "move" water molecules (heat them up).

LAWS OF THERMODYNAMICS

Several basic principles of energy change have been discovered. Two of these, the First and Second Laws of Thermodynamics, are of particular value in understanding life processes.

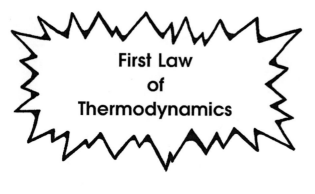

First Law of Thermodynamics

The amount of energy does not change; only the form of energy changes.

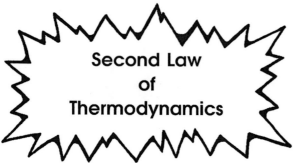

Second Law of Thermodynamics

Heat is always produced whenever one form of energy is converted into another form.

Imagine that the Engineering Department decided to build a campus wind generator for capturing and storing energy in batteries that could be used later to run electric motors. The size of the energy boxes in the diagram on the next page represents the amount of energy available at each step along the way. The numbers in the boxes represent energy units.

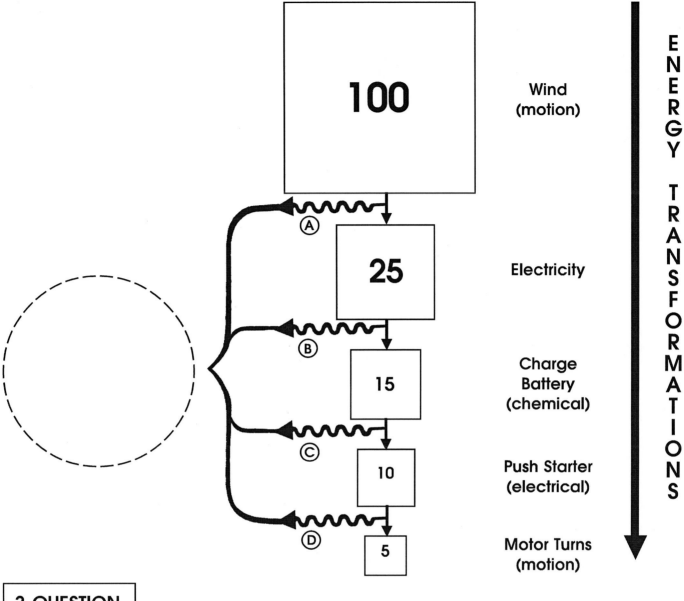

100 — Wind (motion)

25 — Electricity

15 — Charge Battery (chemical)

10 — Push Starter (electrical)

5 — Motor Turns (motion)

ENERGY TRANSFORMATIONS

Ⓐ Ⓑ Ⓒ Ⓓ

? QUESTION

1. What form of energy is represented by Ⓐ,Ⓑ,Ⓒ, and Ⓓ?
Write the name of this form of energy inside the circle on the left side of the diagram.

2. Which Law of Thermodynamics is used to answer question #1?

3. Using the First Law of Thermodynamics, calculate the amounts of energy released at . . .

   Ⓐ ＿＿＿＿＿   Ⓑ ＿＿＿＿＿   Ⓒ ＿＿＿＿＿   Ⓓ ＿＿＿＿＿.

4. What is the total amount of heat in the big circle? ＿＿＿＿＿＿＿＿＿＿

5. A biology student who learned about the Laws of Thermodynamics, suggested that the school's Engineering Department should have designed a wind machine that directly turned the campus motors. How would her suggested change improve efficiency?

6. Imagine there is an "unknown thing" giving off heat. What can we conclude is going on inside the "unknown thing"?

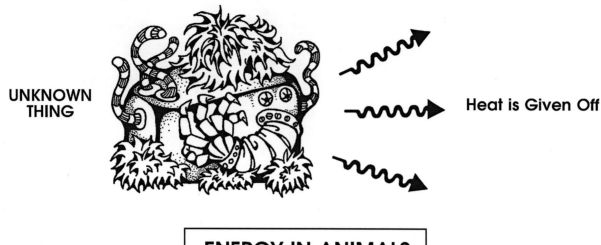

UNKNOWN THING

Heat is Given Off

ENERGY IN ANIMALS

We can measure the amount of energy in food. Also, there are machines designed to record the heat that an organism gives off during the day. Assume that the *size* of the boxes in the diagram below represents the amounts of energy for one day.

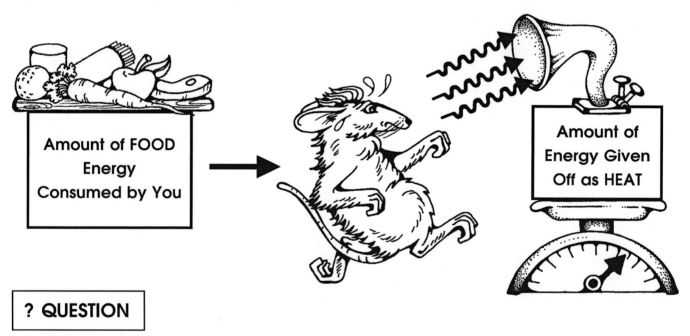

Amount of FOOD Energy Consumed by You

Amount of Energy Given Off as HEAT

? QUESTION

1. Use the First Law of Thermodynamics to analyze the energy transformation diagram on the previous page. Has the size of the boxes changed? But, what does the First Law say about that?

2. Where is the rest of the energy? (This refers to the difference in the size of diagram boxes.)

The process of FOOD ENERGY ⟶ YOU ⟶ HEAT is called *Respiration*. We will outline the substances that are changed during respiration in Activity #3.

ENERGY IN PLANTS

We can measure both the amount of light energy absorbed by a plant during a day and the amount of heat released by the plant. Assume that the size of the boxes represents amounts of energy.

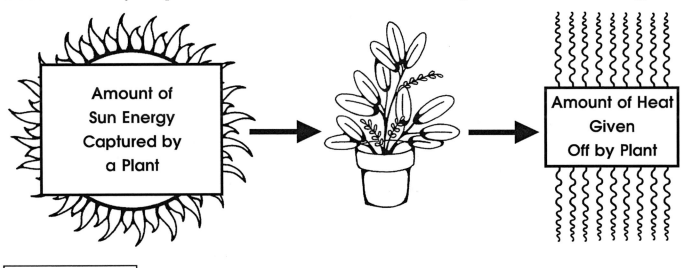

? QUESTION

Considering the First Law of Thermodynamics and the difference in the sizes of the diagram boxes, where is the rest of the energy? (**Hint:** What does a healthy plant do during the day?)

The process of SUN ENERGY ⟶ PLANT is called *Photosynthesis*. We will describe the substances that are changed during photosynthesis in Activity #2.

ENERGY IN ECOSYSTEMS

The Laws of Thermodynamics help us to understand conversions of energy within ecosystems. Energy of sunlight is first converted into the chemical energy of plants. This conversion occurs with about 1% efficiency. This means that photosynthesis requires about 100 units of sun energy to produce one unit of sugar energy.

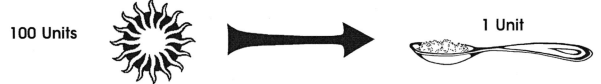

100 Units   1 Unit

The animal that eats plants is called a *herbivore*. The animal that eats herbivores is called the *first carnivore*. The *second carnivore* eats the first carnivore, and so on. At each step from the plant outward, the energy conversion efficiency is about 10%. (For example, 100 kg of plant are required to produce 10 kg of rabbit.) The diagram on the next page shows the amounts of energy at each food level in the ecosystem.

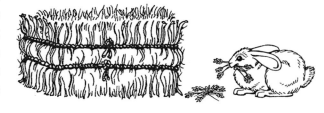

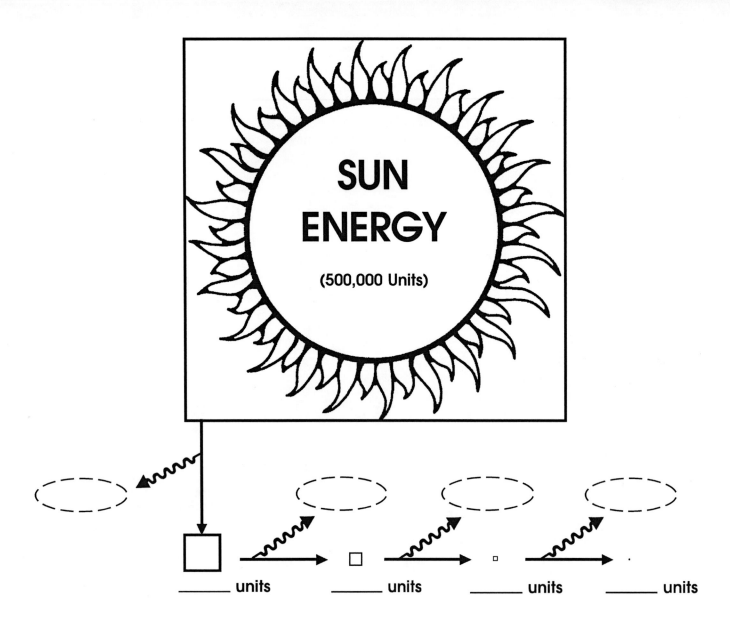

SUN
ENERGY

(500,000 Units)

_____ units   _____ units   _____ units   _____ units

? QUESTION

1. Each of the four boxes represents a food level. Write the name of each food level (from plants ⟶ second carnivores) below the boxes.

2. Starting with 500,000 units of sunlight energy, calculate and record the number of energy units (on the lines below each box) for each of the energy levels in the diagram.

3. What form of energy is given off during the conversion from one ecosystem level to the next? *Hint:* Remember the Second Law of Thermodynamics.

4. Record the amount of energy (question #3) given off at each step in the ecosystem diagram. (Put your answers in the dotted ovals at the ends of the wavy arrows.)

5. Assume that humans are the second-level carnivores, and that each energy unit in their level represents 25 people. How many people can be supported in the ecosystem?

6. Assume that we eat herbivores only. As first-level carnivores, how many humans can now be supported in the ecosystem?

7. If we ate plants only, how many humans could be supported by the ecosystem?

8. If we ate plants only, what would happen to the amounts of energy available for the other herbivores and carnivores in the ecosystem?

9. Let's look at energy conversion another way. It takes about 0.5 kg of meat to support a human for one day. Assuming that beef is the only available nutrient, how much meat energy (kilograms of meat) will it take to get you to 20 years old?

10. How much plant energy (kilograms of plant) will it take to feed the beef that gets you to 20 years old? (Refer to question #9.)

11. Your digestive system is very efficient at digesting meat, but is not as efficient at getting all of the available nutrition from plants. Now, assume that you were raised on plants instead of meat. Plant material has about 40% of the per-kg food value as meat. How much plant energy would it take to get you to 20 years old?

Do you get the general idea of how the Laws of Thermodynamics give us a better understanding of ecosystems?

The next Activities present how matter is changed by energy in both photosynthesis and respiration.

ACTIVITY #2

"PHOTOSYNTHESIS"

Activity #1 presented photosynthesis from the energy perspective. In this Activity we consider the changes in *substances* (matter) during photosynthesis.

HISTORICAL DISCOVERY PROCESS

The chemical changes that occur during photosynthesis have been investigated for the past 300 years. The general highlights of these discoveries help us to understand the basic process of photosynthesis.

Three centuries ago people wondered where plants came from. They knew that plants grew out of the ground, but *how* that happened was a complete mystery to them. The first step in answering the question was to plant a small tree in a large pot supported off the ground. They did this so that the soil of the container was separated from the soil of the earth. Only the dirt in the pot was available to the plant.

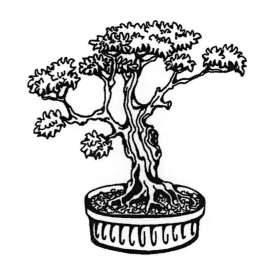

The people cared for the plant during one year. At the end of the year the small tree had gained 100 kg. (*The actual data from this experiment have been changed to simplify the discussion.*)

? QUESTION

1. What do you think the experimenters considered as two possible sources for the substances (matter) that became incorporated into new tree growth? (This experiment was performed nearly 300 years ago. People didn't know very much about chemistry, and air was thought to be a non-substance.)

   _____   _____

2. When the experimenters measured the weight of the two substances (question #1) given to the plant, they found 35 kg of one and 2 kg of the other. Where do you think they thought the rest of the plant's weight came from?

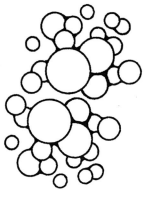

People guessed that there must be some invisible substance in light or somewhere else that was added to the plant. It took another century for humans to discover the chemical makeup of air. Once humans invented accurate scales, they could measure small changes in the weight of air.

Experimenters put a plant into a sealed jar with air that had been weighed. After the plant was exposed to light for a few hours, the air lost weight. They had discovered another source of matter for the new plant growth—the air! The basic equation for photosynthesis was complete:

$$CO_2 + H_2O + \text{a little soil} \xrightarrow{\text{Light Energy}} \text{New Plant Tissue} + O_2$$

heavy air $\qquad$ $C_6H_{12}O_6$ and its variations $\qquad$ light air

? QUESTION

1. Look at the molecular formula for plant tissue. Where does the carbon come from?

2. Where does the hydrogen in $C_6H_{12}O_6$ come from?

3. When radioactive isotopes of oxygen atoms are put into CO_2 molecules and the plant is allowed to photosynthesize, only new plant tissue ($C_6H_{12}O_6$) is radioactive and the oxygen gas given off is not radioactive. Draw a dotted line in the photosynthesis equation to show where the oxygen atoms in CO_2 go.

4. Draw a dotted line in the equation to show where the oxygen atoms in H_2O go.

CHLOROPHYLL

All chemical reactions involve changes in the *electrons* of atoms. The key to photosynthesis is a special molecule called **chlorophyll**. This large and complex molecule has electrons that become "activated" when light shines on the molecule.

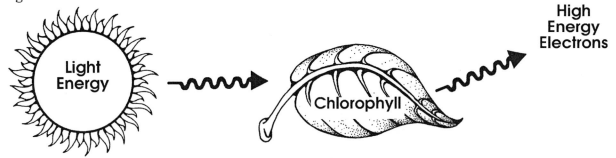

Light Energy → Chlorophyll → High Energy Electrons

This reaction is unusual because most substances only heat up when exposed to sunlight; that is, their electrons aren't "activated" by light energy. But the electrons in chlorophyll are activated by light, and this electron energy is used to make new plant tissue ($C_6H_{12}O_6$).

1. Sunlight contains all of the colors of light in the visible spectrum. Which color do you see reflecting from the surface of plants?

2. Which two primary colors do you *not* see when looking at the plant leaves?

3. Which colors of light probably activate the electrons of the chlorophyll molecule? Explain.

CHLOROPLASTS

All of the unicellular algae and multicellular plants are eukaryotic and have specialized organelles called **chloroplasts**. The chloroplasts contain chlorophyll and enzymes for the photosynthesis process.

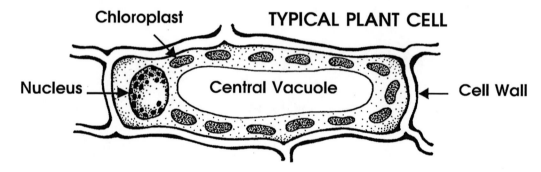

Chloroplast   TYPICAL PLANT CELL

Nucleus   Central Vacuole   Cell Wall

The exceptions to this rule are the photosynthetic bacteria (cyanobacteria). They are prokaryotic; that is, they don't have cell organelles like chloroplasts. However, cyanobacteria *do* photosynthesis, and they *have* chlorophyll.

CYANOBACTERIA

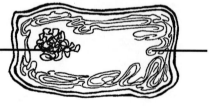

DNA is not in a specialized nucleus.

Chlorophyll is distributed throughout the cell and is not in a specialized chloroplast.

The chloroplast has many specialized structures. Stacks of discs, called **grana,** contain the chlorophyll and act like photoelectric cells. When light shines on these grana, the electrons of the chlorophyll are "activated." This is the first stage of photosynthesis.

CHLOROPLAST

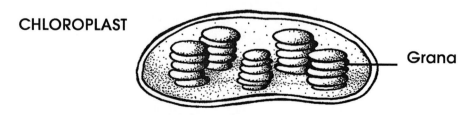

Grana

The second stage of photosynthesis involves the building of sugar molecules from carbon dioxide and water. These two ingredients will not combine unless chemical energy is provided. That energy comes from the "activated" electrons in the chlorophyll reaction. Sugar molecules are made in the fluids of the chloroplasts that surround the grana.

Simple sugars made during photosynthesis are modified into all of the other organic molecules needed by the plant.

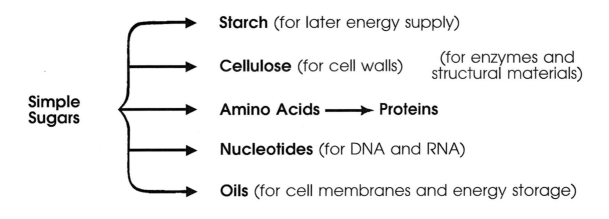

? QUESTION

1. When light energy shines on chlorophyll, the light energy is transformed into . . .

   Light Energy ⟶ **Chlorophyll** ⟶ _____ **Energy**

2. Some biologists refer to the two parts of photosynthesis as the light reactions and the synthesis reactions. Which part do you think that they call the light reactions?

3. Which part of photosynthesis do you think they call the synthesis reactions?

4. The synthesis reactions happen in the daytime, but are sometimes called "dark reactions" because light energy is not directly required. What kind of energy is required to run the synthesis reactions?

   Where does that energy come from?

CHARACTERISTICS OF LIGHT

Our description of energy includes anything that is non-material, travels in waves, and has the capacity to move and change matter. There are many different kinds of energy, and each has its characteristic *wavelength*. When all of these energy waves are arranged on a scale from short waves to long waves, the scale is called the *electromagnetic spectrum*.

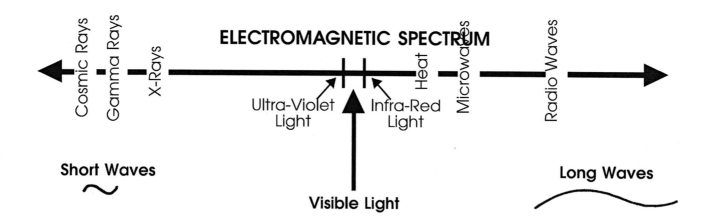

You can see that visible light is only a very small slice of the electromagnetic spectrum. An important feature of electromagnetic energy is that shorter waves have more energy than longer waves. This is the key to understanding why only a narrow segment of waves in the electromagnetic spectrum is ideal for biological reactions like photosynthesis and vision. Some people humorously refer to this idea as the "Goldilocks" principle—the wavelength has to be "just right."

The energy waves just shorter than violet light are called *ultra-violet*, and the waves just longer than red light are called *infra-red*.

Ultra-violet waves are damaging to life. These waves have too much _____. The molecules exposed to ultra-violet waves become over-activated and are chemically changed or destroyed.

When the molecules are exposed to infra-red waves they "warm up," but these waves do not have enough _____ to activate electrons (essential for biochemical reactions).

White light (visible light) is made of different wavelengths of energy (different colors). You can remember where the various colors occur in the visible light spectrum by recalling the image of a rainbow in your mind.

Long Side (long waves)

Short Side (short waves)

? QUESTION

1. Which color is on the short side of the rainbow?

2. Which color is on the long side?

3. Which color is about in the middle?

4. Put these colors in the rainbow diagram above. (The long side of the rainbow is the longer wavelength.)

5. Which color do you see when you look at plants? (The color that you *see* is the color that plants do *not* use in photosynthesis.)

6. Which two primary colors do you *not* see when looking at a plant? (These are the two wavelengths of energy that plants mostly use for photosynthesis, so they are *absorbed* by the plant rather than reflected back.)

_____   _____

There is much more to photosynthesis than is covered in this Activity. You will have to get those details from lecture or your textbook.

ACTIVITY #3

"RESPIRATION"

Respiration was presented from the energy perspective in Activity #1. In this Activity we consider the changes in substances (matter) during cellular respiration. Respiration is the chemical breakdown of food molecules, converting food energy into usable energy (ATP) for the cell.

HISTORICAL DISCOVERY PROCESS

Investigation of the chemical changes during respiration coincided with experimental revelations about photosynthesis. The earliest experiments on respiration were performed about 300 years ago, and involved both plants and animals.

EARLY EXPERIMENTS

Mouse in a sealed jar $\longrightarrow$ Mouse dies in an hour or so

Mouse in a sealed jar
with a large plant in the light $\longrightarrow$ Mouse lives just fine

Mouse in a sealed jar
with a large plant in the dark $\longrightarrow$ Mouse dies in an hour or so

These early experiments revealed several facts:

▶ There was something in the air that animals needed to live.

▶ Somehow plants "regenerated" the air that animals needed.

▶ Light was necessary for plants to "regenerate" the air.

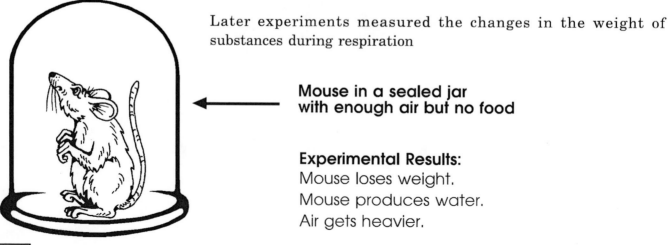

Later experiments measured the changes in the weight of substances during respiration

Mouse in a sealed jar
with enough air but no food

Experimental Results:
Mouse loses weight.
Mouse produces water.
Air gets heavier.

1. Based on this experiment, where did the weight of the mouse go? _____ and _____

2. The air started out light in weight. What was the substance of that air? (Refer to "light air" in Activity #2.)

3. The air ended up heavier in weight. What was the substance of that air? (Refer to "heavy air" in Activity #2.)

4. Write the molecular formulas for each substance in this basic equation for respiration below. (Use the same formula for mouse tissue that we used for plant tissue in Activity #2.)

Mouse Tissue + Light Air $\longrightarrow$ Water + Heavy Air

5. Radioactive isotope experiments have shown that atoms of carbon, oxygen, and hydrogen are rearranged just like in photosynthesis, only the equation is in reverse. (Refer to the photosynthesis equation in Activity #2 on page 353.) Draw a dotted line in the respiration equation (question #4) to show where the carbon atoms in the food molecule go.

6. Draw a dotted line in the respiration equation to show what happens to the oxygen atoms in the air that we breath.

7. Where do the oxygen atoms in CO_2 come from? (Show this with another dotted line in the respiration equation.)

RESPIRATION COMPARED TO A BURNING CANDLE

Experimenters discovered that a burning candle is the same basic chemical process as animal respiration. The burning of any substance is called *combustion*.

Candle + O_2 $\longrightarrow$ CO_2 + H_2O

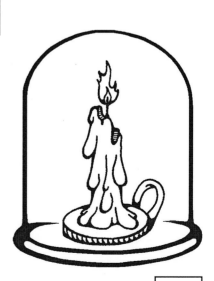

1. Respiration is the opposite of _____.

2. Which must have evolved first—animals that required oxygen or the process of photosynthesis?

3. Assume that all oxygen in the atmosphere came from photosynthesis. Knowing this, what has been happening faster—respiration or photosynthesis?

4. Evidence suggests that the early atmosphere of our planet was very high in CO_2. Based on your answer to question #2, where did the CO_2 go?

5. If your answer to question #3 is true for this planet, then where is all the "extra" plant material that hasn't burned or been eaten? (***Hint:*** think of two major resources.)

   _____   _____

6. If all the resources referred to in question #5 were burned, what change would happen in the atmosphere?

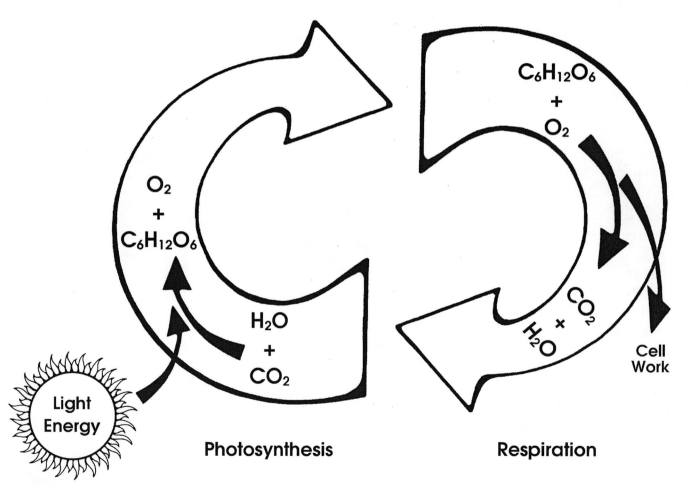

Photosynthesis   Respiration

DOES RESPIRATION HAPPEN IN PLANTS?

Plant in a sealed jar in the dark ➡️

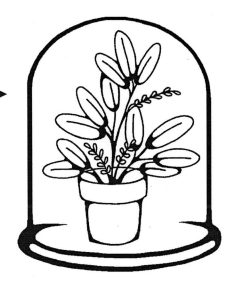

Experimental Results:
Plant loses weight.
Plant produces water.
Air gets heavier.

Conclusion:
Plants do respiration.

? QUESTION

A house plant was kept one month in each of three rooms in the house. Compare the intensity of photosynthesis and respiration by the plant in each of the rooms.

In room #1 the plant lost weight and started to die. _____

In room #2 the plant gained weight. _____

In room #3 the plant survived but didn't gain weight. _____

CHEMICAL BREAKDOWN OF FOOD

Using a few basic rules about chemical reactions, you can understand much about respiration.

Rule: Electrons have energy.

Rule: Sometimes electrons can move from one molecule to another.

Rule: Whenever hydrogen atoms are added to or removed from a molecule in a chemical reaction, assume that the number of electrons also changes (one hydrogen added = one electron added).

Rule: The Second Law of Thermodynamics applies to situations in which the electron energy of one molecule is transformed into the electron energy of another molecule.

Heat

| Electron Energy of One Molecule | ➡️ | Electron Energy of Another Molecule |

1. In the reaction shown, is the molecule gaining or losing energy?

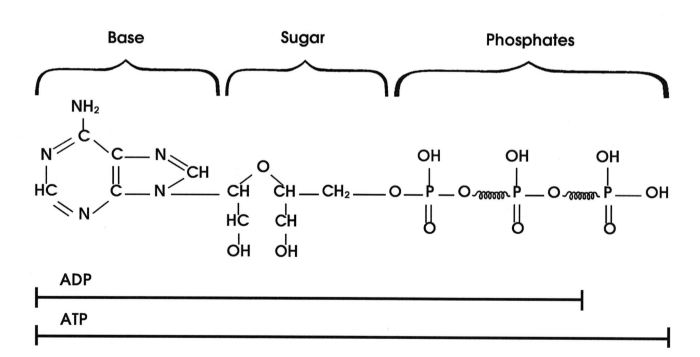

2. Which has more electron energy—$C_6H_{12}O_6$ or $6CO_2$? _____

3. How many electrons are removed from sugar during respiration—$C_6H_{12}O_6 \longrightarrow 6CO_2$?

   _____

4. Cells need a special molecule called ATP to do the work of life. Assume that the energy of one electron from food ($C_6H_{12}O_6$) can be transformed into the energy in 3 ATP molecules. How many ATP molecules are generated during the breakdown of one sugar molecule during respiration? (Refer to your answer for question #3.) _____

ATP

ATP (adenosine triphosphate) is a special high-energy molecule in the cell. This molecule can also exist in a low-energy form called ADP (adenosine diphosphate). ATP has more high-energy electrons than ADP. That extra electron energy comes from food molecules.

ATP delivers high-energy electrons to other energy-requiring processes in the cell. The two processes (ADP $\longrightarrow$ ATP and ATP $\longrightarrow$ ADP) create an energy exchange system in the cell.

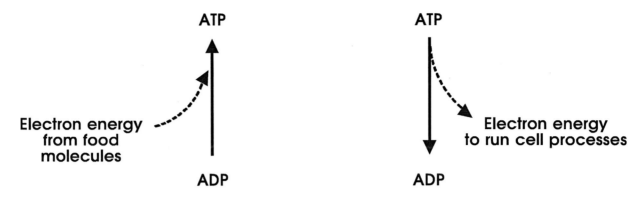

AEROBIC AND ANAEROBIC RESPIRATION

You concluded previously that cells requiring oxygen for respiration must have evolved after photosynthesis. We know that some chemical reactions can happen without oxygen. So, could there have been a form of respiration that might have existed before photosynthesis? The answer is yes. Respiration can occur without oxygen, and there were primitive cells living by this process before photosynthesis evolved.

Respiration without oxygen present is called **anaerobic** (without air). Respiration with oxygen is called **aerobic**. Aerobic respiration occurs inside a specialized organelle called the **mitochondrion**, whereas anaerobic processes (also called *fermentation*) are associated with other membranes in the cytoplasm.

The sugar molecule is only partially broken down during anaerobic respiration. Have all high-energy electrons been removed from the sugar molecule below? _____

Anaerobic Respiration in Human Muscles

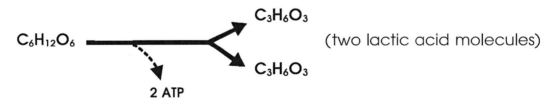

The energy of two ATP molecules is generated when sugar is "split" into the two lactic acid molecules. These two ATP molecules are the *only* energy captured from the food molecule during anaerobic respiration. High-energy electrons remain in the lactic acid. This means that anaerobic respiration is very *inefficient* compared to aerobic respiration. (**Remember:** In question #4 under "Chemical Breakdown of Food," you calculated that 36 ATP are generated during aerobic respiration.)

In humans, anaerobic respiration happens for short periods of time only in the skeletal muscles. During strenuous exercise, this maintains metabolism when oxygen is temporarily depleted. Other organs of your body are incapable of anaerobic respiration, and their cells begin to die when oxygen is used up.

Complete the following table comparing aerobic and anaerobic respiration.

Comparisons	Aerobic	Anaerobic
Is oxygen necessary?		
Which came first on the planet?		
What are the end products?		
How much ATP energy is generated?		
Where in the cell does it happen?		

MITOCHONDRIA

Aerobic respiration is the process in living organisms that extracts electron energy from the chemical bonds in food (organic molecules), and converts that energy into a more useful form of energy (called ATP) to run cell activities. This cell process uses oxygen and produces carbon dioxide. The complete equation is:

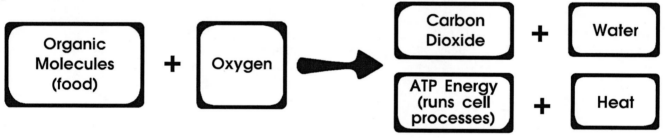

Aerobic respiration occurs inside the mitochondria, which are cellular organelles in both plant and animal cells.

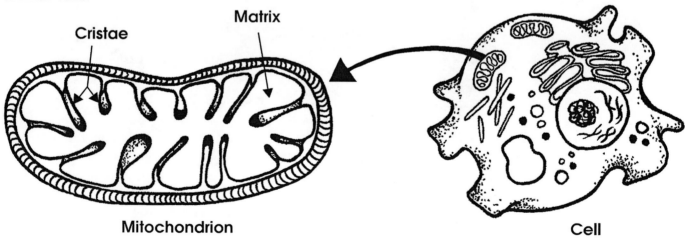

Cristae   Matrix

Mitochondrion   Cell

The mitochondria have a remarkable structure that is somewhat like a factory. The high-energy electrons are stripped off the food molecule in the fluid matrix, and then the energy of those electrons is used to generate ATP energy along the *cristae* membranes.

1. Which cells evolved first—eukaryotic or prokaryotic?

2. Which cells have mitochondria—eukaryotic or prokaryotic?

3. Some of the cells of your body have many mitochondria and other cells have few mitochondria. Why would there be differences?

METABOLISM OF NUTRIENTS

Sugar is not the only type of food molecule that can be metabolized during cell respiration. Fats, proteins, and starch are other energy sources for the generation of ATP.

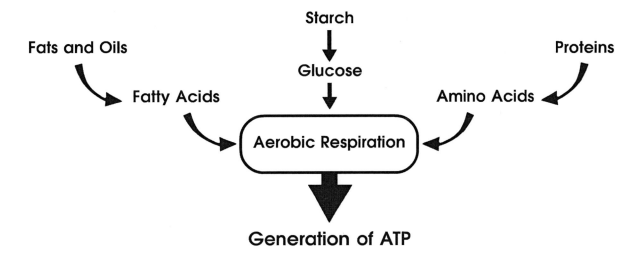

The amount of ATP generated by these nutrients depends on the size of the molecule and the number of high-energy electrons that can be stripped off.

Starches are easy to metabolize because they consist of glucose sugar molecules hooked together.

Proteins must first be broken into amino acids, which are then modified. The nitrogen atoms are broken off the amino acid molecule, and ammonia is produced which is then converted into urea. Urea is dumped into the urine. The part of the amino acid remaining after nitrogen removal can be broken down by aerobic respiration. An amino acid generates about the same amount of ATP energy as does an equal weight of sugar.

Fat molecules have many more high-energy electrons than an equal weight of either sugar or protein. Protein and sugar provide about 4 Calories of energy per gram. Fat provides about 9 Calories of energy per gram. Now you can see why it's so easy for those high-energy electrons to pile up!

1. What factor determines the amount of energy that can be gained from a nutrient molecule?

2. Which nutrient provides the most ATP energy per molecule metabolized?

3. Urea is one of the substances that gives urine its characteristic smell. Urea in the urine means that you have been metabolizing _____. (which nutrient)

This completes our discussion of cellular respiration. Your textbook will present many more details about the process, and applications related to health and nutrition.

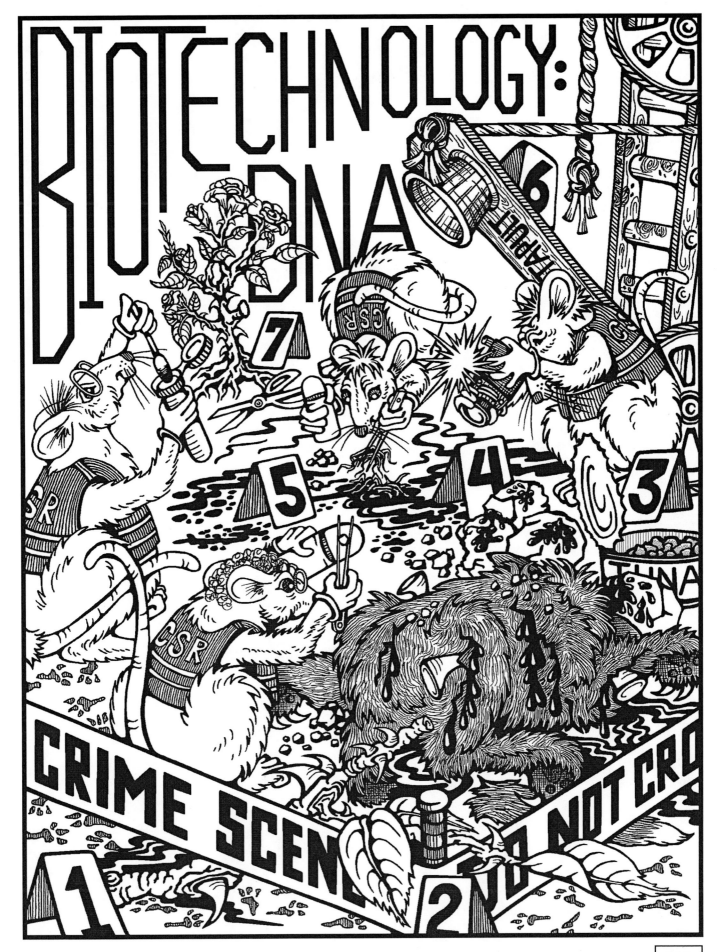

Cases of *chimerism* (in which a person may possess the genetics of two distinct individuals) challenge the irrefutability of DNA testing. Forensic science may not be able to rely on DNA testing as the sole source of evidence, as the criminal or victim may be a chimera.

—HTTP://WWW.SCQ.UBC.CA/THE-TRUTH-ABOUT-CHIMERAS/

BIOTECHNOLOGY: DNA

INTRODUCTION

Biotechnology uses organisms and their biological processes to produce new solutions for medical, agricultural, and commercial problems, as well as many other social and environmental applications.

This research area is advancing rapidly and its applications are expanding contemporary imagination. Its advances can be compared to the invention of the computer with the blossoming information age. Biotechnology is fueled by discoveries of the biochemical events both controlling and controlled by biomolecules, including the structure and function of proteins (enzymes), RNA, and DNA. It is as if we have discovered a basic secret of life—all that it creates, and all that it could create.

Has biotechnology uncorked the bottle and let out the Genie?
For what do we wish?
Which wishes will improve the world or human condition?
How will we avoid making a foolhardy wish?
This lab introduces a small part of
the biotechnology world,
focusing on DNA
technologies and
how they are
valuable to us.

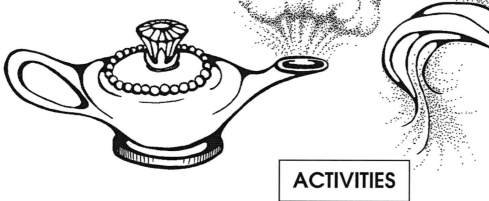

ACTIVITIES

ACTIVITY #1

"DNA FINGERPRINTING TOOLS"

DNA fingerprinting (more accurately called DNA profiling) is a procedure used to identify specific characteristics in DNA molecules. This procedure allows us to distinguish the DNA of different people or of any other organism. DNA fingerprinting has been applied to criminal investigations, paternity cases, genetic-relationship questions, identification of inherited disorders, and the personal identification of individual humans.

The classic use of fingerprints taken from the hand is for identification purposes only, and it lacks the ability to show genetic relationship between people. Identical twins have different hand fingerprints because those prints are partly determined by non-genetic conditions during embryonic development. Whereas classic fingerprints focus on whorls and intersections of ridges on the fingers that are not inherited, DNA fingerprinting identifies actual sequences of nucleotides in the DNA. DNA fingerprinting uses many biotechnology tools, and a discussion of several of those tools will give you a basic understanding of the process.

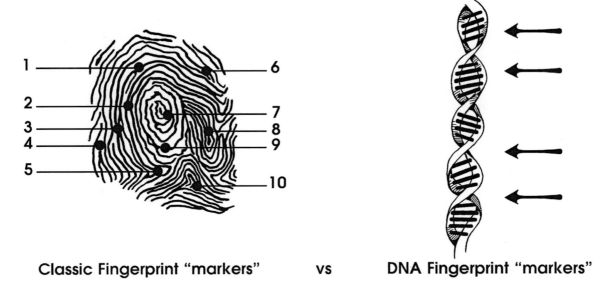

Classic Fingerprint "markers"   vs   DNA Fingerprint "markers"

TOOL 1: PCR—HOW TO CLONE DNA

PCR (polymerase chain reaction) is a method used to make millions of copies of DNA from a small sample. It is sometimes called "molecular photocopying." The DNA is "unzipped" by heating the sample in a mixture of lab-made DNA nucleotides and a special enzyme called *Taq DNA polymerase*. A small amount of "primer" (short piece of RNA that starts the chain reaction) is also added to the mixture. The DNA molecule copies itself (A pairs with T; G pairs with C) under these conditions.

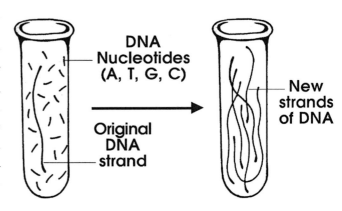

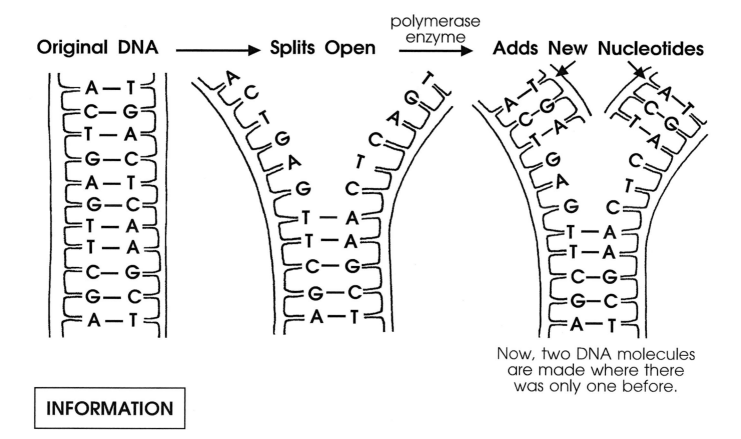

Original DNA → **Splits Open** → polymerase enzyme → **Adds New Nucleotides**

Now, two DNA molecules are made where there was only one before.

INFORMATION

The special Taq polymerase was discovered and extracted from thermal-pool bacteria like those in Yellowstone National Park. The bacteria was named *Thermus aquaticus*, hence the name Taq polymerase. This enzyme is capable of functioning at the high temperatures of the laboratory PCR process. Most enzymes are destroyed by high heat. Use of this enzyme is another example of a biotechnology advancement.

There are a couple of tricks to this procedure. The starting sample is heated to about 95 °C. This causes the DNA molecule to unzip into two complementary halves. When the DNA is cooled to about 50 °C, each half makes a new *complementary* copy of itself from the mixture of nucleotides. Heating again separates the two new DNA molecules and another replication occurs when the sample is cooled for a second time. An automated machine can repeat these temperature change cycles (30–40 times) to produce millions of exact copies of the original DNA. The PCR technique creates plenty of sample for the DNA technician to do specific DNA tests.

? QUESTION

1. What is a simple definition of biotechnology?

2. In which example is the "fingerprint" identical for identical twins? (circle your choice)

    Classic hand fingerprints   or   DNA fingerprints

3. What does PCR produce?

4. What are the ingredients for the PCR process?

5. Where did biotechnology find the special DNA polymerase enzyme used in the PCR process?

TOOL 2: RESTRICTION ENZYMES

When long molecules of DNA are mixed with *restriction enzymes*, the DNA is cut into shorter threads. Restriction enzymes act like "scissors" cutting the DNA at specific nucleotide sequences called *recognition sites*. Let's see if you get the idea of how this biotechnology tool is used.

Start with three examples of restriction enzymes (BamHI, EcoRI, and HindIII). Each enzyme cuts at its own recognition site. A recognition site could be as simple as CCCGGG where the restriction enzyme cuts the DNA between the G and C. There are hundreds of restriction enzymes developed by biotechnology and each has its own technical name. We have used a simple shape to represent the recognition site for each of the three cutting enzymes above. The particular restriction enzyme cuts only where that shape occurs in the long thread of DNA.

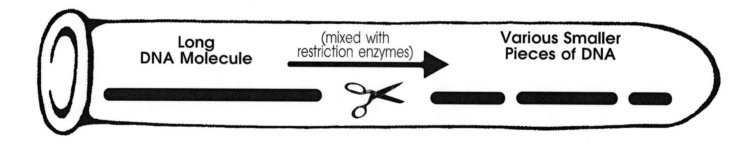

Restriction Enzymes		Recognition Site
BamHI	✂	▲
EcoRI	✂	●
HindIII	✂	■

1. Your job is to analyze the DNA of three subjects. Their DNA was mixed with the three restriction enzymes ("scissors").

2. The long threads of DNA from each subject are cut at the recognition sites. Determine the length of each resulting piece of DNA from the subjects after cutting has occurred.

3. Measure the length of each piece with a cm ruler and make a thick line mark on the graph to indicate each of the pieces.

4. We have done this for the first piece in Subject A. Finish measuring and making marks for all the DNA pieces of Subjects A, B, and C.

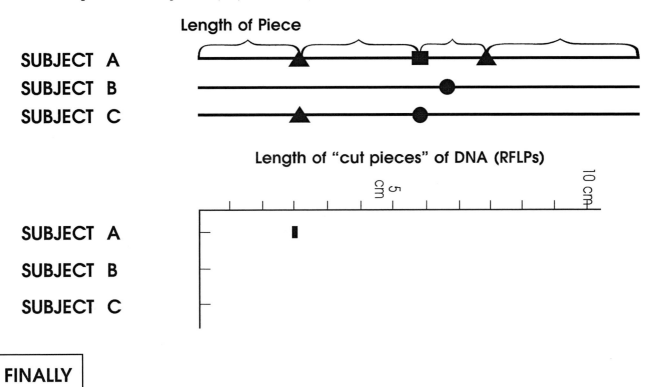

FINALLY

You now have a visual picture of a DNA comparison of Subjects A, B, and C.

INFORMATION

1. The scientific name for these individual pieces of DNA cut up by restriction enzymes is **RFLPs** (Restriction Fragment Length Polymorphism).

2. RFLPs are separated from each other during actual DNA fingerprinting in the process called *gel electrophoresis*, which is the biotechnology tool described next.

3. The length and number of RFLPs is dependent on the restriction enzymes used and the unique DNA code in each person.

4. The forensic use of DNA fingerprinting has particular criteria for selecting restriction enzymes to analyze DNA crime scene samples.

TOOL 3: GEL ELECTROPHORESIS

Gel electrophoresis is a precise method for separating pieces of DNA (called RFLPs) that have been cut by restriction enzymes. It is the most familiar part of the DNA fingerprinting process because it produces a visual gel record similar to the graph in the previous discussion.

INFORMATION

1. PCR amplifies the original DNA sample.

2. Restriction enzymes cut the DNA into smaller pieces.

3. DNA pieces are separated from each other by gel electrophoresis.

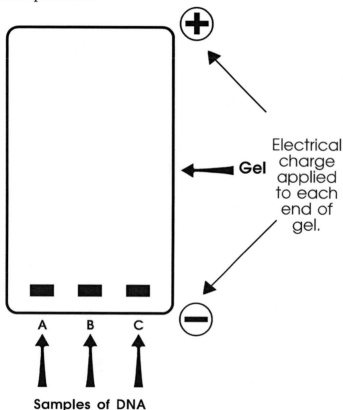

Electrical charge applied to each end of gel.

Samples of DNA

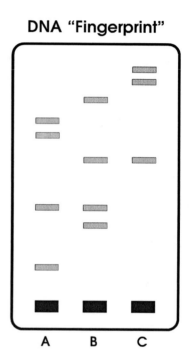

DNA "Fingerprint"

A   B   C

OVERVIEW

1. *Prepare an agarose gel sheet in a casting tray.* Agarose is made from seaweed. This gel-like sheet provides the medium through which RFLPs move. The structure of this gel allows different size pieces of DNA to separate from each other. Think of the gel as a matrix of many small particles suspended in it. The particles form an "obstacle-course" with uniform size openings between the particles. Bigger pieces of DNA move slower through the gel than smaller pieces.

2. *Cover the gel sheet with a buffer solution.* This stabilizes the pH and serves as a conductor of electricity between the gel and the electrodes during the electrophoresis.

3. *Place the samples to be compared into small "wells" at one end of the gel sheet.*

4. *Apply an electrical charge to each end of the gel.* DNA pieces (which have a negative charge) begin to move away from the negative electrode and towards the positive electrode.

5. *Wait for the "DNA fingerprint" to develop.* This might take 30 minutes or so.

This basic technique can be modified to improve the separation of DNA fragments. RFLPs of identical size but different genetic coding (for example, different GC content) will separate into multiple bands in the gel.

? QUESTION

1. What are restriction enzymes?

2. What are recognition sites?

3. What are RFLPs?

4. What is the purpose of the gel?

5. What is the purpose of the buffer?

6. Where do you put the DNA samples?

7. When the electrical charge is applied to the gel, what happens?

8. Why are there different "bands" when the process is finished?

TOOL 4: RADIOACTIVE AND FLUORESCENT PROBES

Radioactive or *fluorescent probes* are special molecules that are designed to combine only with a particular sequence of nucleotides in the DNA sample. The "targeted" sequences are called *genetic markers*. When the marker has combined with a specific probe, that DNA is either radioactive or fluoresces when a special UV light is shined on it. Researchers produce targeting probes to combine with a particular gene, or with a specific gene variation responsible for disease. There are many useful applications of this biotechnology tool.

OVERVIEW

1. Design an appropriate probe to target the genetic marker.

2. Add the probe to the DNA sample you want to test, and incubate at the correct temperature for the probe.

3. Wash the sample. This removes the probe if it has not combined with a targeted gene in the DNA.

4. Test the DNA sample to see if it is radioactive or fluoresces. This will indicate if the probe is attached to the target in the DNA.

? QUESTION

1. What is a genetic marker?

2. Refer to your lecture textbook (or the Internet) to find one clinical use for a DNA probe.

3. Refer to your lecture textbook (or the Internet) to find one forensic use for a DNA probe.

ACTIVITY #2

"DNA FINGERPRINTING SIMULATION"

This exercise will simulate a murder investigation using DNA fingerprinting to identify the perpetrator. There are three suspects: Suspect #1 (S1), Suspect #2 (S2), and Suspect #3 (S3). There is also a DNA sample from the crime scene (CS). Your task is to discover whose DNA matches the forensic evidence collected at the crime scene.

KNOW YOUR EQUIPMENT

You will work in two groups at each table. Each group will perform all the steps.

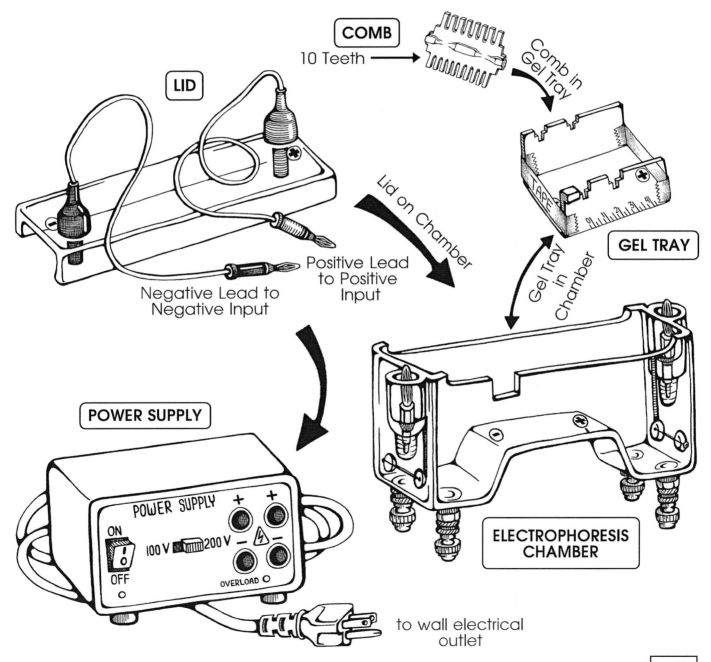

COMB
10 Teeth
Comb in Gel Tray

LID
Lid on Chamber

Positive Lead to Positive Input

Negative Lead to Negative Input

GEL TRAY
Gel Tray in Chamber

POWER SUPPLY
POWER SUPPLY
ON
100 V — 200 V
OFF
OVERLOAD
to wall electrical outlet

ELECTROPHORESIS CHAMBER

Examine the DNA fingerprinting apparatus on the previous page. Notice that there is a main chamber and a small gel tray. The gel tray is notched so that it fits into the main chamber in only one way. The "comb-like" piece hangs vertically, resting in notches of the gel tray. This comb may have two sides—one side with more "teeth" than the other side. (More about that difference later.) The main chamber has a lid with two wires (red and black) projecting from the top. The wires will be plugged into the power supply.

Be sure that you understand the basics of the DNA Fingerprinting Apparatus before you start making the gel. Ask your instructor if you have any questions.

MAKING THE GEL

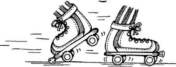

GO GET

1. Masking tape

2. 125-ml flask (for mixing agar)

3. Weighing paper for weigh boat

4. TBE buffer

5. Graduated cylinder (for measuring fluids)

6. Paper tweling (for top of agar flask)

7. Weighing scale

8. Microwave oven

NOW

1. Close off the open ends of the gel tray with masking tape or with rubber dams, whichever is provided. You must do a good job of sealing the ends or the gel pour will fail. Check with your instructor to be sure you are doing it correctly.

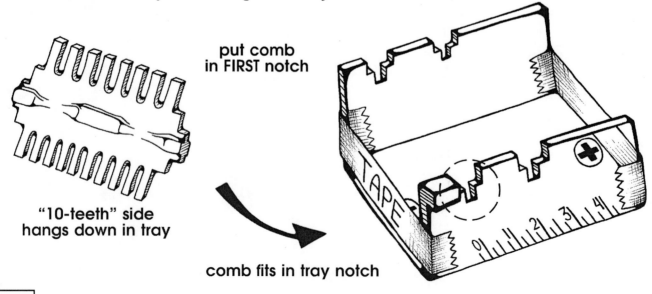

put comb in FIRST notch

"10-teeth" side hangs down in tray

comb fits in tray notch

2. Next, insert the comb into the notches at the *end* of the tray (*not* in the middle). Insert the comb so that the side with 10 teeth faces downward into the tray.

3. The comb will make 10 wells in the gel. You need only four wells for your experiment samples, but you also need a space between each sample and a space along the side of the gel. This assures that each sample won't mix with adjacent samples during the electrophoresis. (The dyes used in this simulation spread more than actual DNA pieces during electrophoresis.)

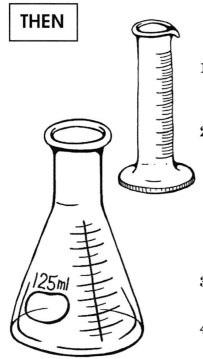

THEN

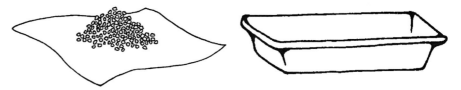

1. Now, prepare the gel solution. *One group of students will work with your instructor to prepare agar solutions for everyone in the lab.*

2. First, determine how many groups are in the class. You need that many 125-ml flasks. Carefully measure 40 ml of TBE buffer and pour it into each flask.

3. Predetermine the weight of a piece of weighing paper or weigh boat and add 0.35 g of agar. This amount of agar is for each flask.

4. Add the agar to each flask and swirl until it dissolves. Give an agar flask to each of the student groups.

5. Each group will heat their agar gel solution. Put the prepared paper toweling over the top of your flask; this prevents boil-over. It also protects your fingers when you remove the hot flask.

6. Set the microwave oven for 15 seconds, place the flask inside, and heat. The solution is not ready until it is clear.

7. You will need to repeat 2 or 3 of these 15-second heatings. Stop the oven if the agar starts to boil.

8. Grab the flask with the paper toweling and move it to a safe place. *Remove carefully. The flask is hot!*

POURING THE GEL

GO GET

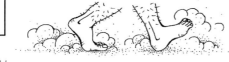

1. Micropipette

2. Micropipette tip

3. Samples from suspects and crime scene

4. Cup of water (for rinsing micropipette tips)

NOW

1. When the flask has cooled to 55 °C, it is ready to pour. A quick way to check for the proper temperature is to carefully touch the bottom of the flask to the back side of your hand. If it is painful, it is still too hot to pour. If it is hot, but not painful, it is ready to pour.

2. Carefully pour the cooled agar into the small gel tray (with the comb in place). You only fill the small gel tray—not the main chamber. Ask your instructor if you get confused.

3. It will take about 15–20 minutes for the gel solution to harden.

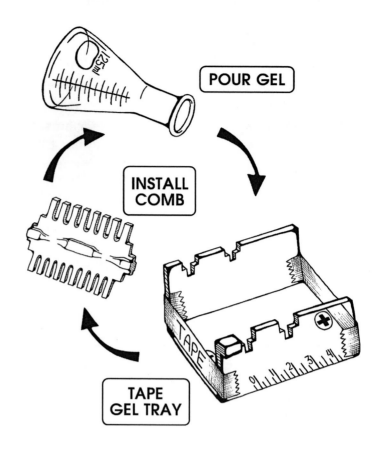

THEN

1. Fill the electrophoresis chamber with 300 ml of TBE buffer. Use the graduated cylinder to measure the proper amount.

2. Carefully remove the tape from the ends of the gel tray and insert the tray into the main chamber so that the "well end" of the tray is oriented toward the negative (black) end of the main chamber (match the notches of the tray and chamber).

3. The gel should be completely submerged.

FINALLY

Next, carefully remove the comb. You are now ready to inject the samples.

INJECTING THE SAMPLES INTO THE WELLS

GO GET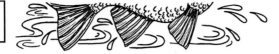

1. Micropipette

2. Micropipette tip

3. Samples from suspects and crime scene

4. Cup of water (for rinsing micropipette tip)

Micropipette

Micropipette Tip

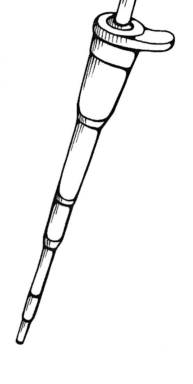

NOW

1. You are going to inject a small sample from each of three suspects and one from the crime scene. These samples are to be injected into the wells of the gel tray. This is very tricky and you will need some practice with the micropipette and tip. Pipette water into and out of the micropipette until you feel confident of your coordination and accuracy. Next, you will fill the wells in the gel tray.

2. The micropipette holds 20 μl (micro-liters). You will inject this amount of each sample into each well. The trick is to dispense the sample into the well (start about half-way down) without piercing the bottom of the agar gel. *You must clean the tip between each sample so that you don't contaminate the next well with two mixed samples. Use the cup of practice water to rinse the tip.*

3. There are four samples: Crime Scene (CS); Suspect 1 (S1); Suspect 2 (S2); and Suspect 3 (S3). Leave empty wells between each sample. Also, leave an empty well on each side of the gel tray. Empty wells keep the dyes (DNA fragments) separate from each other.

4. Mark the order of the samples on your Results Chart.

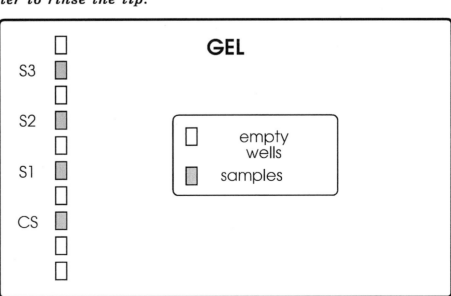

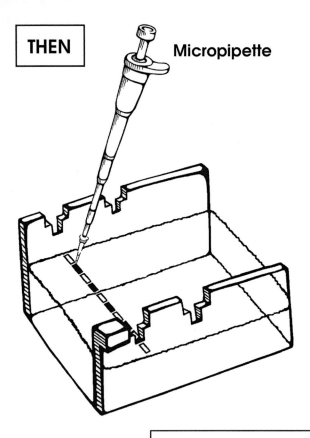

THEN

Micropipette

Gel Tray

1. Now, it's time to inject the samples. Steady your pipetting hand with your other hand and don't poke through the gel sheet.

2. If any sample begins to "float out" of a well, use a disposable pipette to remove the spreading sample from the buffer. If you don't, there could be some color contamination of your results. Ask your instructor for help.

START THE ELECTROPHORESIS PROCESS

NOW

1. Your instructor will demonstrate the way the DNA fingerprinting apparatus is connected to the power supply and turned on. It will take 20+ minutes at 100 V for the fingerprinting to be completed.

2. When the samples have separated into bands, you can remove the gel tray and slide the gel from the tray into a weigh boat filled with water. This will make it easier to see the separations. The gel will remain stable in the water until you can show it to your instructor.

3. Show your results to your instructor.

4. Use colored pencils to record your results. Be sure each sample is labeled.

   Which suspect matched the crime scene evidence? _____

FINALLY

Clean up by throwing out the gel into the trash can (not in the sink). Rinse the gel tray, comb, and 125-ml flask. Do not throw out plastic pipettes, tips, or buffer. Leave the buffer in the chamber for the next class, but do remove any floating bits of gel from the chamber.

ACTIVITY #3

"DNA ISOLATION FROM HUMAN CHEEK CELLS"

DNA occurs inside the nucleus of every cell of your body (except red blood cells) and contains the instructions for all your biochemical processes. If the DNA in a single cell nucleus were uncoiled, it would stretch about 2–3 meters in length. If you collect a small sample of cells and isolate the DNA, you can actually see this "stringy-looking" molecule. You will perform a simple technique for isolating DNA from some of your own cheek cells.

OVERVIEW

1. **Collect cheek cells.** Rinse your mouth, then add more cells by gently scraping the inside of your cheek with a toothpick.

2. **Break open the cheek cells.** Mix cheek cells with a solution of SDS (sodium dodecyl sulfate). It is a detergent that dissolves the fatty cell membrane. This releases DNA from the cells.

3. **Add some salt.** Salt makes DNA less soluble in water by neutralizing some of the electrical charges in the DNA molecule.

4. **Pour a little alcohol over the top of your sample.** DNA is not soluble in alcohol. If alcohol is carefully poured on top of a DNA solution, then a special "interface surface" forms between the alcohol and water. (Chemists use tricks like this to start a precipitation process in a solution.) The DNA will begin to form "strings" along the interface surface between the alcohol and the water.

COLLECTING CHEEK CELLS

GO GET

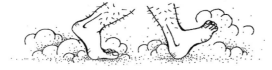

1. 1 disposable drinking cup

2. 5 ml of drinking water

3. 1 toothpick

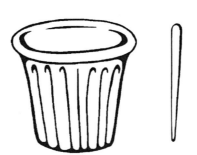

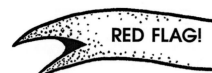

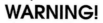

RED FLAG!   **WARNING!**   **WARNING!**

Be sure to use a clean drinking cup, drinking water, and toothpick.

1. Put 5 ml of clean water into a disposable drinking cup.

2. Swish the water vigorously in your mouth for 1 minute, and spit it back into the drinking cup. (This will collect many cheek cells.)

3. Next, use the "blunt end" of a toothpick to gently scrape the inside of your cheeks several times. Don't dig in, but rub firmly to pick up cells. Dab the toothpick in the drinking cup to release more cells. Repeat the scraping and dabbing four times. You now have enough cheek cells.

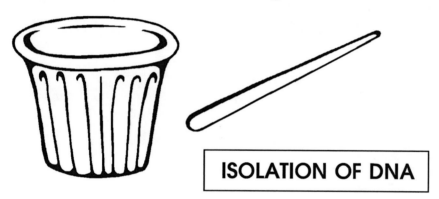

ISOLATION OF DNA

 GO GET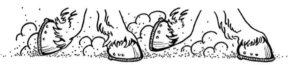

1. 1 regular-size plastic test tube

2. 1 disposable pipette (not the micropipette)

3. Saturated salt solution (NaCl)

4. 10% SDS detergent

5. 1 piece of parafilm

6. Ice cold 95% isopropyl alcohol (get this immediately before you need it)

7. Test tube rack

8. 1 plastic microfuge tube

RED FLAG!   WARNING!   WARNING!

Alcohol is flammable! Keep it away from flame!

NOW

1. Look for the 1-ml graduation mark on the plastic pipette. Put 3 ml of your cheek cell suspension into the disposable plastic test tube.

2. Add 1 ml of the 10% SDS detergent solution to the test tube.

3. Add 1 ml of the saturated NaCl solution to the test tube.

4. Place a small piece of the plastic parafilm over the top of the test tube and gently turn the tube upside down five times. *Avoid making soap bubbles.* Wait about 5 minutes and repeat the gentle inversions five more times.

THEN

1. Get the bottle of ice cold isopropyl alcohol now. *(The alcohol is either in the freezer or in an ice bath in the room).* The next bit is a little tricky.

2. Hold your test tube sample at an angle of 45° while you carefully trickle 5 ml of ice cold alcohol down the inner side of the test tube. Slowly cover the surface of your sample with alcohol.

3. Carefully place the test tube into the rack and wait 10 minutes. Gently tap the side of the test tube several times during the waiting time. You should be able to see something beginning to form between the alcohol and sample. The white strands are DNA (and some RNA also). *Show your instructor.*

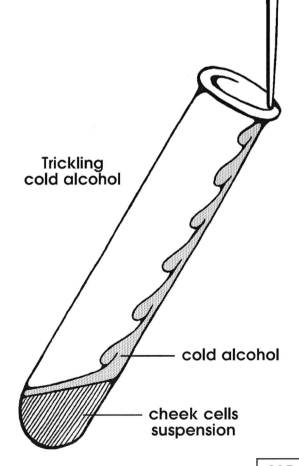

pipette

Trickling cold alcohol

cold alcohol

cheek cells suspension

4. To preserve the sample, use your cleaned plastic pipette, and gently pull up the DNA strands from the test tube and transfer them to the microfuge tube. You should be able to see the floating strands of DNA. The tube is yours to keep.

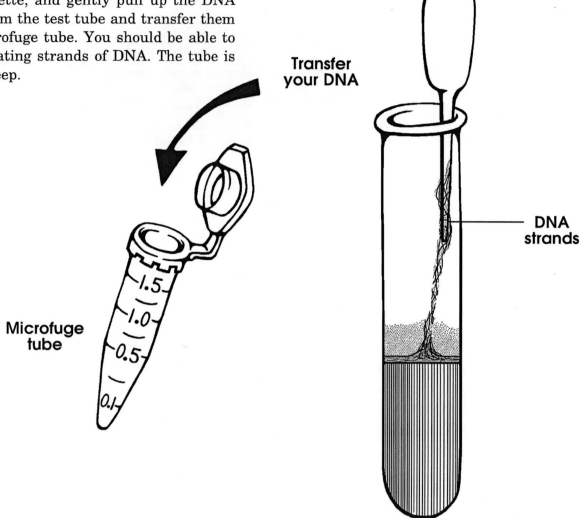

Transfer your DNA

DNA strands

Microfuge tube

1.5
1.0
0.5
0.1

FINALLY

Throw away the drinking cup, toothpick, plastic test tube, and plastic pipette. The liquids are safe to wash down the sink.

There you have it—human DNA!

? QUESTION

1. What is the purpose of adding the 10% SDS detergent solution to your cheek cell sample?

2. What was the purpose of pouring a small amount of alcohol on top of your cheek cell sample?

ACTIVITY #4

"RECOMBINANT DNA"

Recombinant DNA, often referred to as genetic engineering, is the process of combining a gene from one species with the DNA of another species. One example of this technology involves splicing a human insulin gene into a bacterial chromosome. The resulting "genetically engineered" bacteria are able to synthesize human insulin for diabetics. Animal genes can be inserted into plant species, and plant genes can be inserted into animal species. Theoretically, almost anything is possible. A brief description of the procedures will give you a simple understanding of the process.

OVERVIEW

1. The first step is to select a gene to transplant into another species. There are many considerations in this step.

   - What is your end purpose?

   - Which species have this gene?

   - Which species could receive this gene and accomplish your purpose?

2. The selected gene must be cut out of the donor organism's DNA. This is a very complicated and expensive research project. Restriction enzymes must be designed by the biochemists to do the exact cutting needed.

3. Many copies of the donor gene are made through the PCR process.

4. The recipient DNA is cut and mixed with copies of the donor gene. Perhaps the recipient's eggs will receive the donor genes for future fertilizations, thereby altering the next generations. Or, more directly, the gene can be inserted into the first cell of embryonic development.

5. The last step is to wait and see if the DNA recombination is successful.

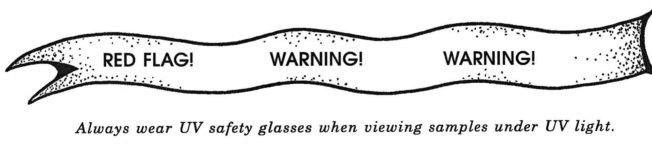

RED FLAG!   WARNING!   WARNING!

Always wear UV safety glasses when viewing samples under UV light.

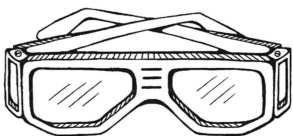

NOW

Your instructor will demonstrate the results of one recombinant project at the college. The gene for "glowing in the dark" from a jellyfish was recombined with the DNA of bacteria using the general techniques described above. The gene codes for a protein called "green fluorescent protein," which fluoresces when excited by UV light. The bacteria were grown on an agar medium, and some of them should demonstrate the new "glowing" gene from the jellyfish. This gene has been inserted into other organisms, too. Try looking on the Internet for "GFP bunny."

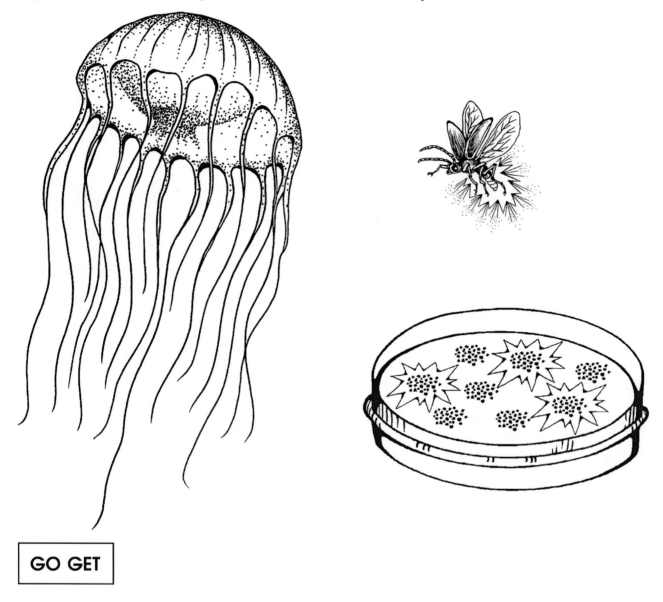

GO GET

1. UV safety glasses.

2. Yourself to the demonstration table.

Go see the demonstration of the "glowing gene" now. If your lab is during the daylight, take one of the plates outside into the sunshine and see what happens. The "glowing gene" from a firefly is not as fluorescent as the gene from a jellyfish, so if your college used a firefly gene for recombination, you may not see any difference in sunlight.

1. Describe your observations. What happened when you took the bacteria into sunlight?

2. What is the name of the gene that was involved in this recombination project?

3. Which species was the "donor" for this gene?

4. Which species was the "genetically engineered" recipient of the gene?

SUMMARY

Recombinant DNA holds an incredible future for us. Agricultural applications include plants with insect resistance, fungal and bacterial resistance, increased protein content, more sweetness, and many other traits that did not previously exist in those plant species. There are many hopeful possibilities for plant "re-engineering," but some people fear that we could produce ecological damage by creating new uncontrollable species. Those fears have led to strict rules for the development of genetically engineered plants.

Genetic engineering projects have also produced drugs for the treatment of diabetes, growth disorders, hemophilia, leukemia, some cancers, ulcers, anemia, heart attacks, emphysema, and other human ailments. The Human Genome Project is well underway to identify the location of every human gene on each chromosome. This project will discover the exact sequence of nucleotides in all human genes. And the genomes of other important non-human research species will be compared to the human genome. Moral and ethical considerations are being considered as science advances this project.

There are many questions for Biotechnology, leading to many unknown and debatable answers. What is done and how it is done are challenges for the next generation.

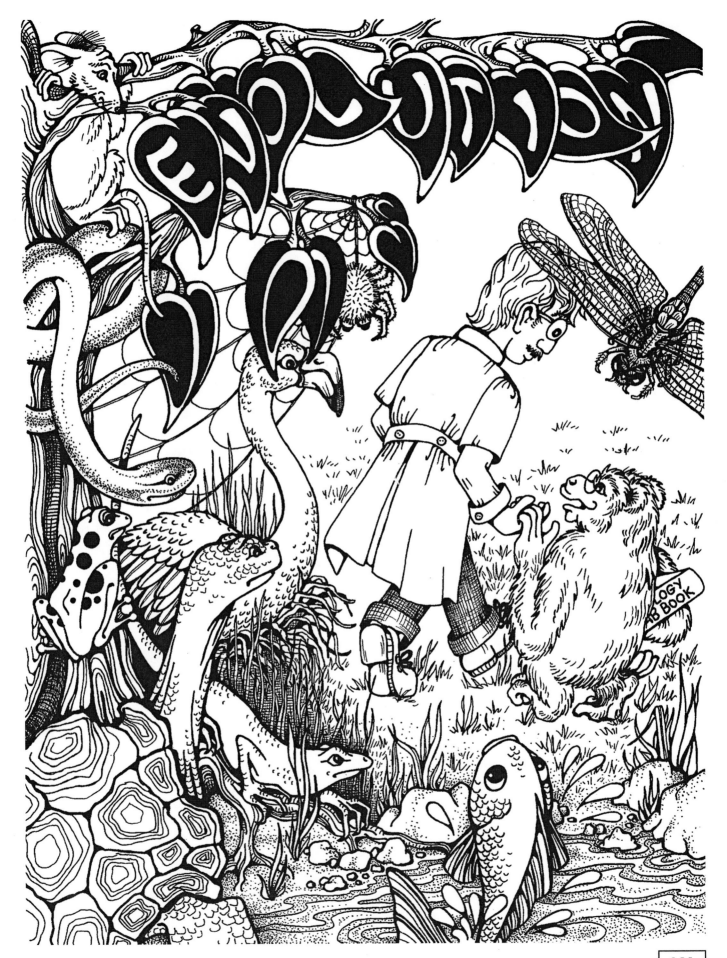

EVOLUTION

Glycolaldehyde, an eight-atom sugar, has been found in an interstellar gas cloud near the center of the Milky Way. Glycolaldehyde can react with a three-carbon sugar to form *ribose,* the basis for both RNA and DNA. The glycoaldehyde found in deep space may be a chemical precursor to life on Earth.

—"20 Things You Didn't Know About Sugar" Rebecca Coffey, *Discover Magazine,* October, 2009, p. 80

Scientists suspect that a large DNA-based virus took up residence inside a bacterial cell more than a billion years ago to create the first cell nucleus. If so, then we are all descended from viruses.

—"20 Things You Didn't Know About Viruses" by Jocelyn Rice, *Discover Magazine,* April 2010, p. 80

Most of our DNA does not reside in the cell nucleus but in the mitochondria, the cellular organelles that produce metabolic energy. Mitochondria are postulated to derive from ancient bacterial inclusions that stayed within cells over millennia.

—"20 Things You Didn't Know About DNA" by Kirsten Weir, *Discover Magazine,* April 2011, p.80

Evolutionary biologists generally agree that accumulation of random mutations leads to novelty and evolutionary change. However, Stephen Jay Gould recognized that the fossil record typically does not show gradualism as expected, but more of a discontinuity in the appearance of new species, which he termed *punctuated equilibrium.* However, there is new and competing evidence that something else may stimulate speciation: *symbiogenesis.* Symbiogenesis asserts that more complex life-forms derived from aggregations of simpler life, and that every life-form is actually a highly complex community of bacteria. This radical idea may not be so far-fetched. We already know that about 8% of the human genome originated in viruses, the integration of which into our own genome took about 40 million years.

—"Discover Interview: Lynn Margulis," *Discover Magazine,* April 2011, p. 66–71

Most DNA is composed of nucleotides, ribose (a sugar), and phosphorus. Nasa scientists have discovered a bacterium that incorporates arsenic instead of phosphorus into its DNA. Life can amaze....

—"20 Things You Didn't Know About DNA" by Kirsten Weir, *Discover Magazine,* April 2011, p. 80

For most species, the longer the generation time, the less likely it will be able to adapt to climate change.

—"Mammals and Climate Change" by Elizabeth Hadley, *FORA.TV online,* 2010

Caught in the act! Scientists have observed a fish species of the cichlid family undergoing evolution in Africa's Lake Victoria and Lake Malawi, splitting into two distinct species. The impetus for the speciation may be pollution, which affects the fish's vision. While evolution may be observed in viruses because of fast generation times, actually witnessing it in a larger species is unprecedented.

—http://ecolocalizer.com/2008/10/07/scientists-discover-fish-in-act-of-evolution-in-africas-greatest-lake/

EVOLUTION

Sceptical scrutiny is the means, in both science and religion,
by which deep thoughts can be winnowed from deep nonsense.
—Carl Sagan, American scientist (1934–1997)

INTRODUCTION

A topic like evolution seems to push everybody's button. Mention it and you're likely to start an argument.

Most people think that the central issue of this controversy is about the descent of humans from other animals. It is not! The argument is not about human ancestry, it is about *change*. In its simplest definition, ***evolution is change***. Disagreements arise because humans both crave and fear change. The social argument about evolution becomes a projection of the dilemma we've created inside our own minds. Religions and philosophies meditate on change, whereas science investigates it. Both ways of thinking are natural, expected by-products of human awareness and curiosity. Both ways of thinking can provide value to people.

Your textbook and lecture class will do a thorough job of presenting the traditional scientific evidence and implications of evolution. The purpose of the following Activities is to start you on the path of understanding evolution, and to offer you some different ways of thinking about it.

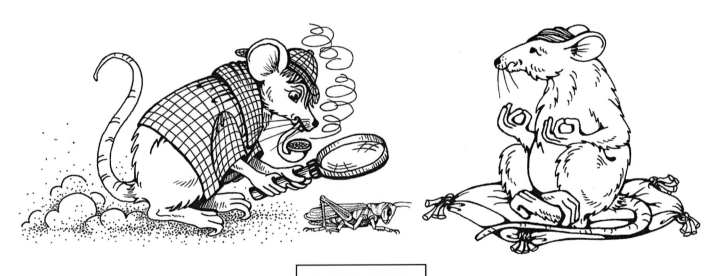

ACTIVITIES

ACTIVITY #1

"GENETIC CHANGE"

Biologists define *evolution* as genetic change in a species over time. Based on what you have learned about DNA, protein synthesis, sexual reproduction, and genetics, you should be able to answer one of the most profound questions about life on this planet:

Is it possible for life to stay the same, or is all life destined to change?

DNA AND TRAITS

In the chapter on "Genes and Protein Synthesis" you learned that small pieces of DNA, called genes, produce *traits* in organisms. These genes contain messages that make amino acids assemble into an exact sequence to produce protein. Proteins are used in cellular structure and as enzymes in an organism's biochemistry.

If it has been more than two weeks since you covered DNA and protein synthesis in lecture, then review Activity #2 and #3 in "Genes and Protein Synthesis" now.

? QUESTION

1. A gene is a long chain of nucleotides. Each group of three nucleotides in a row along the gene is called a _____ , and is responsible for the insertion of an _____ into a protein.

2. Define evolution in the simplest terms from a biological perspective.

3. Does anything stay exactly the same over time? Explain.

MUTATIONS

A *mutation* is a change in the sequence of nucleotides in the gene (DNA). These changes are caused by a variety of natural events.

You might think that your DNA is exactly replicated every time a cell divides or an egg or sperm is produced, but this is not always true. Small amounts of certain chemicals, produced by your own metabolism and in the foods you eat, can chemically alter the sequence of nucleotides. That new sequence will be the model for the *next* replication, and so on.

Nucleotides can also be changed when they are struck by cosmic radiation from outer space or UV rays in sunlight. If these abnormal nucleotides become incorporated into the DNA of an egg or sperm, then a mutation will be passed on to the next generation.

Another mutation event occurs when a nucleotide is accidentally skipped during DNA replication, or when an extra nucleotide is inserted in the DNA. (Accidents do happen!)

Whatever the cause, these mutations will continue to be copied by all future generations of cells.

Mutations can have either minor or major effects in the biochemistry of the organism. Most amino acids have more than one mRNA codon controlling their insertion into a protein. For example, glutamic acid is coded by both GAA and GAG in the mRNA. Therefore, a mutation of GAG to GAA or from GAA to GAG would have no effect on the protein being made. However, a mutation of GAG to GAU would result in *aspartic acid* being inserted instead of *glutamic acid*.

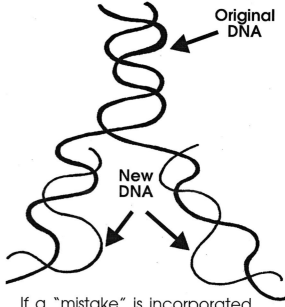

If a "mistake" is incorporated into this new DNA, then that error will be recopied the next time the DNA replicates.

In Activity #3, "Genes and Protein Synthesis," you learned that a single nucleotide change results in sickle-cell anemia. Single nucleotide mutations don't always create radical changes in the protein's basic chemical and physical properties. Sometimes the new protein is equal to the original protein in its performance for the organism. However, if a nucleotide is *deleted* during DNA replication, or if an extra nucleotide is *inserted* into the DNA, then the effects can be major. The following questions will clarify this point.

? QUESTION

1. Define *mutation*.

2. If a three-letter code is changed in the DNA, what happens to protein synthesis? (Be specific.)

3. Does a single nucleotide replacement always create a different protein?

4. Does a single amino acid change in a protein always radically change the properties of the protein?

5. Consider the consequences if an extra nucleotide is inserted into a gene. (The consequence is the same if a nucleotide is deleted.)

Original   **AGATCGGACATAGCCA**

Mutation   **AGGATCGGACATAGCCA**
                    ↑
        Extra Nucleotide Inserted

What happens to all of the three-letter codes in the gene following that one nucleotide change? (Draw brackets around each codon in both the original and mutated gene to illustrate the consequences.)

6. How many amino acids in the protein will be changed by the type of mutation described in the previous question?

7. Researchers estimate that you have 30,000 genes. If the chance of any of your genes being mutated before it ends up in a gamete (egg or sperm) is 1 in 30,000, how many new mutations would be in each gamete you make?

8. Is there any way that the DNA can stay exactly the same from generation to generation?

ALLELES IN A POPULATION

You learned in the "Genetics" chapter that humans are diploid, which means that you have two copies of each gene. When using the word *gene,* we are usually referring to a function—for example, "the *gene* for eye color." The word ***allele*** refers to the particular form of a gene. There is a blue-eye allele and a brown-eye allele. We also know that there are variations of each allele. (Remember our examples of minor mutation events?) In fact, there are many minor variations of the blue-eye allele and the brown-eye allele.

Biologists haven't identified all of the 30,000 individual human genes or the millions of possible alleles of these genes, but eventually they will discover what each of them does. In order to continue our discussion of evolution, the term *gene pool* must be defined. All of the alleles in a species (or a population) alive at a particular time is called the **gene pool**.

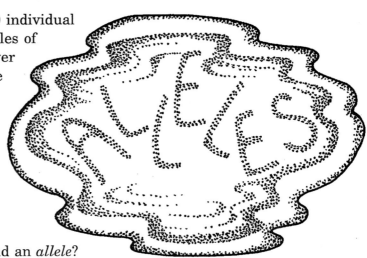

Gene Pool

? QUESTION

1. What is the difference between a *gene* and an *allele*?

2. Assume that a particular human gene is 100 nucleotides long. How many different variations of this gene are possible? (circle your choice)

   a. less than 100

   b. two or three hundred

   c. many thousands

3. Define *gene pool*.

SEXUAL REPRODUCTION

MEIOSIS + FERTILIZATION → **Variety of Offspring**

Certain events during sexual reproduction increase the genetic combinations of alleles in a species. *Crossing-over* recombines chromosomes into new mixes of alleles. *Independent assortment* creates variety in combinations of maternal and paternal chromosomes that are then segregated into separate gametes. *Random fertilization* further increases the mixing of alleles from one generation to the next. Review Activities #6 and #7 in "Sameness and Variety" if you have difficulty remembering the general events that take place during sexual reproduction.

1. What process makes it impossible for all genes to remain unchanged from generation to generation in a species?

2. What process makes it impossible for any one chromosome to be passed on to the next generation with exactly the same set of alleles?

3. You received 23 chromosomes from your mother and 23 chromosomes from your father. What process during meiosis makes it nearly impossible for you to pass on all of those chromosomes to your children?

4. If you don't reproduce, do your genes get passed on to the next generation?

5. Is it possible for one generation of humans to pass on all of its alleles in exactly the same form and frequency (percent) to the next generation?

MICRO-EVOLUTION

Evolution in its smallest scale is called *micro-evolution*. It is a change in the *frequency* of alleles in the gene pool over time. You should have concluded from the previous questions that it is impossible for the gene pool *not* to change over time. Therefore, genetic change (the most specific definition of evolution) does happen—there is no question about it. Two aspects of evolution that should be considered are: "How fast can it happen?" and "How much change can it create?"

? QUESTION

1. Define *micro-evolution*.

2. From a scientific point of view, what is the one question about evolution that is no longer considered appropriate in an argument?

3. From a scientific point of view, what are two questions about evolution that are appropriate to ask?

ACTIVITY #2

"HOW FAST CAN EVOLUTION HAPPEN?"

You learned in Activity #1 that genetic change over time is inevitable. In this Activity you will examine several easy-to-understand events that increase the rate of genetic change in a population. (Your textbook and lecture will spend time discussing more complicated factors related to the rate of micro-evolution.)

MIGRATION

Migration is a simple example of how micro-evolution can happen rapidly in a population. We can represent this situation with two alleles (A and B) of a gene that exists in a species. Assume that the population in one region has a higher frequency of the "A" allele, and in another region there is a higher frequency of the "B" allele.

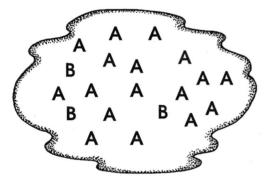

Population of Region 1
(85% have "A" allele).

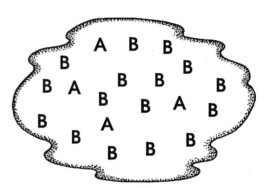

Population of Region 2
(20% have "A" allele).

Now assume that there is a large migration of organisms from Region 1 into Region 2.

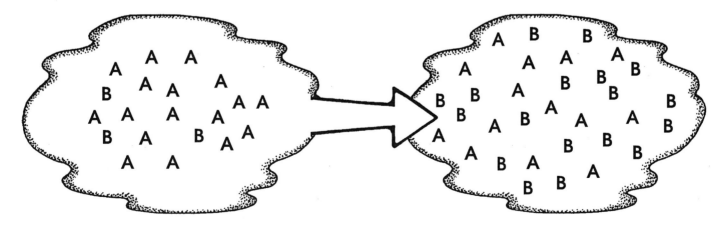

The frequency of alleles changes in Region 2. This change in the gene pool of Region 2 is micro-evolution, and it is a simple example of how genetic change happens on our planet.

1. List some modern examples of micro-evolution created by human migration.

2. Describe a situation in which organisms in one region would suddenly be able to migrate into a new region.

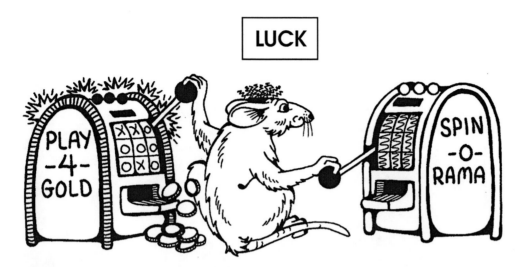

In this example, assume there are three alleles for a particular gene in a species.

Allele "A" is a real "clunker," and organisms with it survive and reproduce, but don't compete well against allele "B." Only a few of them live along the edge of the distribution of this species.

Allele "B" produces a trait that works well for the species, and has been the most common allele for thousands of years.

Allele "C" is a newly evolved mutation, and has been doing fantastically well for the last 100 years. This allele has produced the "best" animal of this species to ever have been on the planet.

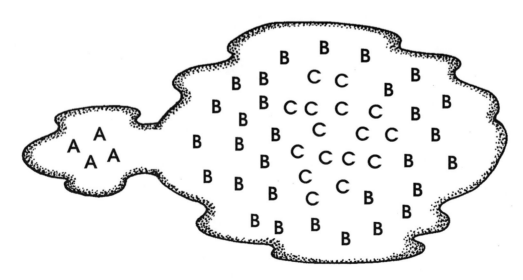

Scenario: An asteroid is heading for the Earth and scientists have calculated it will hit at the black spot. All life in the area will be vaporized for 500 miles in every direction from the impact point.

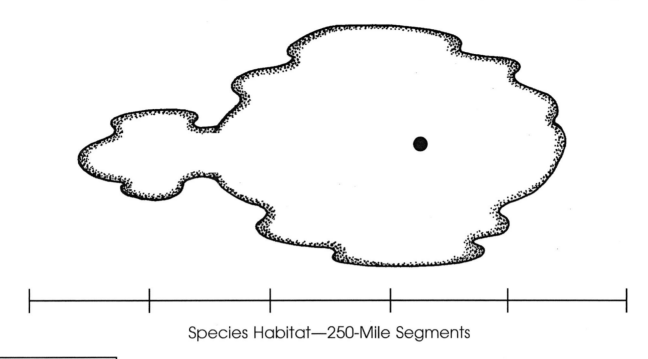

Species Habitat—250-Mile Segments

? QUESTION

1. Draw the asteroid zone of destruction on the species habitat map.

2. Which allele will be passed on to future generations?

3. Did the "best" allele survive?

4. Did the most common allele survive?

5. Which allele had the "good luck"?

6. Does this event represent micro-evolution?

7. Does the idea of "survival of the fittest" explain this example of micro-evolution?

8. How would disasters like fire and flood speed micro-evolution?

SMALL GROUP PHENOMENON

Change can be fast and the direction of change is by chance when small groups are involved. Small groups do not necessarily represent the same percent of alleles found in the total species. *Think about it!* If 30 people got in a boat tomorrow and sailed away to a distant island and started a new population, there is no way that all of the existing human alleles would be in that boat. Furthermore, compared to the total species, it is very likely that there will be a significant difference in the frequencies of alleles that get in the boat (perhaps several red-haired families). The future generations of people on that faraway island won't be like the original group. Micro-evolution occurred because of the *small group phenomenon*.

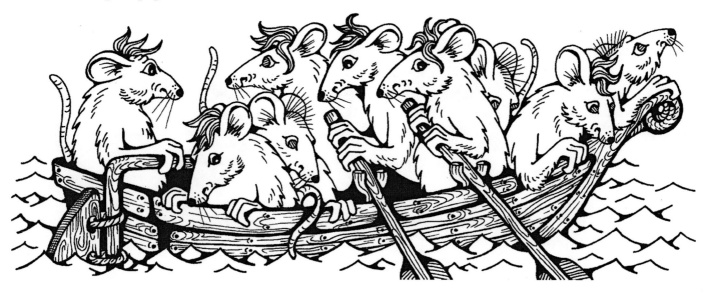

Whenever small groups survive a catastrophe, or a small group migrates to a new region and starts another population, there will be genetic change. Evidence suggests that this type of micro-evolution may be much more common than biologists of a century ago thought.

? QUESTION

1. How does the small group phenomenon lead to fast changes in the gene pool?

2. How could natural disasters like fires and floods influence evolution?

3. What would you expect organisms to look like that live on islands compared to those of the same species living on the mainland?

NATURAL SELECTION

Natural selection occurs when some particular aspect of the environment causes organisms with certain alleles to survive better and reproduce more than organisms with other alleles. It is the situation in which "survival of the fittest" applies. Review the last section of Activity #3 in "Genes and Protein Synthesis." This section covers the natural selection of grasshoppers in different soil habitats.

There are two very important aspects about natural selection that you should remember. First, it does not create new alleles. Mutation does that! Natural selection only changes the frequencies of alleles already existing in the gene pool. Second, there is no "one direction" for natural selection. In the grasshopper scenario, brown alleles do better in areas of brown soil. In areas of red soil, red alleles do better.

Genetic change in the gene pool of a species can be visualized as a young growing bush. Mutation creates many new branches of variety. Some of those branches are pruned back by natural selection, migration, small group phenomenon, or just bad luck. The remaining branches of variety continue to reproduce, and more variety is added to them by new mutations. This process repeats over and over through the eons of time.

← Line Terminated

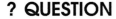

? QUESTION

1. Define *natural selection*.

2. Does natural selection create new alleles in the gene pool?

3. How is natural selection different from the small group phenomenon?

4. Is there one direction to natural selection? Explain.

ACTIVITY #3

"EVOLUTION OF ONE SPECIES INTO TWO SPECIES"

Genetic change is created by random mutations and factors that increase or decrease the frequencies of alleles in future generations. The key to understanding the evolution of one species into many species is the event of *separation*. If two groups become separated, each will change over time, but they will not change in exactly the same way.

GENETIC CONSEQUENCES OF SEPARATION

When the organisms of a species live together, they mate, exchanging and blending their genes over many generations. What happens if one group splits into two separate groups and they migrate far away from each other, never having a chance to interbreed again? As you would expect, the two groups no longer mix their genes or their mutations, and over time they will begin to look somewhat different from each other.

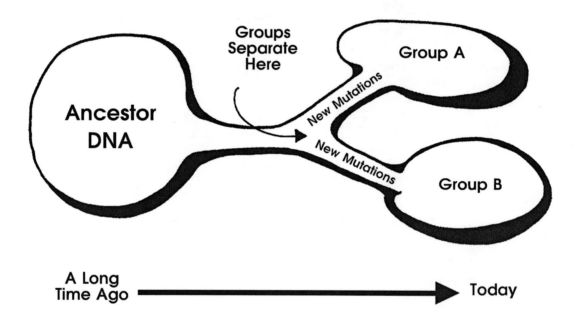

By comparing DNA patterns, chemists can detect the new mutations that have been added to the DNA. If an ancestral group splits into two groups, then both groups will begin to accumulate different mutations from each other. Each group is genetically separated from the other group when they no longer interbreed.

The easiest way to show that two groups have separated in the past is to count the number of new mutations found in the DNA of one group and not found in the DNA of the other group. The greater the number of new mutations, the longer the time span that the two groups have been separated. If however, the DNA of the two groups is quite similar, then the groups have not been separated for very long.

Diagramed below is a comparison of the DNA of three geographically separate human racial groups. Each bar represents a mutation.

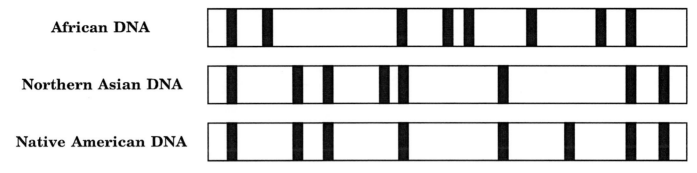

African DNA

Northern Asian DNA

Native American DNA

? QUESTION

1. Which two groups are the most similar?

2. Which of the three groups is the most different from the other two groups?

3. Which group has been separated from the others for the longest time?

4. Which of the two groups haven't been separated from each other for very long?

EVENTS THAT CAUSE SEPARATION

Your textbook and lecture will present several different situations that lead to genetic separation of two populations. One of the situations is created by changes in the geography. *Geographical separation* leads to genetically isolated populations and eventually to different species.

MOUNTAINS, RIVERS, AND HIGHWAYS

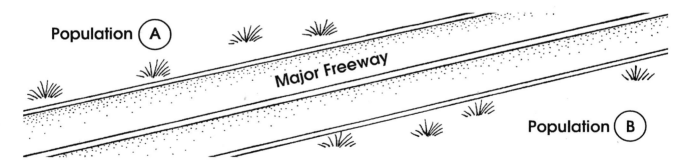

Population (A)

Major Freeway

Population (B)

Graduate students at the local college studied the mouse populations around campus and in the neighboring communities on the opposite side of a major freeway. White-faced mice, purchased for physiological and behavioral studies, routinely escaped from the lab and became part of the campus population of wild mice. For years, the students sampled the neighboring communities across the freeway, but no white-face varieties were collected. The freeway acted as a geographical barrier between the two mouse populations.

The college mouse story is a fun example of small scale isolation, but many studies have been done on populations separated by rivers and mountain ranges. These investigations demonstrate that geographical separation leads to new species. For example, the squirrels on the north and south sides of the Grand Canyon are separate species now. Separation leads to *speciation*.

DRIFTING CONTINENTS—PLATE TECTONICS

Sometimes geological processes create major opportunities for new speciation. North America and Europe were once connected, but following their separation by plate tectonics, the species on each continent evolved in different directions. Today, many species on both sides of the Atlantic are related, but each has evolved new traits that make them separate species.

65 Million Years Ago

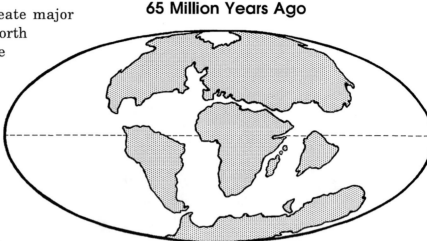

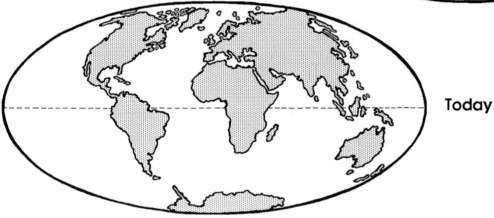

Today

THE AFRICAN EAST-SIDE/WEST-SIDE STORY

A fascinating geological separation event occurred in Africa starting about 8 million years ago. As a result of plate tectonics, a large rift valley and a high mountain range formed, separating East Africa from West Africa. By about 4–5 million years ago, East African fossils of elephants, antelope, rhinoceros, and other animals showed clear adaptations to a drier environment. East Africa was becoming drier, while West Africa remained wet as it is today.

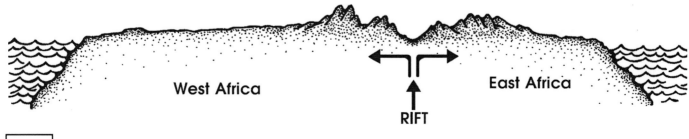

West Africa

East Africa

RIFT

The earliest hominids are called *Australopithecines* although fossils suggest distinct lines within this general category. Most hominid fossils are found in East Africa, some in South Africa, and none in West Africa. The earliest record of *Homo habilis* is also from East Africa.

Genus *Pan* fossils, which produced the chimpanzee, evolved on the West African side of the rift valley. Like the other animal groups in West Africa, genus *Pan* adapted to wet conditions.

Alternatively, the East African hominids were better adapted to a dry environment. This early separation from a common ancestor was evidently caused when plate tectonics split Africa along the rift valley and created a land barrier.

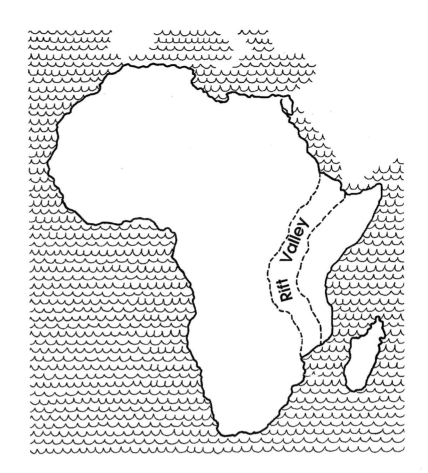

? QUESTION

1. List five geographical changes that could lead to genetic isolation of populations.

   a.

   b.

   c.

   d.

   e.

2. How long would it take for micro-evolution to begin changing geographically separated groups of a species?

3. How much change is required before there would be two distinct species?

4. Explain how the geographical separation of primates in Africa could have led to two separate lines—chimp and human.

ACTIVITY #4

"THE ROLE OF MASS EXTINCTIONS"

UTA'S STORY

Ngoma poked at the curious rock that had been split open by the heat of the fire. Quickly Uta's hands jabbed at a piece until it was positioned near the edge of the cooking pit. Then, she scooped it up and tossed it into the clay water crock where it sizzled and cooled. After a few minutes she removed the rock and held it up to the fire's light. She had seen this rock before in a distant place near the edge of a quiet bay with her fisherman father. Tonight, the story was hers.

Uta pointed at the mushroom shaped rock. The edge of her nail traced each of the inner layers of the mushroom shape. With the flames reflected in her eyes she began her tale.

"This rock is long dead! There are rocks like these today that are alive at a place where my father and I go to fish." She paused. "Each layer is a different age, like the rings of a tree. The parts towards the center are the oldest, and each new layer grew over the top of the inner layers."

Masango and Ngoma looked at each other enthusiastically. This would be a great night! Uta was telling another one of her astounding stories.

THE SCIENTIFIC ACCOUNT

Uta's story, as far as we have told it, agrees with modern scientific research. These same layered rocks have been found by scientists, and are part of the fabric of a new story emerging from the fields of geology, archeology, and biology. The scientific account tells about creation itself, fantastic life-forms, mass extinction, opportunities gained, and opportunities lost. A textbook would be required to summarize the many known details of the history of life, but we can consider some general facts.

Life has been shaped and reshaped by many processes. Four of the processes include: 1) plate tectonics, 2) impacts by objects from outer space, 3) new species evolving and replacing previously existing species, and 4) the process of habitat destruction by people.

PLATE TECTONICS

The interior of the earth is extremely hot. This heat is generated by radioactive decay as well as other physical processes. Heat creates a circulation cycle of compressed molten rock moving slowly beneath the Earth's crust.

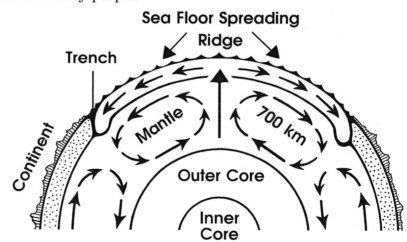

Convection currents of magma crack the Earth's crust into pieces, called **plates**, that are moved around by the convection currents beneath them. Molton rock rises through some of the cracks to form oceanic ridges where new material is continually pushed to the planet's surface. This is called **sea floor spreading**. The movement of the Earth's plates is called **plate tectonics**, a very important factor in the history of life. Plate tectonics forms and changes continents while moving them around on the surface of the planet.

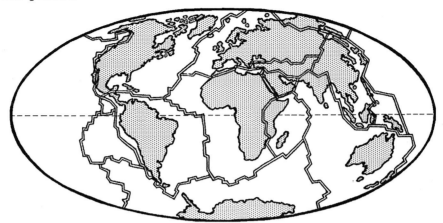

The location of a continent determines its climate. If a continent moves, then the environment will change for the organisms living there. When continents are scattered as smaller chunks of land surrounded by water, or are clumped in a large land mass (such as Pangaea of 240 million years ago), the climate conditions are profoundly different for life on land. If a continent drifts over a pole, then glaciation will occur and the sea level will drop, which transforms the environment for life at the edge of the seas.

IMPACTS FROM OUTER SPACE

The evidence for asteroid impacts as a force for mass extinction comes from the discovery of the element **iridium** in layers of sediment and rocks. Iridium is a heavy metal rarely found on the surface of the planet. However, iridium is abundant in asteroids and meteorites. When an asteroid impacts the Earth, most of it is vaporized and scattered as dust in a thin layer around the impact zone and around the Earth. Iridium deposits tell us when and where the impacts have occurred.

Asteroid and comet impacts also explode huge amounts of debris into the atmosphere. The resulting plume blocks sunlight. Their is also evidence that large impacts trigger ongoing volcanic activity for a period of time, creating even more atmospheric dust. The resulting darkness drastically shuts down the world ecosystem, and can create a mass extinction. This type of extinction closes the door of opportunity for some species, but opens it for others. Evidence is accumulating that most of the major extinctions were triggered by impacts from outer space.

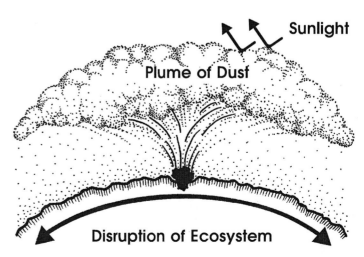

? QUESTION

1. What is the energy source that moves the crustal plates across the surface of the Earth?

2. How does plate tectonics influence the history of life?

3. What specific evidence suggests that an asteroid impact has occurred in the past?

4. How is an asteroid impact catastrophic to life?

IN THE BEGINNING

The dream world of humans has created thousands of stories about the origin of life. These are fascinating tales, but little of what they say is testable from a scientific perspective. Although science cannot provide all of the details of how life began, a general understanding has emerged that is supported by a growing record of scientific evidence.

The first life on earth evolved in an environment without oxygen. There was no oxygen in the air because it had combined with other elements like hydrogen, nitrogen, and carbon to form molecules. This meant that early lifeforms had to gain their energy from a type of metabolism that did not require oxygen. The oldest fossils are found in rocks nearly 4 billion years old. These fossils were originally living mats of bacteria, and look similar to the anaerobic bacteria that are found in today's world. Two contemporary types of anaerobic bacteria are the iron bacteria and the sulfur bacteria. These are examples of organisms that can derive energy by metabolizing minerals. They do not require oxygen. Simple *anaerobic bacteria* are proof that life really can exist in an environment similar to that of the early Earth.

Some questions arise. If anaerobic bacteria were the first lifeforms, then why aren't they the only type of organism on the planet now? And, where did the oxygen in our atmosphere come from?

The answer to these questions is one of the first big lessons of life: *Somebody else can put you out of business*! In biology, this is called extinction.

Now let's finish Uta's story of the mushroom rocks.

UTA'S ROCKS

Anaerobic bacteria had this planet to themselves for a billion or more years. Then, about 3 billion years ago new kinds of organisms evolved in the shallow seas. These colonial micro-organisms produced rocklike deposits. They included two new types of bacteria called *cyanobacteria* and *aerobic bacteria*. The cyanobacteria produced oxygen gas during their biochemistry, and aerobic bacteria used oxygen during theirs. These bacteria grew in layers. Each new generation covered the previous one, eventually forming a large mushroom-shaped deposit that we call a *stromatolite*.

STROMATOLITES

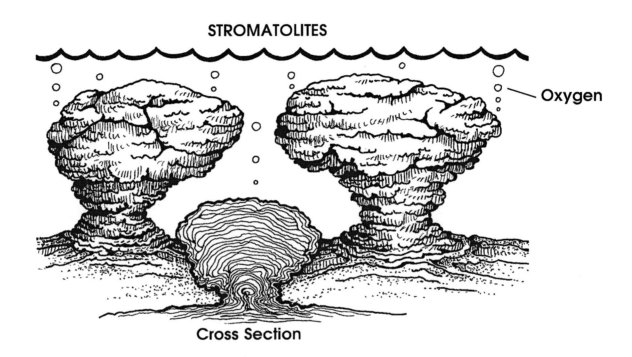

Cross Section

Once the stromatolites appeared, the anaerobic bacteria began to decline in the fossil record. These "newcomer" stromatolites changed the world. The cyanobacteria transformed the atmosphere by using a kind of energy-trapping process called *photosynthesis*. Photosynthesis produces oxygen, a substance that is *poisonous* to anaerobic life. This new gas killed all the early anaerobic life-forms except those living in areas of the planet where oxygen gas could not reach. The anaerobes were restricted to these limited habitats. Today we can still find these very old types of anaerobic bacteria (called archaebacteria) in the black mud of swamps, in salt marshes, and in volcanic hot springs. These smelly, hot places might seem disgusting to us, but they are a paradise for anaerobes. To the anaerobes, the whole planet was once a wonderful smelly place—until stromatolites evolved.

As stromatolites oxygenated the world, they changed it. They covered the floor of shallow seas until about one billion years ago. Then another new group, the *invertebrates*, evolved. These multicellular animals became very diverse and included some that ate stromatolites. What the stromatolites did to the anaerobes was done to them by the invertebrates, and today there are only a few places where stromatolites can exist. We find them in isolated salty bays where they are protected from the appetites of invertebrate predators. This is the scientific story of Uta's rocks—alive for billions of years, and still living reminders of a previous chapter in life's long history.

1. What were the first organisms and where do they live today?

2. About 3 billion years ago, there was a huge reduction of anaerobes. What gas in the atmosphere was responsible?

   What biological process produced that gas?

   Which organisms evolved that process?

3. How do stromatolites form, and what two groups of bacteria are part of their formation?

4. There was a huge reduction of stromatolites between 500 and 700 million years ago. Which group of organisms was responsible for eating stromatolites and out-competing them?

   Where can living stromatolites be found today?

GLACIATION AND SEA LEVEL

When thinking of life in the ancient seas, we usually visualize sharks and fish. But those early seas were filled with organisms beyond the imagination. Again, the history of life is best told by examining the fossil record. Invertebrate animals first evolved as very simple creatures somewhat like today's sponges and jellyfish. By about one-half billion years ago they blossomed into many varieties and bizarre forms. They shared the seas with a strange chordate group, the *jawless fish*. One hundred million years later, *cartilaginous fish* and *bony fish* evolved to join the story. Millions of species lived in the rich continental shelf zone. Today there are only a few jawless fish, and many of the early invertebrates are gone. What happened to them?

A mass extinction of many invertegrate species and most of the jawless fish occurred about *370 million years ago*. Following this event we find new creatures in the fossil record—early types of amphibians. What could cause trouble for invertebrate sea life and jawless fish, yet open up opportunities for amphibians? Here we get some help from geologists.

The oceans of the world are deep bowls with ridges and thin shallow rims. These rims are actually 200 feet below the water surface and are called *continental shelves*. Ocean life is concentrated in the continental shelf waters. The shelf zone is the richest nutrient area in the oceans because ocean currents and runoff water from land constantly stir the bottom sediments. These two processes increase the availability of inorganic minerals that are necessary for photosynthesis. High nutrient levels are resources for plants—the basis of the food chain.

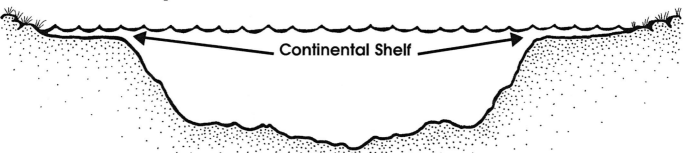

What would happen if the sea level dropped 200 feet? All of the continental shelf zone would be exposed, and the species that lived in that environment would vanish.

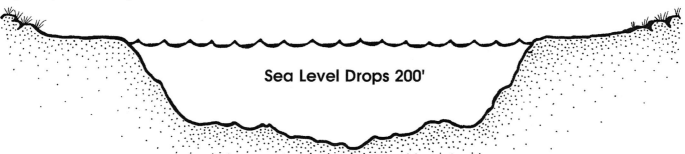

What would cause the sea level to drop? The answer begins with understanding the *water cycle*. First, sunlight evaporates water from the oceans forming large clouds. Next, those clouds rain somewhere on the planet. This rain creates rivers that eventually return to the sea, and the cycle repeats.

WATER CYCLE

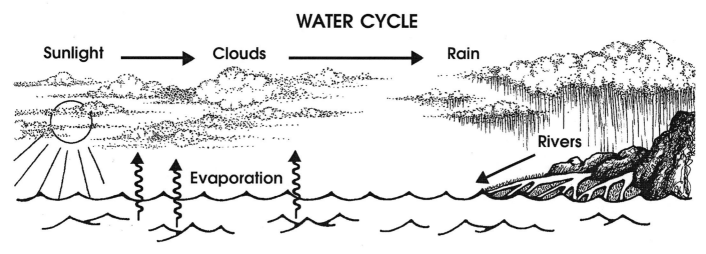

Now, consider how the position of continents might affect the water cycle and the sea level. In this planet's history, continents were sometimes scattered, and at other times continents were crunched together into bigger pieces. About 370 million years ago, a large continental mass drifted into position over the South Pole. With a continent over the South Pole, the snow that fell into the ocean.

now fell on land. The snow piled up forming huge *glaciers*. This interrupted the water cycle. (If water doesn't return to the ocean, then sea level will drop by the amount equal to the mass of the glacier.) There was a significant reduction of invertebrates and marine fishes. It is also worth noting that changes in the location of continents can alter ocean currents and global climate patterns. Furthermore, there is evidence that a meteor or asteroid impacted the Earth and played a role. So, it seems that both cataclysmic and gradual processes contributed to the changes in evolution about 370 million years ago.

However, what was bad for invertebrates and jawless fish was a great opportunity for whomever was left behind. The surviving groups included some of the *cartilage fish* and *bony fish*, from which many new species began to evolve. One group that adapted to the slowly changing conditions was an air-breathing fish with simple limbs. These became the *early amphibians*. The amphibians populated swamps, freshwater lakes, and shallow sea environments until the next big calamity on the planet.

PANGAEA—THE BIGGEST DESERT THAT EVER WAS

The amphibians of *240 million years ago* were challenged by a continent bigger and drier than anything in our modern experience. Geologists call this mega-continent *Pangaea*. Pangaea formed as land masses drifted and merged together from the forces of plate tectonics. The position of Pangaea probably created large scale glaciations, sea level changes, and other global climate changes hostile to existing species.

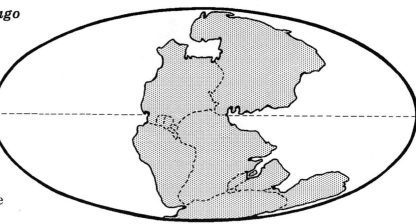

When continents are small and surrounded by water, the rain clouds can reach most of the land and the environment is moderate. The smaller, scattered continents before 240 million years ago were suitable for early land vertebrates like amphibians. But, Pangaea was a huge land mass. Most of it was far from the ocean and the rain clouds. This supercontinent was the largest dry land environment that we know of in the last half-billion years of the Earth's geologic history.

The change from small swampy continents into one huge mass of dry land produced the first big land extinction during which ninety-five percent of the land animals were eliminated. All of the larger amphibians died. An impact from outer space and volcanic activity may have contributed to cataclysmic events, while plate tectonics created climate changes from a swampy to a dry land environment. Climatic shifts directed evolution to a highly modified amphibian——one that had dry skin and a different method of reproduction. These animals could mate and raise their young on dry land. The new traits evolved from the old traits of the amphibians, and produced a *reptile*. The innovation was so profound for land habitats, and the opportunities for reptiles on dry land were so great, that every new species flourished.

With this new game, it seemed as if nothing could go wrong—well almost nothing—unless you are unfortunate enough to be hit by a 10–mile-diameter rock traveling at 150,000 miles an hour.

1. Explain how the extinction of many continental shelf species can be explained by plate movements, glaciation, the water cycle, and sea level.)

2. Which group evolved and flourished in the swampy environments after the 370 million year ago extinction?

3. Does the sea level have to drop thousands of feet before sea life is affected? Explain.

4. What did the land mass look like 240 million years ago, and how did that influence the direction of evolution?

5. What name is given to the supercontinent of 240 million years ago?

6. Which animal group was greatly reduced by the elimination of most swampy environments?

7. Which new animal group greatly benefited from the large amount of available dry land on the planet and the lack of competitors?

BAD TIMES FOR REPTILES

We know that many asteroids struck our planet during its history, including one at about **200 million years ago**. The crater made by this impact is located in eastern Quebec, Canada. It measures nearly 50 miles across. The crater has been dated near the time that an extinction event occurred for many of the early reptiles.

So, approximately 30 million years after the opportunity first developed for reptiles, about 60% of them became extinct. The reptiles that remained alive after this extinction would have the next big opportunity. Several groups, including crocodile, turtle, and snake-lizard types, remain until today. But, the first group to flourish were the predecessors of the **dinosaurs**, and dinosaurs did very well indeed. There was every type and every size of dinosaur that you could imagine during their 150-million-year dynasty. But, their days of being the dominant land vertebrate were numbered.

Scientists now have evidence that about **65 million years ago**, a huge object from outer space hit the earth. Preliminary evaluation of the evidence suggests that the dinosaur extinction was partly caused by the impact. Whether the object was a comet or an asteroid, there is a one-hundred–mile-diameter crater at the tip of the Yucatan Peninsula dated near the time of this extinction. An impact that large would create total destruction within at least 1,000 miles from ground zero. In addition, several thousand cubic miles of vaporized rock would be carried into the atmosphere, blocking sunlight and photosynthesis for months or longer. During this dark time the world's ecosystem was radically interrupted, destroying many species. Dinosaurs, except for the bird line, and about 75% of all marine species were eliminated near the time of this asteroid impact. Many of these species disappeared at the time of impact, while others died out during the years that followed.

As with previous extinctions, whatever species survived had a special opportunity for new evolutionary experiments. Almost anything will work when there are few competitors. The next two successful land groups that flourished were **mammals** and **birds**. From 65 million years ago until today, these two groups and the **flowering plants** have taken advantage of the land environments.

HUMAN HUNTERS

The previous examples are large-scale events that have radically affected the evolution of life. Fossil evidence also suggests that thousands of **small-scale extinctions** have happened on this planet. One such small-scale extinction of large mammals about 20,000 years ago followed the migration of humans from the Eastern Hemisphere into the Western Hemisphere. Hunting artifacts are dated at the same time that a dozen or so large mammal species disappeared. This type of extinction occurs whenever a new species moves into a region where there is easy prey. This is also an example of how much impact one successful species can have on another species, and serves as a warning to us concerning our destructive actions of today.

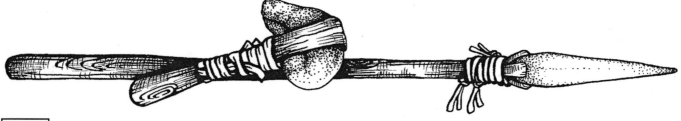

HABITAT DESTRUCTION

The most recent extinctions have been caused by humans eliminating the natural habitats of other species. When habitats are destroyed, the species that depend on those habitats are also destroyed. This process is occurring at an alarming rate wherever there are dense populations of humans in or near geographically smaller or isolated habitats. One example is islands. But there are many small and strange habitats and their associated species around the world that are vulnerable to human development (e.g., Madagascar).

Today there is an even faster rate of extinction occurring in the tropical rain forests of the world. These are the richest ecosystems on land. Experts conclude that many species face extinction as rain forests are cleared and burned for their wood, to grow crops, and to graze cattle. The fragile top soil washes away within a few years, and all the benefits are lost for indigenous people as well as for the world ecosystem.

? QUESTION

1. Explain how the presence of the element iridium in sediment is related to asteroid impacts.

2. About 200 million years ago, an asteroid or meteorite hit the Earth (creating the crater in Quebec), and about 60% of the existing species became extinct. Many early reptiles were eliminated, which allowed one of them the opportunity to become very successful. What group was that?

3. Explain how asteroid impacts can cause extinctions.

4. Another asteroid hit the planet (creating the crater in Yucatan) about 65 million years ago. Which reptile group was eliminated?

   Which two vertebrate groups benefited from the reduction of reptilian competitors?
   a.
   b.

5. What caused the extinction of most of the large mammal species in the Western Hemisphere beginning about 40,000 years ago?

6. What specific change accounts for today's increasing rate of species extinction?

SUMMARY

Science has discovered many truths about how life has evolved on Earth. This short story covers only a partial description of all we know and are still investigating. The example events we have discussed in this chapter include:

- ▶ the addition of oxygen to the atmosphere (photosynthesis),

- ▶ plate tectonics,

- ▶ glaciation and the lowering of sea levels,

- ▶ what happens when swamps dry up,

- ▶ impacts by asteroids and comets,

- ▶ the effects of early human hunters, and

- ▶ the damage to ecosystems and habitats by people.

Thanks to the discoveries of science, what once began as exciting stories around the fire pit has expanded into a complex understanding of the Earth's remarkable history. Now, the challenge for humanity is to find a balance between short-term interests and long-term stability. If we don't, the planet will continue to experience changes in evolution because of us. And the direction that evolution takes could lead to our own decline, and possibly extinction.

SELECTED READINGS AND FILMS

The following references offer expanded discussions about some of the topics mentioned in *Biology Lab Book*. We hope that you view your life as an adventurous game, and enjoy exploring some of our selected readings and films.

BOOKS

Adam Hart-Davis, Editor. *Science: The Definitive Visual Guide*. D.K. Publishing, 2009.

Adams, Douglas, and Mark Carwardine. *Last Chance to See*. Harmony Books, New York, 1991.

Buchanan, Mark. *Ubiquity: Why Catastrophes Happen*. Broadway Books, 2002.

Burke, James. *The Day the Universe Changed*. Little, Brown and Company, 1985.

Campbell, Joseph. *Myths to Live By*. A Bantam Book by Viking Press Inc., 1972.

Campbell, Joseph. *The Power of Myth*. Anchor Publishing, 1991.

Carse, James P. *Finite and Infitite Games*. The Free Press, A Division of Macmillan, Inc., 1986.

Cavalli-Sforza, Luigi Luca. **"Genes, Peoples and Languages."** *Scientific American,* November 1991, 104–110.

Cook, Theodore Andrea. *The Curves of Life*. Republication by Dover Publications, Inc., 1979.

Coppens, Yves. **"East Side Story: The Origin of Humankind."** *Scientific American,* May 1994, 88–95.

Coppens, Yves. *Human Origins: The Story of Our Species*. Hachette Iluustrated. UK, 2004.

Dawkins, Richard. *The Greatest Show on Earth: The Evidence for Evolution*. Free Press (Simon and Schuster, Inc.), 2009.

Feynman, Richard P. *What Do You Care What Other People Think?* W.W. Norton & Company, 1988.

Gazzaniga, Michael S. *Human: The Science Behind What Makes Us Unique*. HarperCollins, 2008.

Gleick, James. *Chaos: Making a New Science*. Penguin Books, 1987.

Gould, Steven Jay. *Wonderful Life: The Burgess Shale and the Nature of History*. W.W. Norton & Company, Inc., 1989.

Hawking, Stephen W. *A Brief History of Time: From the Big Bang to Black Holes*. Bantam Books, 1988.

Hildebrandt, Stefan and Anthony Tromba. *Mathematics and Optimal Form*. Scientific American Books, Inc., 1984.

Kahneman, Daniel and Paul Slovic and Amos Tversky—editors. *Judgement Under Uncertainty: Heuristics and Biases*. Cambridge University Press, 1982.

Levitt, Steven, and Stephan Dubner. *Super Freakonomics: The Illustrated Edition*. Harper-Collins, 2009.

Lomborg, Bjorn. *Cool It: The Skeptical Environmentalist's Guide to Global Warming*. Random House, 2007.

McKean, Kevin. **"Decisions."** *Discover Magazine,* June 1985, 22–31.

McMahon, Thomas A. and John Bonner. *On Size and Life*. Scientific American Books, Inc., 1983.

Moore, John A. *Science as a Way of Knowing: The Foundations of Modern Biology*. Harvard University Press, 1993.

Morrison, Philip and Phylis Morrison. *Powers of Ten*. (About the relative size of things in the Universe.) Scientific American Books, Inc., 1982.

Piattelli-Palmarini, Massimo. *Inevitable Illusions: How Mistakes of Reason Rule Our Minds*. Wiley and Sons, Inc., 1994.

Pollan, Michael. *The Omnivore's Dilemma: A Natural History of Four Meals*. Penguin, 2007

Rock, Irvin. *Perception*. Scientific American Books, Inc., 1984.

Rosenblum, Lawrence D. *See What I'm Saying: The Extraordinary Powers of Our Five Senses*. W. W. Norton & Company, 2011

Saarinen, Eliel. *The Search for Form in Art and Architecture*. Republication by Dover Publications, Inc., 1985.

Seethaler, Sherry. *Lies, Damned Lies, and Science: How to Sort Through the Noise Around Global Warming, the Latest Health Claims, and Other Scientific Controversies*. FT Press/Pearson Education, Inc., 2009.

Shubin, Neil. *Your Inner Fish: A Journey into the 3.5-Billion-Year History of the Human Body*. Vintage, 2009.

Silver, Lee M. *Challenging Nature: The Clash Between Biotechnology and Spirituality*. Harper Perennial, 2007

Stevens, Peter S. *Patterns in Nature*. Little, Brown and Company, 1974.

Stewart, Ian. *The Mathematics of Life*. Basic Books Inc., 2011.

FILMS

Abbott, Edwin A. *Flatland*. DVD. Flat World Productions, LLC, 2007.

Burke, James. *After the Warming*. Http://www.Video.Google.com. Directed by Mike Slee. Film Australia, 1989.

Campbell, Joseph. *The Power of Myth*. DVD. Six-hour PBS miniseries with Bill Moyers. USA: 1988.

Cohen, Chad. *The Human Family Tree*. DVD. Directed by Chad Cohen. Human Origin Project—National Geographic, 2009.

Davis, Mark, and Hobson, Mark. *NOVA: The Doomsday Asteroid*. Produced by John Angier. Chicago: WGBH Educational Foundation, 1995.

Friedman, Peter, and Brunet, Jean-François. *Death by Design: Where Parallel Worlds Meet*. DVD. Directed by Jean-François Brunet and Peter Friedman. USA: Independent Television Service (ITVS), 1997.

Holt, Sarah. *NOVA: Alien From Earth*. DVD. Chicago: WGBH Educational Foundation and Essential Media & Entertainment, 2008.

Jampel, Barbara. *National Geographic's Mysteries of Mankind*. DVD. National Geographic, 1988.

Linklater, Richard. *Fast Food Nation*. DVD. Directed by Richard Linklater (inspired by Eric Schlosser's 2001 nonfiction book of the same name). Los Angeles: 20th Century Fox, 2007.

Lomborg, Bjorn. *Cool It*. DVD. 1019 Entertainment, in association with Interloper Films, 2010.

PBS. *NOVA: Dimming the Sun*. DVD. Directed by Duncan Copp. Chicago: A DOX Production for NOVA/WGBH and BBC, 2006.

Talcott, Richard. *Stephen Hawking's Universe* (6-part PBS series). DVD. Directed by Philip Martin. New York: Thirteen/WNET/Uden Associates/David Filkin Enterprises Co-Production in association with BBC-TV, 1997.

Townsley, Graham. *NOVA: Becoming Human*. DVD. Directed by Graham Townsley. Shining Red Productions for NOVA, WGBH Educational Foundation, 2009.